D1461745

032568

PIG DISEASES

Sixth edition

PIG DISEASES

Sixth edition

D. J. Taylor, MA.Vet.MB.PhD.MRCVS,
Reader in Veterinary Microbiology
Glasgow University

1995

ISBN 0 9506932 5 1

First edition 1979
Second edition 1981
Third edition 1983
Fourth edition 1986
Reprinted November 1986
Fifth edition 1989
Sixth edition 1995

Published by and copies obtainable from the author:

Dr. D. J. Taylor
31 North Birbiston Road
Lennoxtown
Glasgow G65 7LZ

Design and production in association with
Book Production Consultants PLC, Cambridge

Printed in Great Britain by
St Edmundsbury Press, Bury St Edmund's, Suffolk

CONTENTS

FOREWORD

The first edition of this book was written as student notes, but demand from veterinarians, veterinary students and farmers led to its publication. It is intended primarily to describe diseases of pigs present in the UK and Europe, those that threaten the European pig industry or those which may yet be identified here. It deals mainly with conditions found in intensive units and can, therefore, be used worldwide. Conditions which are uncommon in such intensive units may be dealt with in less detail.

Treatment is only described in general as the book is intended for the use of Veterinary Surgeons who, in Britain, are supplied annually with the NOAH Compendium of Data Sheets for Veterinary Products. These data sheets give details of the veterinary products cited In other countries, similar books exist and provide local trade names for the therapeutic agents and vaccines named. Prescribing practice and the availability of medicines and vaccines differ from country to country and those using the book should take account of this and adhere to local requirements, particularly with regard to withdrawal times and legislation. Feeding, housing and management techniques are adequately described in existing books such as those published by Farming Press, Ipswich, UK. Further information about disease may be found in 'Diseases of Swine' edited by A.D. Leman and others and the other books listed in the Introduction.

The descriptions of diseases and the measures adopted for their control are based on a mixture of personal experience, review of the literature and, in the case of the newer syndromes, word of mouth. This edition reflects the increasing concern of the veterinary profession and public in the UK about welfare, meat quality and general safety. The account of each disease has been supplemented with an opinion on the humane endpoint for slaughter, and no risks to man be expected from each disease and its therapy.

The normal nutritional requirements of the pig given on pages 263-265 are reproduced with some amendments from Tables 5:1, 5:3 and 11:8 in "Practical Pig Nutrition" by C.T. Whittemore and F.W. Elsey with kind permission of the publishers, Farming Press Ltd of Ipswich. I would like to thank the colleagues who commented on the previous editions of this book and, in particular, those who wrote to provide further information. This edition was typed and edited by Mrs. M. Riddell to whom I am extremely grateful.

D.J. Taylor, MA, PhD, Vet.MB, MRCVS.
31 North Birbiston Road
Lennoxtown
Glasgow G65 7LZ

April 1995.

INTRODUCTION

The UK pig industry with 774,000 sows (1944) and 7,704,000 (19) pigs (14,600,000. million slaughter pig in 1994) is small when compared with the total pig populations of the E.C. (11,737000 sows and 110,000,000 pigs). The current trend in E.C. is for pig numbers to decline slightly and for pigmeat supplies to decline also. The continued high price of grain within the E.C. compared with world markets is unlikely to change significantly but, for the moment, the projected decline in supply means that margins for pig producers are improving. Prices for pigmeat are broadly similar throughout the major E.C. pig keeping countries and any further expansion must come through an increase in consumption or in exports.

The historic freedom of the UK from diseases such as swine fever, African swine fever, foot-and-mouth disease, brucellosis, swine vesicular disease, and Aujeszky's Disease, coupled with the development of hybrid breeding stock, has led to a flourishing export trade in British pigs with most of Europe and with other parts of the world. The increasing specialisation in the industry and the requirements of exporters demand an ever increasing degree of technical knowledge from the veterinarian. This book is intended to form a foundation on which such expertise can be based.

Structure of the industry in the UK

Herd sizes in Britain are increasing. The average number of sows per breeding unit is now over 52 and the total number of pigs per unit averages more than 400. The total number of holdings (21,000) is still falling. The concentration of pigs in large herds is reflected in the trade in breeding stock; 75% of all gilts and 65% of all boars sold are supplied by companies, most of them by the 4-8 large breeding companies.

In some areas of the country the pig herds are now large and scattered particularly where there have been closures of slaughterhouses. In future, however, the industry will be organised much as at present but with fewer small scale producers and still fewer units. The organisation of the industry and the type of units and enterprises found are important factors in the diseases which occur. Traditional patterns of husbandry - the single fattening pig or breeding sow, the mixed farm with a few sows and a boar producing weaners for sale or to fatten on the farm, still persist. Organic farming, wild boar farming, the maintenance of rare breeds, the pet pig, transgenic pigs and the experimental pigs used in veterinary and biomedical science all represent new types of animal for the veterinarian.

The use of adapted or old-fashioned buildings and the practice of home mixing rations still give rise to the husbandry, nutritional and parasitic problems which have often disappeared from the larger units. The larger enterprises may be divided into several groups from a health stand-point. The larger breeder-weaner or producer/fattener may run a closed herd apart from purchases of boars and has a variable incidence of disease. Breeding companies may belong to the class described above but sell breeding stock widely. They may use extensive systems for health reasons and parasitism may result. In many cases, they are organised in a pyramid with a nucleus herd supplying multipliers with grand-parent stock and these then produce the parents of the slaughter generation which are sold to the farmer. Constant genetic turnover in the nucleus herd results in the use of young boars and gilts with attendant health problems and the movement of animals from nucleus to multiplier to farm creates a channel by which disease in the nucleus or in a multiplier can rapidly spread to a large number of farms. Finishing may be run on a large scale by feeding companies who own pigs, rent buildings and labour from farmers and supply their own feed. They frequently populate sites on an all-in, all-out basis but purchase their weaners from a number of sources and mix them, a practice which frequently results in disease. Swill feeders still exist, many purchase stock from a number of sources and disease can result from this practice. The difficulty of balancing swill of varying quality and the destruction of nutrients by heating may result in nutritional problems not seen elsewhere. Both in-feed and water medication is difficult to administer on such farms. The husbandry system within a farm also affects the disease pattern and the productivity of the unit. The age at which pigs are weaned is the most important factor. Traditional 8-week weaning is now uncommon. Six week, and 5-week weaning occur but 3-week weaning is now widespread. Weaning at 1 day of age, followed by cage rearing is feasible in experimental situations but weaning at this age is not allowed on welfare grounds. After 3-week weaning, housing in large groups in flat decks or kennels is common with attendant respiratory and behavioural problems. The size of subsequent groups of weaned pigs and the nature of the floors and dung disposal (slats, continuous dunging channel, deep straw) also affects the incidence and nature of disease. Airspace, its size and the type of nutrition - floor fed meal, skim milk, liquid feed, trough feeding are also important. The additives used as growth promoters also have a bearing on the diseases seen. Finally, the way in which breeding stock are housed and handled is important when considering reproductive problems.

Health programmes and health status in the Pig Industry

Pigs may have "conventional" health status i.e. are normal farm stock although perhaps free from some diseases or they may be hysterectomy-derived (primary S.P.F.) or bred from such animals (secondary S.P.F.). The latter class of animals is normally maintained behind some type of barrier and is known as "S.P.F.", "Minimal Disease" (M.D.) or "High Health Status" in advertisements. Several pure bred herds are descendants of hysterectomy-derived pigs and the nucleus herds and multipliers of some breeding companies are also of this type. Health schemes include single farm programmes and those applied to all the farms belonging to one breeding or feeding company. A state-run programme known as the Pig Health Scheme monitors the health of herds involved by means of quarterly veterinary inspections, record collecting and advises on welfare and the control of disease amongst the herds concerned.

Disease and its investigation

The recent identification of the virus of the porcine respiratory and reproductive syndromes (PRRS, PEARS, SIRS) has focused attention on respiratory disease in the pig and the existing pathogens are now being re-evaluated. the effect of the disease on individuals herds is now well documented, but its long-term effects on trading patterns are not yet clear.

The application of molecular biology, genetics and immunology has revolutionised many aspects of the study of pig diseases. The production of DNA probes and the polymerase chain reaction (PCR) enable the frequency of single genes to be determined in pig populations and will allow the selection of disease-resistant stock. Similar methods and user-friendly peroxidase-linked immunoassays such as ELISA tests, have allowed a new sensitivity and specificity in diagnosis. This in turn has been reflected in an extension of the veterinarian's ability to study the pathogenesis and epidemiology of disease. The application of molecular techniques has created new vaccines and treatments which are currently being introduced. Their specificity is often high and they are often very effective against the target agent. Diseases such as *E.coli* enteritis, enzootic pneumonia, swine dysentery and pleuropneumonia may all be controllable as a result of these novel vaccines.

Herd medication and disease eradication procedures

The advances in the understanding of disease and the ability to detect and control it have consolidated the ability of the veterinary profession to eradicate disease from individual herds, pyramids or areas. Combined programmes of treatment and or vaccination, disinfection and restriction of movement or isolation, have been developed for the eradication of Aujeszky's Disease, swine dysentery, enzootic pneumonia, mange, atrophic rhinitis and pleuropneumonia. The widespread availability of artificial insemination (AI) and of disease-free breeding stock (from the high health nucleus and multiplier herds of major companies) has meant that disease-free status can be maintained, particularly where herds are scattered.

The effect of free movement of livestock across national borders within the E.C. on the disease status of individual herds and countries remains to be seen. In general, those purchasing stock from distant units should satisfy themselves that the testing programme carried out prior to certification is adequate and that animals are transported in such a way that they are not exposed to disease en route. Incoming stock should always be quarantined. Where production animals are brought from a distance, vaccination programmes for disease such as Aujeszky's Disease in the herd of origin should be continued in the herd of destination.

Computer programmes for monitoring productivity

Recording of herds by commercially-available computer programmes is now widespread. Many large farms can now produce figures for their days to bacon, weaning to service intervals, numbers born and whether born dead or alive, feed conversion rates and mortality rates. Individual growth rates may be available where on-farm performance testing is carried out. These records can be used to interpret at a glance the recent reproductive and growth performance of a herd and to identify problem areas in production. They are now giving information about the performance of finishing herds and are able to provide individual sow health records. They should always be consulted before assessing a production problem.

Welfare

The welfare of pigs continues to be a matter of considerable concern to the Veterinary Profession, the farmer, Parliament, the E.C., the Press and the Public. Pressure to replace intensive systems of management is continuing in the U.K. and some other countries in Europe.

Particular concern has been expressed over the behavioural requirements of piglets on cage and flat deck systems, especially after early weaning (3 weeks) and those of the confined sow. The question of comfort for all classes of stock has been studied and the Welfare Code amended to give certain recommendations for the humane housing of livestock. The castration of piglets is considered unnecessary on both economic and welfare grounds provided they reach slaughter within 160 days. The handling of pigs in transit and at abattoirs is also the subject for new legislation and it is likely that public pressure will increasingly affect husbandry practices on the farm. The recent requirement for sows to be loose-housed in groups and not in stalls or tethers introduces welfare problems of its own because of fighting on batching, difficulties with individual feeding and difficulties in detecting and managing sick animals. Recent studies of sow behaviour have provided guidance on their requirements and new, economical loose housing systems are being developed and installed which allow individual feeding, adequate comfort, exercise and proper inspection. The limitations of electronic sow feeders and single space feeders are more clearly understood.

Welfare criteria are now being applied more objectively to outdoor sows which represent 20-25% of the UK sow herd. This trend to outdoor pig husbandry has re-introduced problems of foxes and parasitism not seen for many years.

A general increase in slaughter weights or the effects of disease and reduced growth rate can lead to over-crowding and increase welfare problems.

Improvements in welfare have arisen from the requirements for the certification of casualty slaughter animals. The criteria for humane endpoints and the best methods for humane slaughter have reduced suffering. Training of farm staff in nursing and techniques for humane slaughter has also helped and is becoming increasingly important.

Meat quality

Recent attention to meat quality has introduced meatier pigs growing to higher slaughter weight and using Duroc components to improve marbled fat content. The requirements by supermarkets (they purchase in the UK) has influenced breeding, husbandry, medication and slaughter policy considerably. Recent concern about residues of antimicrobials and other therapeutic substances in meat has improved the strict observance of withdrawal times. Monitoring for carcase residues is widely practised in the U.K. and in other E.C. countries. The use of antimicrobials in feed is strictly controlled in the U.K. and E.C. Regulations on prescribing, particularly the Veterinary Written Directive and the licensing of units allowed to incorporate medication into feedstuffs are in place . These controls, coupled with the maintenance of Treatment Records on farms in the U.K. have reduced the likelihood of residues reaching meat. The ban by Sweden on antimicrobial growth promoters may have implications for production in E.C. countries where political (socioeconomic) decisions of this type were made for hormonal substances and are being proposed for all new production enhancers including porcine somatotrophin (PST).

Veterinarians in the Pig Industry

(a) Private Practice

A few veterinarians specialise entirely in pigs and at least two U.K. practices deal solely with pigs. Many practices, particularly in East Anglia and Yorkshire have several members with an interest in pigs. These members may act as consultants to feed firms and other organisations owning pigs. Some practices have their own diagnostic laboratories. A specialist diploma and certificate course is run by the Royal College of Veterinary Surgeons, Belgravia House, Horseferry Road, London.

(b) Industry

Veterinarians are employed by feed firms to service their pig enterprises and by pharmaceutical companies concerned with products for the pig industry. Some breeding companies also employ their own veterinarians to handle health problems both in the U.K. and worldwide. Many other veterinarians based in practice or University offer consultations on a part-time basis for these companies and for the Profession. Increasing numbers of veterinarians are being employed in public health, food hygiene and by the new Meat Hygiene Service.

(c) Ministry of Agriculture (State Veterinary Service)

Veterinarians specialising in pigs are to be found in the Field Service, in the Investigation Service and at the Central Veterinary Laboratory, Weybridge, the Lasswade laboratory and the Veterinary Research Laboratories, Stormont. The requirement for laboratory methods in diagnosis or the confirmation of diagnosis in many pig diseases means that a number of these people are in the Investigation Service, particularly in Centres at Thirsk, Bury St. Edmunds and Winchester, and the Scottish Agricultural College V.I. Centres at Aberdeen and Edinburgh, serving the pig rearing areas. In addition, veterinarians with pig expertise may be employed by the Meat and Livestock Commission and other Government sponsored bodies.

(d) Research

Research Institutes including those of the BBSRC, Industry and the Universities provide most opportunities for research into pigs in this country and a few posts exist in Universities for teaching pig diseases. The use of pigs in biomedical research is increasing and may offer opportunities for the veterinarian particularly as a named veterinary surgeon.

Information about pigs and the pig industry (Bibliography)

Many pig farmers in the U.K. read the following journals:-

Pig Farming, Farming Press Ltd., a monthly.
Pig International, Watt Publishing, Illinois, a monthly
Pigs, Misset International, a bi-monthly.
International Pig Letter. Pig World Inc. Box 662, South St. Paul, Min. 55075 U.S.

and pig articles which appear in less specialised journals.

The following books and videos published by Farming Press deal with pig housing, husbandry and diseases:-

Outdoor Pig Production, K. Thornton.
Practical Outdoor Pig Production, K. Thornton (video)
Housing the Pig, G., Brent
Practical Pig Nutrition, C. Whittemore and F. Elsey
The economics of Pig Production, Bob Ridgeon.
The Sow, Improving her Efficiency, P.R. English, W. Smith and A. MacLean.
Pig Ailments Recognition and Treatment.
P.R. English, V.R. Fowler, S. Baxter and W. Smith.
Stockmanship: Improving the care of the pig and other livestock. P.R. English, G. Burgess R.S. Cochrane, J. Dunne

Other books about pigs include:-

The Science and Practice of Pig Production, C.T. Whittemore   (1993), Essex Longman
Digestion in the Pig, D.E. Kidder and M.J. Manners (1978) Scientechnica, Bristol.
Reproduction in the Pig, P. Hughes and M. Varley (1980) Butterworths.
Pig Health Recording Production and Finance - A Producers' Guide. Pig Veterinary Society, c/o T. Heard, Grove House,
Corsham, Malmesbury, Wilts.
Intensive Pig Production, Seaton Baxter, 1984.Granada books.
Wolfe Colour Atlas of Pig Diseases. W. Smith, D.J. Taylor and R.H.C. Penny. (1989). Wolfe Medical.
M.L.C. 1994 Pig Yearbook. Meat and Livestock Commission (Annu).
A handbook on pig disease. Walton, J.R. Liverpool University Press (1987)

Further information about pig diseases may be obtained from:

Diseases of Swine 7th edition. Edited by A.D. Leman, B.E. Straw, W.L. Mengeling, S. D'Allaire and D.J. Taylor. Iowa State University Press 1992
Veterinary Medicine, Blood, D.C. and Radostits, O.M. 7th Ed. (1989), Balliere Tindall.
A.R.C. Index of Current Research on Pigs (Annual) lists papers published worldwide and current research topics.
Pig News and Information (Quarterly), Commonwealth Agricultural Bureau lists papers on porcine subjects and these are also available on CD ROM.

The UK Pig Veterinary Society meets twice a year and publishes proceedings currently The Pig Journal, previously The Pig Veterinary Journal twice a year. Editorial Committee, c/o T.W. Heard, Grove House, Corsham, Malmesbury, Wilts. Members are informed about International Pig Veterinary Society meetings which are held biennially. The next meeting is in Bologna in June 1996 and the following one will be in Birmingham in 1998. Tape slide programmes on pig topics are obtainable from I.B.V.E.A., Department of Veterinary Medicine, University of

Queensland, Brisbane, Australia and the Audiovisual Library, Royal Veterinary College, Royal College Street, London, NWl OTU.

The Pig: Some Basic Information

Breeds UK Large White, Landrace, rarely Saddleback Tamworth, Berkshire, Middle White and Gloucester Old Spot).

Imported: Pietrain, Hampshire, Duroc, Meishan and others from time to time.

Clinical Information

Body temperature : 39°C (102°F)
  Lower critical point 38.4°C (101.2°F).
  Upper critical point 40°C (103.5°F).
Respiratory rate, resting, 18°C: 20-30 per minute, more in young (up to 50), less in old (to 13-15) in sows.

Pulse (resting) :70-80 per minute, more in young (200-280, newborn).

Packed Cell Volume (PCV)	0.42	(0.37-0.46)	1/1
Red Blood Cells (rbc)	7.0	(6.5-8.0)	$\times 10^{12}$ /1
White Blood Cells (wbc)	18.0	(10.0-23.0)	$\times 10^{9}$ /1
Platelets	400.0	(250.0-700.0)	10^{9} /1
Haemoglobin (Hb)	140	(110-142)	g/l

For blood levels of ions or plasma enzymes, see appropriate section. All blood parameters may change with age. These are adult figures.

Husbandry factors

(a) **Minimum temperature requirements:-**

Adults: In service areas,
  dry sow houses and yards.   15-20°C, 59-68°F
  In farrowing houses   15-18°C, 59-64°F

Piglets to 5 kg.   25-30°C, 77-84°F

Early weaned, 3 weeks and over (5-18kg)   27-32°C, 81-90°F
Weaned pigs (6 weeks and over)   21-24°C, 70-75°F
Growers (19-45kg)   15-21°C, 59-70°F
Finishing pigs (45-95kg)   13-18°C, 55-64°F
Heavy hogs (90-115kg)   10-15°C, 50-59°F

These temperatures should not fluctuate.

(b)   Productivity data

Sexual maturity*:   8-9 months male, 7 months female
Oestrus period   21 days
Gestation length   112-116 days, usually 114 days
* may be younger for Meishan crosses

Levels for some commonly recorded productivity parameters are given below. The values given here may be low when compared with the actual results achieved by top herds in the U.K., using some of the most prolific sow lines and the most recent hybrid stock.

Parameter		Target Level	(Top 10% MLC herds (1994)	Interference level
Weaning: Service Interval:		7 days		9 days
Farrowing to first service		87%		80 days
Returns to service		6%		12%
Abortions		1%		2.5%
Failure to farrow		1%		2%
Sow mortality		2.2%	3.7%	3%
Sow culls/100 sows/yr		30	39%	35%
Total mean numbers born		11.5	12.73	11.0
Mean numbers born alive		11.0	11.81	10.5
Mean numbers born dead		4%	7%	6%
Litter scatter		10%	9.6%	18%
Mean numbers weaned/litter		10.0	10.5	9.0
Pre-weaning mortality		8%	11%	12%
Weaning weight 21 days		5.6kg	6.2 at 23	
35 days		10.0kg		
42 days		11.0kg		
Litter/sow/yr		2.4	2.44	2.3
Piglets/sow/yr		24.0	25.7	22
Days to slaughter Pork	59-68 kg (av. 64)	112		
Cutter	72-82 (75)	126		
Bacon	86-93 (89)	147		
Heavy	100 kg			
Feed conversion	6.2-68 kg		2.04	
efficiency	6.2-76 kg		2.08	
	6.7-90 kg		2.33	
Daily liveweight gain	6.2-85 kg		562	
	6.2-76 kg		590	
	7.7-90 kg		610	

Additional parameters may be found in the MLC Pig Yearbooks and Pig Health, Recording and Finance - A Producers' Guide.

Check list for clinical examination

History

Age, breed or supplier, sex, weight, animal's number, number in batch or litter, number affected, number died, diet + additives. Signs observed, treatment given. Sows - last litter/date served.

Examine in general

1. Housing of animals: type and arrangement of house
                          environmental temperature
                          ventilation
                          drainage
                          flooring
                          drinkers
                          feeding arrangements
                          and type of food
2. Attitude and behaviour of group
3. Is any feed left?
4. Appearance of dung
5. Respiratory rate

In detail

6. Skin colour and lesions/udder
7. Feet/legs and gait
8. Mouth, nose and eyes
9. Rectum for diarrhoea
10. Vagina or prepuce for discharge
11. Respiratory rate/auscultate chest/heart (especially sows)
12. Rectal temperature
13. Nervous signs such as convulsions or tremor
14. E.C.G. may reveal cardiac abnormalities.

Sampling

Blood samples should be taken from the jugular vein, anterior vena cava or ear. Fine needles should be used for neonates. Milk can be obtained in quantity after oxytocin injection. Clean udder.

Nasal secretion. Cotton-tipped fine nasal swabs can be used. The external nares should be cleansed if possible. Inoculation of plates on site improves recovery of respiratory pathogens.

Tonsillar swabs. A pig gag of metal shaped like a tuning fork with an appropriate-sized gap can be used to hold the mouth open and swabs can be taken from the tonsil. In neonates, a tube may be placed on the tonsil and the swab inserted for sampling.

Vaginal inspection can be carried out using a speculum and samples can be taken. If no speculum, use a guarded swab.

Urine. Urination frequently follows disturbance in resting sows. Samples for biochemistry and microbiology can be taken midstream. Dip slides can be used for bacteruria.

Faeces. Rectal faeces for parasitology, rectal faeces diluted in saline for E.M. examination for viruses, toxins, heat-resistant sporulating *C.perfringens* type A and phase contrast microscopy for spirochaetes, rectal swabs for culture and air-dried faeces smears for immunofluorescence or for cryptosporidium.

Skin scrapings for fungi and mites and ear wax for mites, swabs for bacteriology and vesicle fluid or swabs for virology.

Submission of samples (with full history).

For virological examination, swabs should be submitted in transport medium and chilled. Some can be frozen. Faeces should only be chilled.

For bacteriological examination, swabs should be submitted in transport medium without antibiotic and all samples chilled not frozen.

For parasitological examination, chilled never frozen.

Blood samples clotted for serum. Serum itself may be frozen, other blood samples must not be frozen. Unclotted blood for bacteriology or for biochemistry in the appropriate anticoagulant.

Samples should be sent first class post or rail, marked "Pathological Specimen" and packed according to the Postal Regulations or delivered chilled by hand. For specialist examinations the laboratory concerned should be consulted before samples are sent.

Humane endpoints

U.K. farmers and veterinarians are always aware of the requirement of the consumer that animals produced for human food should not be kept alive if they have an injury which is not treatable and which is causing suffering. Both are aware of their legal and moral duty to prevent animal suffering. As a result of the clinical assessments described above, it may be necessary to decide whether each sick animal will -

a)   recover naturally
b)   can be treated and expected to recover fully or
c)   must be killed to prevent further suffering.

A decision must then be taken for all animals in categories b) and c) whether it is economic for them to be treated and fed to slaughter weight or kept until free from residues or whether the animal would be suitable for human consumption of killed. If the animal is to be killed for human consumption, then its fitness to travel must be decided. If there is any doubt, the animal must be killed on farm and not transported regardless of whether the carcase can be salvaged.

To assist the decision process, some suggested humane endpoints are listed below and detailed ones are provided under the individual conditions in the main text. This list is provided also for the guidance of those concerned with welfare and for named veterinary surgeons under the Animals (Scientific Procedures) Act 1986.

General conditions for which euthanasia is advised:

Sows:

Prolapsed uterus, rectum or vagina which cannot be repaired or is already damaged.
Wounds from fighting or accidents of such severity that healing is in doubt.
Severe and extensive burns.
Multiple open sores or wounds.
Cardiac failure from old age or endocarditis.
Lameness from a broken leg, paralysis of hindlimbs, acute or chronic lameness such as from epiphyseolysis/osteochondrosis dissecans or arthritis.
Paralysis
Emaciation with condition score 1.
Dystocia which cannot be treated or where piglets remain.

Growing and finishing pigs:

Wounds as above including open wounds from tail-biting.
Lameness as above including severe claw damage.
Rectal prolapse as above.
Strangulated hernias.
Paralysis
Emaciation.
Severe or terminal septicaemia, pneumonia or enteritis.

Piglets:

Those with congenital deformities incompatible with life such as epitheliogenesis imperfecta, kyphosis and atresia ani.
Emaciation.
Multiple arthritis and lameness.
Weakness at birth.
Umbilical abscessation (severe).
Wounds and overlaying.
Paralysis
Severe and terminal septicaemia, pneumonia or enteritis.

This list is not exhaustive, but provides a general guide
Euthanasia

Rapid and humane slaughter is routine in all pig units and the pig veterinarian frequently kills pigs for welfare reasons and for post-mortem examination. This section provides a brief guide to methods of humane destruction. A guide to appropriate humane endpoints is given for each condition in which death or chronic disability might occur. The methods actually used will depend upon the person carrying out the procedure, the availability of barbiturates or firearms and whether the carcase will be used for pathological examination, human or animal consumption. Euthanasia should be rapid and painless regardless of the method used. As all methods can fail on occasions, always be prepared to repeat the procedure. Remember that large injured pigs may be violent.

Location: Euthanasia must be carried out as soon as practicable after a decision has been taken about the animal. Pigs should only be moved to a convenient site if it is humane to do so. The requirement to kill *in situ* will restrict the methods used as free bullets should not be used in confined spaces or on concrete floors in case you or an assistant are injured. Any firearm may startle pigs and where possible euthanasia should take place out of sight and hearing of other pigs. Animals which are to be shot and those to be bled may bleed copiously and should be taken to an area which can be disinfected or cleaned if necessary.

Methods of humane destruction.

a)   Trauma

Only suitable for small piglets of less than 3 weeks of age and weighing up to 5kg. The pig should be held firmly by one person and killed by a second using a heavy blunt instrument directed downwards over the brain (between eyes and ears in the midline). If the animal does not appear to be dead, repeat the blow. The brain cannot be examined post mortem, so another method should be used. Swinging the pig by the hindlimbs and smashing the head against a wall or rail is not controllable or aesthetic.

b)   Barbiturate

Suitable for pigs of all ages but depends upon the availability of barbiturate solution of appropriate strength (20% sodium pentabarbitone weight/volume, w/v) and skill in administration. As a controlled drug (Schedule 3, U.K.) and prescription-only medicine (POM), users must be qualified to hold and administer the product. Pigs killed by this method are unfit for human or animal consumption and should not be left accessible to wildlife. It is the method of choice for most pathological examinations.

Young pigs 0-6 weeks of age (to 10kg).

Intravenous injection into the anterior vena cava is the preferred method. When 1-5ml is given rapidly, death is instantaneous. Restraint involves holding the pig on its back in a bleeding cradle if available with the forelimbs held vertical by an assistant. The operator should hold the chin down with one hand and locate the thoracic inlet with the other. The needle (at least 3cm) should be inserted at 45° to the vertical in a caudal direction (towards the heart) and when inserted to 2-3cm, the plunger should be withdrawn to ensure that the needle is in the vein. The barbiturate should be injected smoothly. Pigs should die instantly, but injection into the trachea or lung may result in coughing and into the pericardial sac in cardiac tamponade. If injected elsewhere outside the vein, the animal will gradually lose consciousness but will usually pass through a stage of anaesthetic excitement with paddling which may make repeated injection difficult. As barbiturate suppresses respiratory movements in the pig, the heartbeat should be absent before the pig is left. Pigs killed in this way may be bled out to facilitate post-mortem examination. This process should not be carried out too soon after injection.

Intravenous injection by way of the ear vein is possible but sometimes difficult because of the small diameter of the veins. See below for method. Intracardiac injection may also be used, injecting 2-3cm cranial to the apex beat and 2cm dorsal to it on the left side. Blood should be withdrawn before barbiturate is administered.

Older pigs

The ear vein is the route of choice. The pig should be restrained by the snout by a snare, the ear to be used should be cleaned and the ear veins assessed. The most prominent vein (usually that on the lateral side) should be selected. A needle of appropriate size should be used. It may be helpful to raise the vein by manual pressure or using a rubber band held by artery forceps, but any pressure should be released as soon as the needle is seen to be in the vein as pig ear veins are very fragile and tear easily. Infection should be slow and smooth for the same reason. Successful injection can be monitored by examination of the vein. The blue-purple colour is replaced by a clear colour in white pigs. Any problem results in interruption of the injection and the process should be stopped immediately. Haematomas occur rapidly and the injection site can no longer be used. For best results, begin at the periphery of the ear. Not only is it easiest, but it is possible to use the same vein further down if a blockage occurs. In very large pigs, be prepared for collapse of the animal and leave the needle in place as it may be necessary to administer more than one syringe filled with barbiturate. Death may occur rapidly, but, in larger pigs, it may require 20-50ml of solution to kill the animal. Apnoea usually follows barbiturate injection in pigs and it is particularly important to confirm death in large animals before leaving them or to bleed them out once anaesthetised. Bleeding should be carried out after complete anaesthesia has developed by cutting into the thoracic inlet with the edge of a sharp knife along the jugular channel lateral to the trachea. One or more reflex gasps may follow this procedure.

It is also possible to use the jugular route, but the potential for movement at this site is considerable and, although suitable for bleeding, injection may be more difficult. For the approach, see jugular bleeding.

c)   Shooting

Pigs other than piglets can be killed by shooting and the method must be used for farm slaughter for human consumption. A variety of weapons can be used, but they fall into the following general classes: humane killers using a captive bolt; free bullets from rifle or pistol and shotguns. All these weapons are controlled in the U.K. under the Firearms Regulations and police permits are required for their purchase, carriage and use. Training in their safe handling, use and cleaning should be sought before use on live animals. All pigs which are shot may thrash around and this may be distressing, disruptive and dangerous. After humane killers and free bullets have been used, the animal should be pithed using a stiff wire or, if for human consumption, a stiff nylon/plastic pithing cane. This can be done in the period of quiet after the shot and before the onset of reflex movements. The cane is inserted into the hole and fed into the spinal cord through the foramen magnum. As this method destroys the spinal cord and much of the brain, the method is unsuitable if the carcase is required for neuropathological examination.

Humane killers

These operate by means of a bolt which penetrates the skull and brain, withdrawing automatically after firing. Before use, the cartridge size should be confirmed to be adequate for the size of pig (0.22, 3 grain green cartridge, U.K.) and a second cartridge should be ready for use if failure occurs. A pithing cane and knife should be available before starting. Pigs of up to 24 weeks of age may be killed directly, but older animals may be merely stunned. All should be pithed after shooting and may be bled out as described above.

Animals to be stunned/killed should be restrained by means of an easily released snout snare. Restraint by an assistant holding both ears is unwise because of the risk of movement and accidental damage by the bolt. The same applies to use of humane killers on piglets. The muzzle should be placed on the head in the midline 2cm above a line between the eyes and angled slightly upwards to hit the brain.

Free bullets

These may be provided by free bullet humane killers, 0.22 rifles (pigs less than 24 weeks only) and some handguns. In all cases a soft nosed lead bullet should be used and the operation should be carried out outdoors as the bullet may pass through the pig and ricochet on walls or floor. Any assistants or observers should stand behind the operator, but their number should be restricted to the minimum because of the risk. With the humane killers, the muzzle may be applied to the pig's head, but the other kinds of weapon should be held at least 2-5cm from it in the position described for humane killers above. Free bullets should not be used if there is an alternative and handguns and rifles should be used only in an emergency.

Shotguns

Shotguns used to kill pigs are usually 12 bore, but 0.410 guns may also be used. Restraint is by snare. The muzzle should be held 5-25cm away from the head and the gun may be aimed at the same point as the weapons described above, but are more usually aimed at a point behind and below the ear pointing inwards towards the brain. A neat round hole results with some smoke staining and little blood. The brain and skull bones are smashed but shot remains under the skin at exit and the method is less dangerous than free bullets. The same precautions should be observed. Pithing is difficult with this method and may not be necessary. Post-mortem examination of the pharynx, brain and posterior nares may be impossible.

d)   Commercial slaughter

This is by electric stunning or killing, humane killer or by carbon dioxide inhalation. Stunned pigs are then shackled and bled out.

Check list for post mortem examination

General

History as above, condition of carcase, weight for age, chilled, fresh, frozen. Length of time since death. Method of killing.

External features

Appearance of skin, presence of ectoparasites. Snout normal or twisted, discharge, eyes, normal or discharge, ears congested, bitten/mange, oral cavity, feet and coronary band, udder, rectum and vulva. For stillborn piglets note membranes on skin, gelatinous hoof tips and soft moist cord. Note post-mortem change indicating death *in utero*

Post mortem examination

Abdominal cavity. Umbilicus, peritoneal cavity, fluid or adhesions present, liver, gall bladder, spleen, kidney, adrenals, ureters, uterus, ovaries and bladder. Check mammary glands, and testes and preputial diverticulum. Examine foetuses for placental necrosis, crown rump length, transudates, gross abnormalities, weigh thyroid and X-ray for growth arrests.

Alimentary tract. Pharynx, open and examine oesophagus, open and note restrictions/mucosal ulceration, stomach, open and record feed present, and appearance of mucosa, and examine greater curvature for oedema, small intestine, check villus height at several sites at least 10 cm from duodenum if enteritis present. Record contents and mucosal appearance. Ileum, caecum, colon - note contents and mucosa. Examine mesenteric nodes. Pancreas. Rectum examine mucosa.

Thoracic cavity. Pleura and pleural cavities, the lungs, thymus, pericardium, pericardial cavity, heart - open to check valves. Examine bronchi, trachea and larynx including epiglottis. Bronchial lymph nodes. Oesophagus.

Head. Tonsils, retropharyngeal lymph nodes, teeth, saw snout at premolar 1 for nasal cavity, septum and turbinates, remove brain in cases of meningitis and spinal cord in cases of paralysis. Take CSF before removing head. Note any cerebellar coning and obtain whole brain: cerebellar weight ratio in piglets

Carcase muscle, joints and lymph nodes not so far checked should be examined and any relevant nerves or ganglia dissected out and fixed.

Laboratory examinations should be carried out as described under individual conditions.

For a detailed acount of technique, see Wells, G.A.H.1977, Proc.Pig Vet.Soc. 2, 19-25. Pictures of lesions can be found in the Colour Atlas of Pig Diseases, Smith, Taylor and Penny, Wolfe Medical.

Carcase disposal

Safe and effective disposal of clinical wastes such as carcases follows from post-mortem examinations. Carcases must be examined on washable and waterproof surfaces and drainage from those surfaces must not contaminate surface waters. Disinfection of the site with an appropriate disinfectant is essential. Sharps from euthanasia and the post mortem must be discarded into sharp safes and taken back to the practice for disposal or placed in the farm sharp safes for later disposal.

Carcases may be collected by traditional knackers for onward processing or may need to be buried, incinerated or composted. Storage until collection by knackers is best carried out in a separate building or depot (which may be refrigerated) sited on the periphery of the farm so that the knacker does not enter. It should have appropriate drainage and be capable of disinfection. Burial should only be carried out where the carcases do not contaminate water supplies or surface water and should be deep enough not to cause nuisance to neighbours. Incineration should only be carried out in licensed incinerators capable of incinerating the quantity of material generated by the farm. Composting is possible, but again, the composting bins should be sited so as not to contaminate water courses or cause offence. When high mortality occurs, special plans may have to be made to dispose of carcases safely as ordinary farm mechanisms may be unable to cope. Planning is particularly necessary on sites with little land attached.

Safety on the farm

Pig farms contain a number of hazards to human health and all U.K. farmers should have carried out hazard analysis to reduce the risk to the workforce or visitors. The veterinarian is, however, in charge of hazards during procedures he/she initiates. The following hazard areas specific to pig farms are listed below and should be considered in particular:

Trauma: Pigs may be aggressive and injuries can kill. Restrain or tranquilise mature animals and ensure that an escape route is available. Avoid pig bites and needle stick injuries or cuts from knives or scalpels.

Electrocution: Power should be turned off prior to investigating electrocuted pigs. Avoid old electrical equipment.

Gassing: May occur in poorly ventilated houses.

Drowning: May occur in standing water or slurry lagoons.

Fire: This is a hazard in straw-filled units. If it occurs, evacuate buildings first, consider rescue of other humans next and of the pigs last. Do not endanger human life.

Allergy: Farm dusts are allergenic. Straw, hay, feed and pig urine may all provoke sensitisation. Wear masks or respirators to avoid sensitisation and carry antidotes if sensitised.

Infection: Some pig pathogens are zoonotic and infection should be avoided. Masks and gloves are essential at post mortem and disinfectants should always be available. Zoonotic conditions are listed in the text. Remember that farm rodents etc., also pose a hazard.

Medicines: Some affect human health and should be used carefully. They should be stored carefully, labelled correctly, used only after instruction and their use recorded. Used containers or unused drugs should be discarded as clinical waste. Prostaglandins are hazardous to female staff. Spills should be treated according to data sheet suggestions. Medical advice should be sought after ingestion of medicines and self-infection.

Public health

a)   On farm

The practitioner visiting farms on a regular basis may give advice on management practices which can affect the quality and safety of meat and the risks posed by the disposal of manures and effluent. He can provide early warning of diseases which may be zoonotic such as salmonellosis and monitor the use of medicines and their withdrawal.

b)   At the abattoir

Ante-mortem and post-mortem inspection are vital elements in safeguarding the quality of meat and meat products. The health of the workers in the industry may also benefit from advice about zoonoses.

c)   In onward processing
A knowledge of the production systems used can be invaluable in tracing and eliminating public health hazards from food.

VIRUS DISEASES

A large number of viruses cause clinical disease in pigs and infections with many others have been recorded. The recent occurrence of the Porcine Reproductive and Respiratory Syndrome (PRRS) has highlighted the importance of being able to recognise viral disease and to take any measures appropriate to the disease concerned.

Viral diseases may be recognised as such by the identification of clinical signs, post-mortem findings or epidemiological picture with those of familiar or recorded diseases. These are described below and listed under the appropriate age group in the section on Differential Diagnosis. Appropriate laboratory tests can then be used to confirm their identity and control their identity and control measures such as vaccination can be initiated. The infections which have been described in pigs are listed as an aid in the recognition of unknown syndromes. Others may also occur.

Virus diseases frequently spread from affected animals to susceptible animals after a recognisable incubation period. They are therefore recognisable as infectious. They may be recognisable as virus infections by:

a) the presence of clinical signs suggestive of viral disease such as vesicles

b) the failure of any antimicrobial to affect the course of the disease i.e., not a bacterial condition

c) the presence of specific pathological findings including the presence of syncytia and inclusion bodies

d) viral particles may be identified in lesions or extracts of lesions by electron microscopy or my immunofluorescence using recovered sera

e) virus may be isolated in cell cultures such as established cell lines, primary cultures such as pig kidney cells or alveolar macrophages

f) experimental animal transmission with bacteria/parasite-free inocula may also confirm.

Parvovirus

Definition

Porcine parvovirus (PPV) infection causes infertility, mummified foetuses, stillbirths and small litters in sows. It may be associated with poor growth in the postnatal period. Parvovirus particles have been demonstrated in, and isolated from diarrhoeic faeces and skin lesions.

Incidence

Porcine parvoviruses occur worldwide. Reports of individual surveys indicate that from 76% (Finland), 82% (U.S.), 93% (UK) and 95% (Switzerland) of herds may be infected. One survey of 499 herds in the UK indicated that 7% were negative for antibody to parvovirus and 30% contained both seronegative and seropositive animals. 18% of all sows, 44% of all gilts and 47% of all boars surveyed were seronegative. These figures are similar to those found in other countries and in subsequent surveys in the UK A recent US survey suggests that at least 11% of all litters contain parvovirus-infected foetuses. An antigenically distinct enteric parvovirus has been shown by serological surveys to be widespread in Japan, the only country to be examined, but enteric parvovirus has also been detected in UK and US studies.

Aetiology

Porcine parvovirus is a small (20nm) non-enveloped DNA virus which appears to be stable over a wide range of pH (3-10 for 1 hour at 37°C) and can resist heating at 56°C for 2 days but is killed after exposure to 80°C for 5 minutes. The virus is not affected by ether or a number of proteolytic enzymes. The virus haemagglutinates guinea pig, human and chicken red cells. One antigenic type of the virus exists although isolates with different pathogenicity have been reported. The antigenicity appears to reside in the three capsid proteins, VPl (81kDa) VP2 (66kDa) and VP3 (62kDa). The virus replicates in cells about to divide and may be grown in vitro in primary pig kidney cell monolayers or continuous cell lines. C.P.E. (intranuclear inclusions and cell rounding) may be transient on primary isolation and infected cells may have to be identified using fluorescent antibody, DNA probes, haemadsorption, haemagglutination reactions or ELISA.

Another parvovirus has been reported from the faeces of pigs with diarrhoea in several countries. It has 4 viral proteins and resembles bovine parvovirus. growing best in porcine thyroid and swine embryo kidney cells taking 9 days to C.P.E.

Pathogenesis

Porcine parvovirus enters by the oronasal or venereal routes. A viraemia ensues followed after 10 days by a transient, barely detectable leucopaenia. Viraemia results in passage of the virus into the reproductive tract taking 10-14 days from infection to cross the placenta. In boars it may be found on spermatozoa from days 5-9 post-infection and in seminal vesicles and testicular tissue from days 8-21.

The virus adheres to the zona pellucida of eggs and infects and kills embryos and foetuses until they reach immunocompetence at 67 days' gestation. The virus does not affect the products of conception in animals infected 1-4 weeks prior to service but crosses the placenta in those infected at service and for at least 90 days thereafter. Embryos and foetuses dying before 33-35 days may be resorbed completely while those dying later may become mummified, stillborn or, occasionally, aborted. Infection may spread from piglet to piglet along the uterus. In dams infected later in gestation, piglets which do not die from infection may develop high levels of neutralising antibody or become immunotolerant and remain infected for up to 8 months after birth. Recovered infected piglets may be stunted. Infection of the immuno-incompetent foetus appears to cause endothelial damage, perivascular haemorrhage in the brain and kidney and placental damage. In immuno-competent foetuses, meningoencephalitis with perivascular cuffing appears to develop but more extensive lesions have been described following infection with the Kresse (skin) strain. Maternal endometrial vessels may become surrounded by mononuclear cells. Serum antibody appears at 7-10 days after infection and rises rapidly. Virus is shed in low concentrations in urine, faeces, tonsillar debris and nasal secretions from 2 weeks after infection and pigs remain infectious for approximately 2 weeks. Recovered pigs are solidly immune and passive immunity is passed in colostrum to piglets and can be detected for 4-6 months after birth. The use of PCR and DNA probes may extend these periods.

Clinical signs

Returns to oestrus, failure to farrow, the production of small litters, mummified pigs, stillbirth and, rarely, abortion are the main clinical syndromes associated with parvovirus infections in pigs and are particularly prominent in newly introduced and first litter gilts in which a mean loss of 1.1 pigs per litter results from parvovirus infection. Farrowing rate to first service may be as low as 36% (first litter); small litters (especially those containing 5 or less) and the presence of mummified and stillborn pigs may all occur. Pseudocyesis and irregular returns to oestrus may also be seen. Clinical signs may occur in a whole susceptible herd if disease is introduced. Infection in boars is asymptomatic and appears to have no effect on semen quality or fertility. The virus has been recovered from a vesicular skin condition and from diarrhoeic faeces after weaning. Reports of the experimental production of pneumonia, leucopaenia, diarrhoea and encephalitis in piglets exist.

Pathology

Gross lesions are restricted to the uterus of the sow. Embryos may be shrunken and may die to appear as small areas of necrotic material on the uterine wall. Foetuses may be reduced in size, congested and oedematous prior to death. Dead foetuses become mummified. Mummified foetuses may increase in size along the uterus until stillborn animals are found. For microscopic lesions see Pathogenesis.

Epidemiology

Infection occurs most commonly in young sows and gilts or in susceptible animals introduced into an infected herd. Boars may transmit the virus in their semen for up to 2 weeks after infection and both semen and embryos are potential sources of infection in clean herds as are congenitally-infected pigs. The disease is most common in herds where sows are stalled or tethered, especially where gilts have no contact with older animals. The brief period of virus shedding after infection and the small amount of virus shed in urine, faeces and nasal secretions prevents the rapid and thorough spread of infection from pig to pig. There is persistent environmental contamination for up to 4 months with virus from faeces, secretions and the products of parturition. The products of parturition may be the major source of infection in housed animals and lack of hygiene is important in spread. Piglets of immune sows which do not have active immunity at birth are protected from natural infection and may become susceptible, seronegative gilts or sows. In some herds, immune sows may form a majority and infection may die out. Introduction of infection by pigs, germ plasm or fomites to such susceptible herds can lead to outbreaks of returns to service, small litters and increases in stillbirths and mummified piglets. Virus can infect rats which in turn can shed infective virus for 2-3 weeks but subsequent transmission of infection to pigs is difficult.

Diagnosis

The occurrence of returns to service, small litters, mummified and stillborn pigs in gilts rather than sows with little or no abortion and no history of maternal illness suggests parvovirus infection. The diagnosis may be confirmed by the demonstration of virus in mummified foetuses of less than 70 days' gestation age, by isolation or more commonly, by the demonstration of parvovirus antigen in frozen or histological sections of lung and liver by specific immunofluorescence, immunoperoxidase or using radiolabelled, digoxin or biotin labelled DNA probes. Extracts of foetuses may be tested for viral antigen by latex particle agglunination and recently UK) by ELISA. A number of polymerase chain reaction primers have been used successfully. Neutralising antibody may be detected in the sera of infected sows, of newborn piglets and in foetal fluids including exudates and transudates in stillborn piglets from infected litters. A haemagglutination inhibition test using guinea pig red cells has been used. Sera for this test should be absorbed with kaolin and the erythrocytes used in the test. Antibody levels may reach 1:10,000 or more. Titres greater than 1:256 indicate infection. ELISA tests are now widely used in the UK for the detection of serum antibody and antibody in foetuses. A rise in serum antibody level indicates infection in the absence of vaccination.

Control

Vaccination of susceptible stock is the best way to prevent losses from parvovirus infection. Killed adjuvanted vaccines inactivated with acetylethyleneimine, formalin or ß-propiolactone appear to be capable of preventing the disease if given i/m at least two weeks prior to service. Live viruses attenuated by passage and growth at low temperatures have been used as vaccines. An acetyl-ethyleneimine-inactivated oil-adjuvanted vaccine prepared from virus grown in utero and administered 5-9 weeks before farrowing produced life-long immunity and overcame waning passive immunity. Only killed vaccines are currently in use in the UK (Suvaxyn Parvo, Duphar, Delsuvac Parvo Mycofarm, Parvovax Rhone Merieux and Pig Parvovirus Vaccine, Pitman Moore). Vaccination appears to protect even if low levels of serum antibody are present. Typical vaccination schedules involve a first injection in gilts about 8 weeks before service, followed by booster vaccination at least 2 weeks before service. Sows should be revaccinated after farrowing at least 2 weeks before service. Boars should also be vaccinated at 6 months of age, 6 months later and then annually. Maternal antibody may not disappear until 6-7 months of age and the ability of any vaccine used to overcome this will affect the vaccine schedule for gilts. Subunit vaccines based on capsid protein VP1 are under investigation. In countries where vaccines are not available 'feed back' may be practised. The foetal membranes and other products of parturition and faeces from weaned pigs are ground and administered to susceptible gilts 3 weeks before service. Variable amounts of virus are present in this material. Mummified foetuses represent the best source, followed by stillborn piglets (which may contain antibody) and the products of abortion. The procedure must be licensed under the Waste Foods Order in the UK and is not advisable where vaccine is available.

In herds with solid immunity it is not cost-effective to vaccinate, and vaccination should only be undertaken if the whole herd, a significant portion of the younger stock or introduced gilts are seronegative. About 20 samples are needed and should be identified by parity of the sow sampled to give a profile of herd immunity. Herd immunity should be checked at intervals. Where a seronegative unvaccinated herd exists, and vaccination is not to be carried out, incoming stock should be vaccinated and disinfection practised. Where seronegative and seropositive stock exist, the control of rats and hygiene may reduce the spread amongst pregnant sows. The virus can be destroyed within 5 minutes using sodium hydroxide and sodium hypochlorite. Glutaraldehyde 2% and Formaldehyde 8% are also effective but take longer. Steam cleaning may be used. Commercial disinfectants such as Virkon may also be effective.

References

Bachman, P.A., Sheffy, B.E. and Vaughan, J.T. (1975). Infection and Immunity 12, 455-460. Experimental in utero infections of foetal pigs with a porcine parvovirus.
Cartwright, S.F., Lucas, M. and Hick, R.A. (1969). J.Comp.Path 79, 371-377. A. small haemagglutinating porcine DNA virus I. Isolation and Properties.
Cartwright, S.F. and Lucas (1971). J.Comp.Path. 81, 145-155. II Biological and serological studies.
Jenkins, C.E. (1992). J.Virological Methods 39, 179-184. An enzyme-linked immuno-sorbent assay for detection of porcine parvovirus in fetal tissues.
Kresse, J.I., Taylor, W.D., Stewart, W.N. and Eernisse, K.A. (1985). Vet.Microbiol. 10, 525-531. Parvovirus infection in pigs with necrotic and vesicle-like lesions.
Mengeling, W.L., Brown T.T., Paul, P.S. and Gutenkunst, D.E. (1979). Am.J.Vet.Res. 40, 204-207. Efficacy of an inactivated virus vaccine for the prevention of porcine parvovirus induced-reproductive failure.
Mengeling, W.L., Paul, P.S. (1986). J.Am.Vet.Med.Ass. 188, 1293-1295. Survival of virus.
Meyers, P.J., Liptrap, R.M., Miller, R.B., and Thorsen, J. (1987). Am.J.Vet.Res. 48, 621-626. Hormonal changes after infection.
Molitor, T.W., Oraveerakul, K., Zharg, Q.Q., Choi, C.S. and Ludemann, L.R. (1991). J.Virological Methods 32, 201-211. Polymerase chain reaction for the detection of porcine parvovirus.
Nash, W.A. (1990). Veterinary Record 126, 175-176. Porcine parvovirus survey
Oraveerakul, K., Choi, C.S. and Molitor, T.W. (1990). J.Veterinary Diagnostic Investigation 2, 85-91. Detection of parvovirus using non-radioactive nucleic acid hybridisation.
Robinson, B.T., Cartwright, S.F., Danson, D.L.G. (1985). Veterinary Record 117, 611-612. Porcine parvovirus: a serological survey in the United Kingdom Jan. 1984-Jan. 1985.
Wrathall, A.E., Wells, D.E., Cartwright, S.F. and Frerichs, G.N.1984). Research in Veterinary Science 36, 136-143. An inactivated oil emulsion vaccine for the prevention of porcine parvovirus-induced reproductive failure.
Wrathall, A.E. (1988). Veterinary Record 122, 411-418. Field trials of an inactivated oil-emulsion porcine parvovirus vaccine in British pig herds.
White, M.E.C. (1984). Pig Veterinary Journal 22, 93-99. Some thoughts on vaccination.
Yasuhara, H., Matsui, O. et al. (1989). Japanese J.Vet.Sci. 51, 337-344. Characterisation of parvovirus isolated from diarrhoeic faeces of a pig.

Enterovirus Infections

Infection with enteroviruses may be asymptomatic, is associated with polio-encephalomyelitis and less frequently with abortion, stillbirth and infertility. They are also associated with myocarditis and have caused pneumonitis and transient diarrhoea in experimental animals. Swine vesicular disease is also an enterovirus.

Incidence

Porcine enteroviruses occur worldwide and the infection rate in pig populations is high. Individual strains such as Teschen virus may be restricted in their distribution.

Properties of porcine enteroviruses

Porcine enteroviruses are spherical RNA viruses 25-31nm in diameter and are resistant to chloroform and ether. They are relatively heat stable and survive heating at 56°C for 3 hours relatively well, persist in infected tissue culture fluids for weeks or months at room temperature and have been shown to survive for up to 168 days at 15°C. They are stable between pH 2.0 and 9.0 and are relatively resistant to some disinfectants, e.g. lysol and cetrimide, but can be inactivated by formaldehyde, sodium hypochlorite, 70% ethanol and modern iodophors.

Porcine enteroviruses grow readily in cultures of pig kidney cells and produce cytopathic effects (C.P.E.) of three types. Isolates are classified according to the type of C.P.E. produced and on antigenic grounds. Strains of serogroups 1-7 and 11 e.g. Teschen produce Type 1 C.P.E. in which focal areas of rounded cells occur and those of serogroup 8, e.g. V13 produce Type II C.P.E. in which cells become granular with cytoplasmic protrusions. Up to 8 serogroups were described by serum neutralisation and isolates (other than swine vesicular disease) fall into 11 serogroups by complement fixation. Original isolates from infertility cases were identified by letters as follows: SMEDI (Swine mummification embryonic death and infertility) A-E etc. SMEDI A belongs to serogroup 8, B to 3, C to 1, D to 8 and E to 6.

Porcine enteroviruses multiply in the intestines of pigs but do not readily infect laboratory animals.

References

Knowles, N.J. (1983). Br.Vet.J. 139, 19-22. Isolation and identification of porcine enteroviruses in Great Britain 1979-1980.
Knowles, N.J., Buckley, L.S. and Pereira, H.G. (1979). Arch.Virol. 62, 201-208. Classification of porcine enterovirus as by antigenic analysis and cytopathic effects on tissue culture.

Polioencephalomyelitis
(Teschen disease, Talfan disease, Benign enzootic paresis)

Definition

Infection with Serogroup 1 porcine enteroviruses can be asymptomatic or cause polioencephalomyelitis with varying degrees of fever, convulsions, tremors or paresis.

Incidence

Teschen is not seen in Britain but may still occur in Central and Eastern Europe. Talfan is reported from time to time in the U.K. and less pathogenic Serogroup 1 infections may also occur in all pig-iology

Caused by Teschen virus (Group 1 C.P.E., Serogroup 1) and other members of Serogroup 1.

Pathogenesis

The pathogenesis of the condition is similar to that of polio in man. Infection leads to multiplication in the ileum and large intestine and the associated lymph nodes, and, in non-immune animals, this is followed by viraemia associated with the pyrexia of 40-41°C, 104-106°F, and by localisation of the virus in the brain and spinal cord where it affects the neurones of the grey matter to give rise to the clinical signs, within 7-10 days of infection.

Virus is shed from multiplication sites in the reticuloendothelial tissue of the lamina propria of the intestine, especially in the ileum and the large intestine, for several weeks and may be isolated from the faeces. Recovery is associated with the development of systemic antibodies and with local IgA immunity in the gut. Passive immunity from the dam protects sucking pigs from infection until after weaning and infection is common as this immunity wanes at 5-8 weeks of age.

Clinical signs

Two clinical syndromes are recognised, the severe form (Teschen disease) which occurs in Central Europe and the mild form: Talfan disease, (G.B.); benign enzootic paresis (Denmark); or polio-encephalomyelitis (Canada, U.S., Australia).

Severe form: Affected animals develop fever of 40-41°C, 104-106°F, and show slight incoordination of the limbs, lassitude and anorexia. This stage is followed by irritability and then by stiffness, tremors, convulsions and paralysis often ending in death in 3-4 days. Mildly-affected animals may recover. This form affects non-immune pigs of all ages in herds where the disease is enzootic.

Mild form: This form affects young, unweaned and weaned pigs. 50-100% of a litter may be affected. Elevated temperature, diminished control of the hind legs and ataxia are succeeded by paresis or recovery. Mortality is unusual. Animals are frequently seen in the "dog-sitting" position.

Humane slaughter of animals with total paresis, or any degree of paresis which prevents eating and/or drinking, prevents use of all 4 limbs or leads to pressure sores or erosions. As neurones have been destroyed recovery is unlikely.

Pathological findings

Gross lesions other than muscle wasting in chronic cases are not apparent. Encephalomyelitis is found on microscopic examination and is more severe in the grey matter than in the white. Neuronal degeneration, perivascular cuffing, neuronophagia and meningitis may all be seen. The ventral columns of the spinal cord, the brain stem and the cerebellar cortex are chiefly affected. In mild forms, the lesions are milder and less extensive and have been restricted to the spinal cord in recent cases in the UK.

Epidemiology

Severe disease is only found in Central Europe. Mild forms are most common elsewhere. Inapparent infection is widespread and, in Britain, the clinical signs are rarely seen and are sporadic when they occur in a herd. Recovering pigs may pass infective faeces for several weeks. Manure and natural waters may remain contaminated for weeks. There is no documented risk to man.

Diagnosis

A presumptive diagnosis may be made on the basis of the clinical signs, epizootiology and the pathological findings. Confirmation may be obtained by examining for a rise in complement fixing, ELISA or virus neutralising antibody levels but isolation of the virus from the brain and spinal cord is necessary for a conclusive diagnosis. Chronically-affected pigs may not yield virus from the CNS.

Control

Vaccination using live attenuated vaccine is practised in Central and Eastern Europe, but the milder forms of the disease are usually not treated or controlled in Britain. If the severe form should appear here, a slaughter policy might be used to control it coupled with isolation. The disease is notifiable under the Teschen Disease Order (1994) in domestic and EC legislation.

Reproductive Failure, Stillbirths and Infertility (SMEDI)

Definition

Infection with enteroviruses may cause mummification (M) embryonic death (ED) and infertility (I).

Incidence

Infection is widespread in Britain but the reproductive effects are difficult to distinguish from parvovirus infections without laboratory tests.

Aetiology

The enteroviruses concerned have been called SMEDI viruses. Examples include V13 and F34, serotypes 3 and 8.

Pathogenesis

Infection of the foetuses takes place after viraemia in the sow or via infected spermatic or ovarian fluids. Infection of the litter is rarely complete and may never occur in immune animals, although maternal immunity cannot protect against intra-uterine infection.

The results of infection vary according to the period of gestation in which infection occurs. The most common sequelae of infection are death and resorption of the embryo if infection occurs before 35 days' gestation, resulting in delayed returns to service or death, mummification, abortion or malformation of the foetus and stillbirth if infection occurs after 35 days' gestation.

Clinical signs

Delayed returns to service, abortions and the production of litters containing variable numbers of mummified, dead or stillborn piglets or litters containing few piglets may follow the introduction of fresh breeding stock to a farm. Affected sows normally farrow satisfactorily on subsequent occasions. Reproductive failures due to enterovirus are rarely associated with clinical signs in the dam.

Epidemiology

Reproductive failure usually results from the introduction of a fresh strain of enterovirus to a non-immune herd and affects sows of all ages once only.

Diagnosis

Several other micro-organisms cause infertility of this type, especially porcine parvovirus and sometimes Aujeszky's disease virus, in countries where it still occurs. Leptospiral infection should be ruled out, also erysipelas and other systemic infections. If possible, virus should be isolated from the lungs of foetuses or stillborn piglets for confirmation. Frozen or chilled foetuses should be submitted for diagnosis. Paired serum samples may be of use in confirmation of the agent involved. Serum samples or samples of transudates from thoracic or abdominal cavities of piglets may also be used for antibody determination. A titre of 1:32 or more may indicate active infection.

Control

Isolation is probably the only method of prevention. When an outbreak occurs in a herd, the full economic effects can be mitigated and the immunity of the general population raised by dosing sows and gilts with ground faeces, foetal membranes and mummified foetuses at least 3 weeks prior to service. There are risks to health in this practice, but if used with care, it may maintain immunity to these viruses at a high level. In the UK the Waste Foods Order must be observed.

Reference:

Huang, J., Gentry, R.F., Zarkower, A. (1980). Am.J.Vet.Res. 41, 469-473. Experimental infection of pregnant sows with porcine enteroviruses.

Encephalomyocarditis

Definition

A condition of viral aetiology in which pigs of varying ages are found dead. Mortality varies between 10 and 100% and rates are highest in young pigs. Depression and staggering may occasionally be seen before death. The same virus is also associated with stillbirths and the birth of mummified foetuses of uneven size.

Incidence

Reported from the U.S., where 89% Iowa herds, 13.8% breeding stock and 8.5% finishing pigs had antibody in 1992, Central America and Australasia but the rodent viruses are found worldwide. Antibody to the virus has been found in pigs in the UK but neither clinical syndrome has been identified. Clinical disease has been identified in most European countries and 69% sera were positive in one Italian survey.

Aetiology

The condition is caused by encephalomyocarditis (E.M.C.) virus, a picornavirus of rodents assigned to the cardiovirus group. This virus is ether-resistant and resistant to a wide range of pH. Most isolates are inactivated at 60°C for 30 minutes. The virus haemagglutinates guinea pig red cells. There are four major viral proteins.

Pathogenesis

Infection is oral and follows exposure to infected rodents such as rats or consumption of their entrails. Virus multiplies in the pig intestine, becomes systemic and multiplies in heart muscle. Transplacental infection also occurs as soon as 2 weeks post-infection. Foetuses of all ages can be affected.

Clinical signs

Sudden death, particularly in piglets. Pigs with sub-lethal infections may show signs of fever to 41°C (105°F), cyanosis of extremities, depression, staggering or dyspnoea. Sows and gilts may be fevered and abort at 107-111 days' gestation. Failure to farrow and the birth of litters containing stillborn piglets and mummies of different sizes may occur over a period of 2-3 months.
Animals with cardiac failure should be killed humanely. Heart damage is unlikely to resolve.

Post mortem findings

Carcases may be congested. Excess clear fluid is present in the thoracic, pericardial and peritoneal cavities and pulmonary oedema and hepatic enlargement are common. The heart is soft and pale with white areas 2-15 mm in diameter suggestive of necrosis, commonly on the right ventricular epicardium and extending for varying distances into the myocardium. Necrosis of the myocardium with lymphocytic and macrophage infiltration is seen in acute cases. Fibrosis of these lesions occurs in recovered animals. Mild meningo-encephalitis may be present. Affected foetuses may be mummified or have non-suppurative encephalitis including perivascular cuffing and focal myocarditis in addition to gross lesions of myocardial haemorrhage and excess pericardial fluid.

Epidemiology

Found in a wide variety of species but the main reservoir of infection is rats. Feed is contaminated by rats or their faeces. Pig-to-pig transmission has not been confirmed. Antibodies have been found in man, but have not been associated with heart disease.

Diagnosis

The clinical picture and post-mortem findings are suggestive of encephalomyocarditis but other causes of sudden death such as Vitamin E deficiency may need to be considered. Encephalomyocarditis reproductive disease must be distinguished from parvovirus and other infectious forms of reproductive failure.

Virus demonstration by isolation on PCR and/or detection of serum neutralising or haemagglutination inhibition antibodies are necessary for confirmation of a diagnosis. Foetal transudates may contain antibody and can confirm intra-uterine infection.

Control

Prevention of exposure from rodents or pigs from infected farms. Disinfection with chlorine (0.5 ppm) disinfectants. An inactivated oil adjuvanted vaccine has been described and appears to prevent reproductive failures in experimental studies.

References:

Acland, H.M., Littlejohn, I.R. (1975) Aust. Vet. J. 51, 409-415. Encephalomyocarditis virus infection of pigs. I. An outbreak in New South Wales.

Coulson, A. and Carlson, J. (1992). Proc. IPVS 12, 103. Encephalomyocarditis in Europe and America.

Joo, H.S., Kim, H.S. and Leman, A.D. (1988). Arch. Virol. 100, 131-134. Detection of antibody to encephalomyocarditis virus in mummified or stillborn pigs.

Joo, H.S., Kim, H.S. and Leman, A.D. (1988). Arch.Virol. 100, 131-134. Detection of antibody to encephalomyocarditis virus in mummified or stillborn pigs.

Koenen, F., De Clercq, K. and Strobbe, R. (1992). Proc. IPVS 12, 104. Isolation of encephalomyocarditis virus in the offspring of swine with reproductive failure in Belgium

Littlejohn, I.R. (1984). Aust.Vet.J. 61, 93. Encephalomyocarditis virus from stillborn pigs. Encephalomyocarditis antibodies in sera from apparently normal pigs.

Zimmerman, J.J., Owen, W.J., Hill, A.T., Beran, G.W. (1991). J.Am.Vet.Med.Ass. 199, 1737-1741. Seroprevalence of antibodies against encephalomyocarditis virus in swine of Iowa.

Vomiting and Wasting Disease

Definition

A disease of neonatal piglets caused by a Haemagglutinating Encephalomyelitis Virus (H.E.V.) and characterised by vomiting, constipation and anorexia leading to wasting and death as a result of encephalomyelitis and viral damage to gastrointestinal neurones.

Incidence

The disease was first recorded in Canada, but is now known in the U.K. and most of Europe, the U.S., Japan and Australasia. Clinical signs of infection are uncommon in Britain, and the other countries but antibodies to the virus occur widely in the pig population (up to 95% of sows although a recent survey in Japan suggested a lower figure there).

Aetiology

The disease is caused by infection of young piglets with H.E.V., a coronavirus. This RNA virus is ether and chloroform and heat sensitive, stable from pH 3-10 and agglutinates and becomes adsorbed to chick, rat and hamster erythrocytes, unlike T.G.E. virus. The mean size of H.E.V. is 120 nm with projections of 19 nm. There may be some antigenic similarity between the 2 viruses, but they are distinct in serum neutralisation tests. The virus grows in pig kidney cells to form syncytia within 12-16 hours. CPE is complete in 48 hours. There is only one serotype.

Pathogenesis

After oronasal infection, clinical signs develop within 3-5 days. Primary viral multiplication takes place in epithelial cells of the tonsil, lung, nasal mucosa and lungs. Virus spreads along nerves to the trigeminal, inferior vagal, superior cervical, solar and dorsal root ganglia and to the intestinal nervous plexuses. The trigeminal and vagal sensory nuclei in the brain stem become infected followed by other nuclei, the cerebrum, cerebellum and the spinal cord. Viral replication in the gastric nervous plexus causes damage and leads to delayed gastric emptying and eventual starvation. Passive colostral immunity protects against infection.

Clinical signs

Piglets aged between 5 days and 3 weeks are affected. The first signs to be noted are vomiting, huddling of the piglets which may be associated with a rise in temperature, depression, anorexia and constipation. Some affected animals may show signs of encephalomyelitis, e.g. hind leg weakness or difficulties in swallowing. Affected piglets die within 36-48 hours or become progressively emaciated. The contrast between affected and unaffected piglets in the same litter is striking. Clinical signs in piglets may be preceded by transient fever (to 40.6°C, 105°F) in the sows. Most infections occur in older pigs after maternal antibody has disappeared and are inapparent. Young pigs with progressive wasting or nervous signs should be killed by 7 days after development of clinical signs.

Post mortem lesions

No specific lesions are seen. The intestinal tract is normally empty with scanty faeces and there is pronounced wasting. In 25% of cases a non-suppurative encephalomyelitis is found in which perivascular cuffing with mononuclear cells, glial node formation, neuronal degeneration and meningitis are seen in the grey matter of the mesencephalon, pons, medulla oblongata and in the upper spinal cord.

Epidemiology

A few litters may be affected in a herd at any one time (between 16 and 95% of the piglets at risk) and most of the clinically affected piglets die. Infection (monitored by serological means) spreads throughout the herd in nasal secretions. Frequently the clinical disease appears only in the litters of bought-in breeding stock and not in the herd at large. Maternal immunity is transferred in the colostrum but has disappeared by 15 weeks of age. The virus also spreads amongst weaned fattening pigs and active immunity develops within 8-16 weeks. The virus is rapidly destroyed by UV light.

Diagnosis

The disease occurs in piglets less than 21 days of age and may be suspected when vomiting, depression and constipation is followed by wasting and hairiness compared with uninfected littermates. Diagnosis may be confirmed by virus isolation from the respiratory tract, hindbrain and spinal cord of early cases. The C.P.E. can be confirmed as specific by haemagglutination, haemadsorption, serum neutralisation or immunofluorescence. Demonstration of antibody in the sera of wasting piglets and in sera from the dams of affected litters 14 days after the clinical signs are first noted is also of use. Enteroviruses and Aujeszky's Disease may also cause encephalitis but are more severe and usually also affect older pigs. T.G.E. causes profuse diarrhoea and no encephalitis.

Treatment and control

There is no treatment and control in non-infected herds depends upon the maintenance of a closed herd or the purchase of stock from herds known to be free from the disease. In infected herds the only preventative measure is to ensure access to colostrum. It is possible that immunity may be stimulated in non-pregnant gilts by feeding affected piglets or the faeces of weaned pigs to them. This would require permission under the Waste Foods Order in the U.K. Disinfection is possible using lipid solvents.

References:

Andries, K. and Pensaert, M.B. (1980). Am.J.Vet.Res. 41, 215-218. Virus isolation and immunofluorescence in different organs of pigs infected with H.E.V.
Andries K. and Pensaert, M.B. (1980). Am.J.Vet.Res. 41, 1372-1278. Immunofluorescence studies on the pathogenesis of H.E.V. after oronasal inoculation.
Cartwright, S.F. and Lucas, M. (1970). Veterinary Record 86, 278-280. Vomiting and Wasting Disease in piglets.
Cartwright, S.F. Lucas. M., Cavill, J.P., Gush, A.F. and Blandford, T.B. (1969). Veterinary Record 84, 175-176. Vomiting and Wasting Disease in piglets.
Narita, M., Kawamura, H., Haritani, M. and Kobayashi, M. (1989). J.Comp.Path. 100, 119-128. Demonstration of viral antigen and immunoglobulin (IgM and IgG) in brain tissue of pigs experimentally infected with H.E.V.

Transmissible Gastroenteritis (T.G.E.)

Definition

T.G.E. is a highly infectious viral disease of pigs, the chief clinical signs of which are diarrhoea, dehydration, occasional vomiting and a high mortality rate in young pigs.

Incidence

T.G.E. is of sporadic occurrence in Britain but its effect on individual farms is devastating. Up to 750 outbreaks per annum have been recorded, but more recently fewer outbreaks have been recorded and the disease now appears to be present throughout the year in a few herds with more than 300 sows. U.K. survey data showed 0.6% sows seropositive in 1990. It is absent from Scotland and was first seen in Ireland in 1984. In the mid-West United States it is common.

Aetiology

The causal agent is an ether sensitive, spherical RNA corona virus approximately 135 nm in diameter composed of a filamentous nucleocapsid enclosed within an envelope with spikes or peplomeres 12-25 nm in length. The molecular biology of the virus and its growth in cells has been studied extensively. The RNA has been sequenced and the structure and functions of several genes are known. The major structural proteins are the M or membrane glycoprotein of 29-31 kDa, the S or spike peplomer glycoprotein of 195-220 kDa associated with attachment, membrane fusion and neutralisation. Monoclonal antibodies have revealed a number of antigenic sites on these proteins. The virus is not inactivated at pH 3.0, is partially sensitive to sodium desoxycholate but is fully resistant to trypsin. It is very thermolabile and treatment at 50°C for 45 minutes is sufficient to inactivate virus of pig intestinal origin. The half-life at 37°C is less than 2 hours. Some strains are very sensitive to light, but the virus is extremely stable when frozen. The virus is difficult to isolate as C.P.E. is very slight in the first 4-5 passages. However, more extensive C.P.E., syncytia and round refractile cells are produced in later passages if large amounts of virus are used to initiate infection. Pig kidney or testis cells are used. Serological tests have shown that only 1 serotype of T.G.E. virus exists but there are some relationships (shared peptides) with dog and cat (Feline Infectious Peritonitis) viruses and considerable homology with Porcine Respiratory Coronavirus. Serum neutralisation of tissue culture virus is used to assay antibodies and to compare viral isolates. ELISA tests using monoclonal antibodies have demonstrated minor antigenic differences between isolates.

Pathogenesis

Infection takes place by ingestion or inhalation of infected droplets of faecal material. The virus multiplies in extraintestinal sites such as lungs and lymph nodes but principally in the cells of the alimentary tract, especially in those of the duodenum, jejunum and ileum. The cells chiefly affected are those at the tips of the villi, i.e. mature absorptive cells and their loss due to the effects of viral multiplication leads to their replacement by immature cells from the bases of the crypts. Loss of cells from the tips of the villi leads to lowering of the height of the epithelium, shortening of the villi and to an increase in the depth of the crypts. The ability of the small intestine to digest food (enzymes such as lactase are absent or in low concentration) and to absorb products of digestion is reduced by cell loss and damage. This results in hypoglycaemia and in osmotic diarrhoea which is exacerbated by a reduction in glucose-mediated sodium transport in the small intestine. Colonic absorption of water increases markedly but cannot prevent the diarrhoea and the subsequent in piglets from dehydration. Superinfection with *E.coli* and *Clostridium perfringens* types A and C may occur and affect the clinical signs and pathology.

IgG serum antibodies develop in recovered pigs as do IgA, IgG and IgM antibodies in the lung but local IgA immunity in the small intestine is most important in protection against the disease. Specific IgA antibody in the colostrum and milk of immune sows protects piglets against infection for 36 hours after its withdrawal. Maternal antibody levels rise before and after parturition and maternal antibody can be detected in the sera of piglets for 6-12 weeks after birth. Serum antibody from active infection develops within 7-8 days of infection and may persist for at least 6 months in finishers and 16 months to 2 years in sows. Cold stress has been shown to reduce the rate of antibody formation. Cell mediated immunity develops rapidly and may be important in recovery and immunity. It can last for over 100 days. Recovery from the disease is not always associated with elimination of the virus from the body. Virus can still be demonstrated in the lung 104 days after infection and in the gut for at least 104 days. Virus shedding in the faeces may not, however be easily detectable more than 14 days after infection but may continue for longer.

Clinical signs

The clinical signs of the disease are most characteristic in a non-immune herd. An explosive outbreak of diarrhoea occurs which involves pigs of all ages within a few days. The diarrhoea is profuse, watery and yellowish green in colour, sometimes with a foetid odour and containing curds of undigested milk. Vomiting may occur in piglets under 3 weeks of age and piglets under 1 week of age may show pink flushing of the skin. There is no febrile reaction and no nervous signs occur. Affected pigs become dehydrated - resulting in death in piglets within 24-48 hours and in agalactia in sows. The disease has a short incubation period of 1-2 days and occurs within 3-4 days of birth in susceptible piglets. The pattern of mortality in piglets is characteristic in a non-immune herd where water is not available to the piglets.

Age   0 - 7 days   100% mortality
      8 - 14 days   50% mortality
      15 - 21 days   25% mortality

Mortality is rare in piglets aged 3 weeks or more. Affected adults usually recover within 7-10 days. Some abortions and a reduced conception rate in sows bred after the deaths of their litters have been recorded. Where the disease is enzootic, its effects are most obvious in pigs aged between 10 days and 6 weeks. Diarrhoea and growth depression (F.C.R. may be reduced by 0.2) are the main clinical signs noted. In finishing pigs which seroconvert, growth depression may be the only clinical finding. Where wet feed is given with no supplementary water, pigs may die from salt poisoning and these clinical signs may be superimposed on those of T.G.E.

Recent studies in enzootic infections in large herds suggest that disease occurs one week post-weaning and may persist for several weeks.

Recrudescence of severe disease may occur in piglets aged 6 days or more and give rise to mortality. Such outbreaks rarely last more than 6-10 days. The litters of recently-purchased gilts may be most severely affected in such a herd.

Piglets which are comatose and cannot be treated should be killed humanely.

Pathological findings

Dead piglets are dehydrated but in good condition. The stomach is often distended with curdled milk and the small intestine is distended with foamy yellow fluid and is thin-walled. In some cases yellowish deposits or urate crystals may be seen in streaks in the kidney medulla. Areas of gastritis may also be present. The mesenteric lymph nodes may be enlarged. Villous atrophy may be seen in areas of the small intestine distal to the first 10 cm of the duodenum. Intestinal mucosa is best mounted in saline and viewed X 10 under a dissecting microscope

Histological changes in the small intestine are difficult to detect and consist mainly of alteration of the cell types in the mucosal epithelium, and alteration of the crypt:villus ratio. All lesions may be less obvious in animals nursed by partially immune sows.

Epidemiology

T.G.E. outbreaks commonly occur in winter and, in Britain, originate from foci in East Anglia or Yorkshire, spreading slowly to other parts of the country. The approach of summer limits the spread and the disease has not reached Cornwall, Wales or Scotland. Severe, widespread epizootics of T.G.E. have not occurred for many years. The last epizootic (winter 1969 - summer 1977) was unusual as a few outbreaks occurred in summer. This pattern was repeated in the 1980-88 period and the disease has persisted in finishing herds. The susceptibility of the virus to heat and light inactivation has been thought to account for the seasonal incidence of outbreaks. The severe widespread outbreaks reported in the Mid-West of the U.S. in winter may reflect this. Outbreaks usually last for 3-4 weeks. The virus is present in large amounts in the faeces of affected animals and may be excreted in the faeces of recovered pigs for up to 10 weeks. Carrier pigs may be important in the spread of the disease. Spread of the disease on a farm is by:

(a)   the ingestion of infected faeces by pigs in contact with affected animals.
(b)   inhalation or ingestion of droplets of faeces
(c)   transfer
(d)   indirect transmission of faeces on implements, etc.
(e)   direct transmission in the sows' milk

Spread of the disease between farms is usually by:

(a)   the introduction of affected or carrier pigs (usually weaners)
(b)   indirect carriage of infective material on boots, in contaminated lorries, etc.
(c)   wind transmission for distances of up to 1 mile. (Slurry may be important here)

(d)   the virus may be transmitted passively in the gut of starlings or by dogs. The virus can survive in and remain infective for pigs in dogs for up to 14 days

(e)   virus may persist i25°C for 30 days.

Diagnosis

Diagnosis of T.G.E. is usually made on the basis of the epizootiology of the outbreak and the clinical signs of diarrhoea throughout the herd, deaths in the young piglets and the pathological findings. T.G.E. may be distinguished from E.coli diarrhoeas by the extensive morbidity and mortality, the absence of enteropathogenic E.coli and the degree of inflammation and lack of villous atrophy in the small intestine in that disease. Rotavirus diarrhoea only affects piglets and weaned pigs but Epidemic Diarrhoea can affect all ages, usually without the mortality seen in piglets with T.G.E. In coccidiosis, clostridial and cryptosporidium infections there is marked necrosis of the intestine.

Diagnosis may be confirmed by:

(a)   by serum neutralisation tests, ELISA, or the bentonite agglutination test to detect serum antibodies in recovered pigs. In countries such as the U.K. in which the porcine respiratory coronavirus occurs, only tests such as the blocking ELISA using monoclonals specific for T.G.E. can now be used

(b)   by the use of a specific fluorescent antiserum or, now, specific in monoclonal antibodies T.G.E. virus in frozen sections of the small intestine of freshly-killed piglets. A positive diagnosis is made by finding fluorescence in epithelial cells at the tips or sides of the villi. Fluorescence is patchy in actively-infected pigs. Immunoperoxidase may also be used, DNA probes have been shown to be extremely sensitive in dot hybridisation in faeces and cell culture.

(c)   by virus isolation from mesenteric lymph node, tonsil and small intestine which may be frozen prior to examination. As C.P.E. is poor in initial cultures, virus may be identified by immunofluorescence or DNA probes.

Samples for laboratory examinations should include at least 1 moribund or live affected piglet for immunofluorescence, virus isolation and for examination of the villi.

Treatment and control

T.G.E. may cause massive and spectacular losses amongst young piglets, but acute outbreaks are relatively uncommon and are localised in the U.K. Chronic infection in fattening houses may cause economic loss by affecting growth rate. The disease can be treated symptomatically with electrolyte solutions, e.g. (Beecham Scour formula), given in cube drinkers. Early weaning, especially onto glucose containing artificial feeds, the maintenance of high environmental temperatures and hygiene may all help reduce mortality. Cross suckling of litters onto immune sows may also help if they can be identified reliably e.g. by recording episodes of clinical disease. Water should be freely available to weaned pigs not treated as already described. Antimicrobials may control infections by E.coli and Clostridium *perfringens* in piglets and swine dysentery in weaned pigs. Experimental studies of chemotherapeutics suggest that clonidine may be of value.

Control must be based on prevention by:-

(a) Isolation. Unnecessary visitors or contaminated lorries should not be admitted to susceptible herds and all visitors entering a herd should do so via a disinfectant dip. Stock should not be purchased during epizootics of T.G.E. Stock from infected farms may be non-infectious 40 days after the last clinical signs.

(b) An all-in, all-out policy should be operated in fattening houses in herds where the disease is enzootic. Disinfection and control of rodents and birds may break the cycle of infection.

(c) When outbreaks occur, sows due to farrow within 14 days should be maintained in isolation. The infected buildings may be re-occupied after 3 months.

(d) Deliberate infection of sows. Sows which are more than 14 days from farrowing can be infected with intestinal contents from dead pigs and may develop immunity in time to protect their litters. This would require a licence under the Waste Foods Order but use of faeces does not.

(e) Vaccination. The crude infectious materials mentioned above may be replaced by a number of vaccines. Virus killed by acetylethylenimine, detergent, and formalin has been administered by the intranasal and/or intramuscular routes. Live virus vaccines consisting of related viruses such as Feline Infectious Peritonitis, virulent T.G.E. (given to sows to cause or boost immunity) and varying strains of attenuated virus have been developed. These have been administered by the oral, intranasal, intramuscular and intramammary routes. The oral or nasal route produces the best colostral and lactogenic immunity but virulent virus may infect susceptible pigs on the farm of use or on adjacent farms. Less virulent virus may not produce adequate immunity or even become established.

Strains which infect only a local area of gut and give good protective immunity have been described. The 200 kDa proteins from the spikes on the viral envelope have been engineered into vaccinia and yeasts but have not been tested in the field.

Vaccines are not available in the UK In the US live attenuated virus vaccines e.g. Ambico and dead vaccines e.g. Diamond are available. Vaccination should take place at least two weeks before farrowing to prevent mortality in the litter and more in the case of live virus vaccines. No vaccine has yet been shown to be more than 50% effective. T.G.E. eradication from a chronically infected herd has been described by whole herd vaccination in the US

For differentiation of PRCV from TGE see PRCV section below.

References
Argenzio, R.A., Moon, H.W., Kemeny, L.J. and Whipp, S.C. (1984). Gastroenterology **86**, 1501-1509.

Brown, I.H., Paton, D.J. (1991). Vet.Rec. 128, 500-503. Serological studies of T.G.E. in Great Britain using a competitive ELISA.
Cox, E., Cools, V. and Houvenaghel, A. (1989). Veterinary Research Communication 13, 159-170. Effect of antisecretory drugs on experimentally-induced weanling diarrhoa.
Drolet, R., Morin, M. and Fontaine, M. (1984). Canadian Journal of Comparative Medicine 48, 282-285. Hypoglycaemia: a factor associated with low survival rate of neonatal pigs infected with transmissible gastroenteritis virus.
Fitzgerald, G.R., Welter, C.J. (1990). Agri.Practice. 11, 25-29. The effect of an oral T.G.E. vaccine on eliminating virus from a herd of swine.
Garwes, D.J. (1988). Vet.Rec. 122, 462-463. Review of TGE vaccination.
Pritchard, G.C. (1982). Vet.Rec. 110, 465-469. Observations on clinical aspects of transmissible gastroenteritis of pigs in Norfolk and Suffolk.
Pritchard, G.C. (1983). Pig News and Information 4, 145-149 (Review).
Pritchard, G.C. (1987). Vet.Rec. 120, 226-230. TGE in endemically infected breeding herds of pigs in East Anglia. 1981-1985.
Siegel, J.P., Hungerford, L.C., Hall, W.F. (1991). J.Am.Vet.Med.Ass. 199, 1579-1583. Risk factors with TGE in swine.

Epidemic Diarrhoea

Definition

Epidemic diarrhoea of pigs is a highly contagious disease characterised by vomiting, diarrhoea and inappetence in pigs of all ages. Mortality in young piglets is less common than in TGE.

Incidence

First described in Britain in 1972, it has now been identified in most European countries and Taiwan but antibody was absent from sera from small numbers of pigs from Sweden, Australia, Northern Ireland and the US. Similar diseases not confirmed as epidemic diarrhoea have been identified in Canada, Japan and China. In Austria and Switzerland serological surveys suggest that the incidence is low in contrast to Belgium.

Aetiology

The causal agent is a coronavirus distinct from TGE, PRCV and H.E.V. The virus is 95-150 nm (mean 130 nm) in negative stain and 60 nm in section. The peplomeres are 18-23 nm in length. There are three major protein antigens, the S or spike glycosylated protein of 85-130 kDa, the M protein of 23 kDa and an N protein of 58 kDa with some relationship to Feline Infectious Peritonitis virus. All isolates appear to belong to a single serotype. It can be cultivated in Vero cells with added trypsin and produces syncytia on subculture. The virus is destroyed at >60°C within 30 minutes, is stable at 50°C. At 37°C it is stable between pH 6.5 and 7.5 but at 4°C between pH 5.0-pH 9.0.

Pathogenesis

The virus does not replicate in the respiratory tract but otherwise pathogenesis resembles that of TGE Epithelial cells can shed virus without being destroyed but, by the onset of diarrhoea, epithelial cell shedding has already begun. Six hours later it then occurs in the ileum. Levels of alkaline and acid phosphatase, succinic dehydrogenase and monoamine oxidase fall. In older pigs lactase levels have also been shown to fall. Villous fusion and atrophy are widespread within 24 hours of the onset of clinical signs. In partially-immune piglets, a very localised area of the small intestine may show villous atrophy. Serum antibody levels become detectable 2-4 weeks after infection and rise to levels of up to 1:10,000 declining rapidly to lower levels of 1:20-1:640. Passive antibody has disappeared from the sera of piglets within 5-13 weeks and active immunity then develops. The presence of serum antibody in a nursing sow does not rule out epidemic diarrhoea in her litter. Antibody levels on infected farms peak at 4 months and decline from then onward.

Clinical signs

The disease occurs as an explosive outbreak of diarrhoea in non-immune weaned pigs (Type I) or pigs of all ages (Type II). After an incubation period of 1-3 days, piglets develop a TGE-like watery diarrhoea and may vomit but although morbidity in non-immune pigs approaches 100%, mortality is low. The disease spreads rapidly in the unit. Twenty to thirty per cent of the older pigs may be affected with vomiting and diarrhoea. One hundred per cent inappetence may occur, especially in breeding stock. In Type I, sucking and young weaned pigs under 32 kg liveweight are rarely affected. Affected weaned pigs are dull and unwilling to rise. Pyrexia is rare. The diarrhoea is greenish-brown in colour and very fluid. Signs of dehydration are common. Vomiting is prominent in some outbreaks and less obvious in others. The acute stage of vomiting and diarrhoea lasts approximately 3 days but recovery takes a further 7-8 days. Mortality is rare in the absence of intercurrent disease and where water is freely available. Affected feeding pigs take about 14 days longer to reach 90 Kg due to the effects of inappetence and loss of condition. Clinically-recovered pigs show no after effect. Agalactia may occur in sows and result in some indirect mortality in unaffected litters.

Severely dehydrated, wasted piglets not responding to supportive therapy should be humanely destroyed.

Pathological findings

Few weaned pigs have been examined as mortality is low. The stomach is usually empty or filled with bile-stained fluid, and both large and small intestines are pale, often with fluid contents. Some villous atrophy may be seen in the small intestines of baby pigs affected by this condition and they may have a gastritis

Epidemiology

Separated from TGE on epidemiological grounds in the 1969-1977 TGE outbreak in 1971. The disease continued until spring 1972 and then died down in the summer to reappear in winter 1972-73. Pig contact is important and spread has occurred through markets and by pig transport lorries. Type II disease was first described in 1977. Epidemic diarrhoea is usually introduced by carrier pigs and introduction may be followed by an explosive outbreak. Severe outbreaks involving sows and piglets are now unusual and clinical disease may be confirmed to individual litters or occur in recently purchased grower pigs.

38

Diagnosis

Type I disease may be suspected by its history and clinical signs of an acute, rapidly spreading scour with vomiting and inappetence not affecting sucking pigs. The only similar condition is TGE. which can be eliminated by laboratory tests. Coronavirus particles may sometimes be seen in the intestinal contents or faeces of affected pigs by E.M. Specific fluorescent antibody demonstrates the virus in intestinal epithelium and an ELISA test is available for the detection of specific antibody in the sera of recovered pigs. Only rising titres in paired serum samples are diagnostic. A number of ELISAs have been evaluated. The most efficient appears to be one using whole, tissue culture virus as antigen although the S protein can also be used.

Type II disease may be suspected by the pattern of mortality in a non-immune herd. In a partially immune herd, only a few piglets may develop the disease and differentiation from E.coli (absence of agent, villous atrophy) clostridia, cryptosporidia and coccidia (no blood or necrosis of the small intestinal epithelium) and rotavirus and TGE (laboratory methods including immunofluorescence and ELISA must be carried out).

Treatment and Control

Provide adequate water and provide milk substitute for any piglets of affected sows which may lose their milk and adequate water for all affected stock at all times. Piglets may be treated using glucose: glycine electrolyte solutions (Beecham scour formula). There is no specific treatment, and the effects of an outbreak of the disease may be controlled by isolating all sows within 14 days of farrowing, and by infecting all those due to farrow in more than 14 days. Weaners may also be infected in order to reduce the duration of the outbreak. Where swine dysentery or other intercurrent disease is present, recovery from epidemic diarrhoea is hastened by the treatment appropriate to the intercurrent disease.

References

Bollwahn, W. (1983). Pig News and Information 4, 141-144. Epizootic viral diarrhoea of pigs.
Chasey, D. and Cartwright, S.F. (1978) Res. Vet.Sci. 25, 255-256. Virus-like particles associated with porcine epidemic diarrhoea.
De Bouck, P., Pensaert, M. and Coussement, W. (1981). Vet.Microbiol. 6, 157-165. The pathogenesis of an enteric infection in pigs experimentally induced by the coronavirus-like agent CV777.
Ducatelle, R., Coussement, W., De Bouck, P. and Hoorens, J. (1982). Vet.Path. 19, 46-56. Pathology of experimental CV777 coronavirus enteritis in piglets. I. Histological and histochemical study.
Ducatelle, R., Coussement, W., Charlier, G., De Bouck, P. and Hoorens, J. (1982). Vet.Path. 19, 57-66. II Electron microscopic study.
Egberink, H.F., Ederveen, J., Callebaut, P. and Horzinek, M.C. (1988). Am.J.Vet.Res. 49, 1320-1324. Characterisation of the structural proteins of PED virus strain CV777.
Hofmann, M. and Wyler, R. (1988). J.Clin.Micro. 26, 2235-2239. Propagation of the virus of porcine epidemic diarrhoea in cell culture.
(1989). Vet.Microbiol. 20, 131-142. Quantitation biological and physicochemical properties of cell culture adapted P.E.D. coronavirus.

(1990). Vet.Microbiol. 21, 263-273. ELISA for the detection of porcine epidemic diarrhoea virus antibodies in swine sera. Wood, E.N. (1977) Vet.Rec. 100, 243-244. An apparently new syndrome of porcine epidemic diarrhoea..

Porcine Respiratory Coronavirus Infection

Definition

Infection with porcine respiratory coronavirus (PRCV) causes rapid seroconversion of a herd to some tests for T.G.E. virus and can cause fatal bronchopneumonia with fever coughing and anorexia in experimental pigs. In the field infection can cause a similar syndrome or be subclinical.

Incidence

First reported from Belgium in 1986 it has been found in the UK, France, Germany, Denmark, Canada and The Netherlands. A related virus has been identified in the U.S. In the UK antibody became widespread in 1986 but antibody-free herds still exist.

Aetiology

A coronavirus resembling TGE virus and causing spreading cytopathic effects and syncytia in pig kidney cell cultures has been isolated from the lungs of infected pigs. Antibody to it neutralises T.G.E. virus and the syncytia fluoresce with sera specific to TGE Epitopes common to both viruses have been demonstrated on all virus proteins examined but monoclonal antibodies which react with TGE virus and not with PRCV have been found. The genomic differences between TGE and PRCV are slight and the major antigenic difference appears to be a truncated S protein.

Pathogenesis

Infection is by aerosol and the virus multiplies chiefly in the lungs. Virus has been demonstrated in nasal mucosal epithelial cells, those of the trachea, bronchi, bronchioles and alveoli. Alveolar macrophages are also affected. A viraemia follows respiratory tract multiplication and some viral antigen may be found in the small intestinal submucosa but not in the epithelium. Varying degrees of interstitial pneumonia result from infection. The virus is shed as an aerosol and in nasal secretions for 1-6 days after infection. It does not appear to cross the placenta. Antibody to the virus becomes detectable in sera within a week.

Clinical signs

No clinical signs have been observed prior to seroconversion at 3-5 months in some herds in which maternal antibody is present but coughing and anorexia have been reported in others. Anorexia, reluctance to move, laboured respiration and fever (40°C, 104°F) have been reported 1-5 days following the experimental infection of antibody-free conventional pigs. No clinical signs were noted in gnotobiotes in some studies. Experimental infection with PRCV alone or together with influenza virus has little effect on growth rate.

Pathological findings

No lesions have been reported in some cases and in others severe catarrhal bronchopneumonia has been seen. Lesions are restricted to the lung and bronchi. The lesions include mild interstitial pneumonia, hyperplasia of the bronchiolar epithelium and epithelial cell loss. Syncytia occur in the alveoli and airways.

Epidemiology

Aerosol infection appears to occur within a herd and seroconversion spreads rapidly to pigs of all ages. Maternal immunity appears to persist for up to 3-4 months when active seroconversion occurs. Spread between herds appears to have been by movement of infected carrier pigs. Experimental infections do not protect against TGE infections.

Diagnosis

The clinical signs are not sufficiently consistent to reach a diagnosis on clinical grounds alone. The spread of mild respiratory disease throughout a herd previously free from TGE, coupled with seroconversion to TGE virus in the absence of enteric signs may allow diagnosis. Blocking ELISA tests for serum antibody have been described using monoclonal antibodies specific for TGE The viral antigen can be demonstrated in tissue using immunoperoxidase or biotin labelled monoclonal antibody. PCR primers and DNA probes have been developed.

Treatment and Control

The only indication for control at present is the problem of certification of herds for freedom from TGE This has been approached in the UK by founding and maintaining antibody-free herds by rigorous testing and isolation. Disinfect as for TGE.

References

Brown, I. and Cartwright, S. (1986). Vet.Rec. 119, 282-283. New porcine coronavirus?

Cox, E., Hooyberghs, J. and Pensaert, M.B. (1990). Res.Vet.Sci. 48, 165-169. Sites of replication of a P.R.C.V. related to T.G.E. virus.

Garwes, D.J., Stewart, F., Cartwright, S.F. and Brown, I. (1988). Vet.Rec. 122, 86-87. Differentiation of porcine coronavirus from TGE virus.

Pensaert, M., Callebaut, P. and Vergote, J. (1986). Veterinary Quarterly 88, 2V57-261. Isolation of a porcine respiratory non-enteric coronavirus related to TGE and VWD of pigs.

van Nieuwstadt, A.P. and Pol, J.M.A. (1989). Vet.Rec. 124, 43-44. Isolation of a TGE-related respiratory coronavirus causing fatal pneumonia in pigs.

Rotavirus

Definition

Rotavirus infections are associated with profuse diarrhoea in young piglets and result in varying degrees of mortality. Less severe diarrhoea may occur in weaned animals

Incidence

Infections with porcine rotavirus appear to occur in all pig rearing areas. In both Britain and the U.S. 100% slaughter pigs have antibody to at least one rotavirus group. Groups A, B, C and E are most common.

Aetiology

Rotaviruses contain double stranded RNA arranged in 11 segments and particles are ultrastructurally indistinguishable from calf and human isolates which have been shown to cause disease in gnotobiotic pigs. Particles measure 75nm with the outer capsid (a double-shelled smooth outer layer) and 58nm without it. The two major surface proteins are VP4 non-glycosylated 90 kDa protease sensitive 'P' protein which can haemaggluninate and VP7, a glycosylated protein of 37 kDa. There is also a common core antigen.
Rotaviruses are divided into groups based on antigenicity and polyacrilamide gel electrophoresis banding of the DNA. Groups A, B, C and E have been recorded in pigs. Classification is now expressed as Group (A) strain (OSU) subgroup (II) G protein type (3, 4, 5, 11) and P type (6, 7). The genes for these two proteins have been synthesised and cDNA probes can be used for typing as can monoclonal antibodies.
Rotavirus may resist 60°C for 30 minutes in faeces and survive for 7-9 months at 18-20°C, is stable between pH 3 and 9 but can be inactivated by 3.7% formaldehyde, 70% ethanol, 2% glutaraldehyde, 1% hypochlorite and 0.01% iodine, and heat at 63°C for 30 minutes. It may remain infective for three days in 1% formaldehyde. Rotaviruses may be cultured in calf and kidney cells but require exposure to trypsin and agitation for continued subculture. Cytopathic effects and plaque formation can be produced on monkey cell line MA104 with pancreatin and dextran. Viral antigen can be present in the cytoplasm of cells without CPE. It must be detected by IF, immunoperoxidase or DNA probes.

Pathogenesis

Oral infection with as few as 90 particles results in replication of the virus in the cells of the epithelium of the middle small intestine from upper jejunum to lower ileum. Virus particles enter cells by pinocytosis between microvilli of enterocytes and are then seen in the endoplasmic reticulum. Infected cells do not become vacuolated as in T.G.E. but swell, lose their microvilli and are shed. Replication is most intense 24-96 hours after infection but later becomes restricted to villus tips. Mature absorptive cells are shed and villous atrophy, crypt hyperplasia and villous fusion occur. Lactase levels fall but lactose digestion may not be affected. Recovery may be complete within 7 days of infection. Virus particles are shed in large numbers (10^{7}-10^{8}ml) in the faeces. Other infectious agents are often present and rotaviruses of more than one group or serotype may occur in the same animal. Colostral and milk antibody is important in the development of clinical disease and protects for 3-5 weeks. Passive antibodies have normally disappeared by 7 weeks of age. Active IgA and IgM antibodies first appear 7-13 days after infection and serum antibody, principally IgG, 17-24 days after infection. Antibody is sows passes into colostrum (IgG and IgM) but IgA is the principal class in milk. Sow serum IgG rises with each parity, IgA remains constant and IgM declines progressively.

Clinical signs

The incubation period is 18-24 hours after which depression, anorexia and reluctance to move are noted. Vomiting may be seen. A few hours later, profuse diarrhoea develops and in milk-fed pigs this is yellow with floccules floating in a whey-like fluid, while in others it may be yellow or dark grey. There is a rapid loss of condition. Anorexia continues for 24-72 hours after which appetite returns. Clinical signs regress 4-6 days after infection but loose yellow faeces may persist for 7-14 days. Thirty-three per cent of affected young pigs may die in field outbreaks but mortality can be up to 100% in experimental animals. Weaned pigs may also be affected, but in them no diarrhoea or only transient diarrhoea (mean duration 3 days) results when rotavirus is demonstrated in the faeces. Rotavirus diarrhoea may recur as immunity to one type does not prevent infection with others.

The effects on growth rate range from nothing to at least 5 days to 25kg. Piglets suffering from dehydration and hypoglycaemia such that they cannot rise, should be killed.

Pathology

Dead pigs may appear dehydrated, the stomach is filled with milk and the small intestine is distended with creamy fluid contents. There is desquamation of the epithelial cells of the villi lining the distal three quarters of the small intestine resulting in stunting of the villi and flattening of the remaining epithelial cells with loss of the brush border and the presence of cuboidal cells and multinucleate syncytia. Crypt depth is increased and villous fusion occurs. Infection with other agents such as E.coli, clostridia adenovirus and T.G.E. may also occur, complicating the picture described.

Epidemiology

Infection is transmitted in herds directly from sow to litter as 30% sows pass virus in their faeces over farrowing. Within litters infection begins in one or two pigs and then spreads to the others over a period of 10-14 days, beginning at 19 days and being complete at about 40 days of age. Infection may also be contracted from the environment as rotavirus is stable in faeces for up to 9 months and persists in water.

Groups A infections tend to occur early in life, followed by B and C based on the detection of active immunity. Exceptions are known and Group C infections have been recorded in neonates and Group A infections in pigs of 2-20 weeks in extensive husbandry systems. Piglets of 0-7 days of age may be less susceptible to Group A infections. All infections in a herd may belong to a single electrophoretic type for up to 2 years and then change. Infection may be transferred from group to group in carrier pigs, by man, implements or rodents. Rotaviruses from other species such as calves and man may cause disease in pigs. There is a close resemblance between some pig Group C rotaviruses and human strains but it is not clear whether human infection with porcine strains can occur.

Diagnosis

The clinical signs may suggest rotavirus and are distinct from those of T.G.E. and epidemic diarrhoea in non-immune herds. the ubiquity of rotavirus infection should lead to its consideration as a component of most diarrhoeas of sucking and recently-weaned piglets. Pathological findings may suggest a viral condition and the use of a hand lens or dissecting microscope will reveal the presence of villous atrophy which is often more restricted than in T.G.E. or epidemic diarrhoea. there is no necrosis on the epithelium in uncomplicated rotavirus infections, unlike in cryptosporidial, clostridial or coccidial infections. The presence of rotavirus can be confirmed by the electron microscopical examination of faeces or colon contents for the characteristic particles or by polyacrilamide gel electrophoresis to detect the characteristic double-stranded RNA. These two methods detect all groups of rotavirus. cDNA probes have been developed for virus in tissue, usually based on the VP7 gene and PCR methods have also been described, detecting as little as 5ng of virus. ELISA tests have been described for the detection of faecal antigen and commercial reversed passive latex agglutination tests (RPLA) can be used on faecal filtrates on farm. All serological tests may give false negatives if prepared against individual serotypes of Group A only. Immunofluorescence may be used to detect antigen in frozen sections of intestinal material. Unfortunately, up to 25% of outbreaks of diarrhoea in pigs are said to contain rotavirus particles and mixed infections are common so that it is up to the clinician to decide the relevance of their presence. Serum antibody can be detected by indirect fluorescent antibody and by ELISA tests but serum titres are low. Up to 80% of adults may possess titres of up to 1:80 in serum and 1:640 in colostrum where IgA is more important after 7 days post-partum. Passive antibody levels persist for 2-3 weeks (IgA and M) and 7 weeks (IgG) and active antibody levels increase from 5-8 weeks. IgA antibody is present in the faeces.

Treatment

Withholding milk from affected piglets may enhance recovery. but may have an adverse effect on energy balance. Bacterial and protozoal complications should be controlled. Fluid replacement using glucose:glycine electrolyte solutions (Beecham scour formula) may be of value. Recent studies suggest that glutamine stimulates sodium uptake in damaged intestine. Water should always be available. Growth depression in weaned pigs is reduced if high protein rations are given but milk protein is better than vegetable protein. Prevention may be achieved by stimulating maternal immunity by feed-back of faeces from affected piglets at least 14 days prior to farrowing or by vaccinating. No vaccines are currently available in the U.K. Live vaccines given intramuscularly or orally have been described and may contain serotypes A1 and A2, human rotavirus, or constructs containing viral proteins VP3 and 7 from serotypes 4 and 5 for protection against both serotypes. Significant improvement in performance may result from vaccination of the sow 4 and 2 weeks prior to farrowing followed by oral or i/m vaccination of piglets at 2 or 4 weeks. Viral excretion may not be prevented by dead vaccines and transient diarrhoea may occur. Protection against other rotavirus serotypes or groups may be poor. Cow colostrum containing antibodies to bovine rotavirus will protect if fed to piglets. Disinfection can be carried out using hypochlorite on clean surfaces and proprietary disinfectants such as 'Virkon', Antec, a mixture of surfactant, organic acid, oxidising agents and buffers. Phenolic disinfectants are less effective.

References

Bridger, J.C., Brown, J.F. (1988). Pig News and Information 9, 23-26. Review: Porcine rotaviruses and their role in disease.
Bridger, J.C., Brown, J.F. (1985). Vet.Rec. 116, 50. Prevalence of antibody to typical and atypical rotaviruses in pigs.
Bywater, R.J. and Woode, G.N. (1980). Vet. Rec. 106, 75-78. Oral fluid replacement by a glucose:clycine electrolyte formulation in E.coli and rotavirus diarrhoea in pigs.
Chasey, D., Bridger, J.C., McCrae, M.A. (1986). Arch.Virol. 89, 235-243. A new type of atypical rotavirus in pigs.
Chasey, D. and Davies, P. (1984). Vet.Rec. 114, 16-17. Atypical rotaviruses in pigs and cattle.
Corthier, G., Vannier, P. (1983). J.Inf.Dis. 147, 293-296. Production of coproantibodies and immune complexes in piglets infected with rotavirus.
Fu, Z.F., Hampson, D.J., Wilks, C.R. (1990). Res.Vet.Sci. 48, 365-373. Transfer of maternal antibody against group A rotavirus from sows to piglets and serological responses following natural infection.
Gelberg, H.B., Patterson, J.S., Woode, G.N. (1991). Vet.Microbiology 28, 231-242. A longitudinal study of rotavirus antibody in a closed specific pathogen-free herd.
Gelberg, H.B., Woode, G.N., Kniffen, T.S., Hardy, M., Hall, W.F. (1991). Vet.Microbiology 28, 213-229. The shedding of Group A rotavirus in a newly-established closed SPF swine herd.
Hoshino, Y., Saif, L.J., Sereno, M.M., Chanock, R.M., Kapikian, A.S. (1988). J.Virol. 62, 744-748. Infection immunity of piglets to either VP3 or VP7 outer capsid protein confers resistance to challenge with a virulent rotavirus bearing the corresponding antigen.
McAdaragh, J.P., Bergeland, M.E., Meyer, R.C., Johnshoy, M.W., Stotz, I.J., Benfield, D.A. and Hammer, R. (1980). Am. J. Vet. Res. 41, 1572-1581. Pathogenesis of rotaviral enteritis: A microscopic study.
Rosen, B.I., Saif, L.J., Jackwood, D.J. and Gorziglia, M. (1990). Vet.Microbiology 24, 327-329. Hybridisation probes for the detection and differentiation of 2 serotypes of porcine rotavirus.
Saif, L.J., Terret, L.A., Miller, K.L., Cross, R.F. (1988). J.Clin.Microbiol. 26, 1277-1282. Serial propagation of porcine group C rotavirus (pararotavirus) in a continuous cell line and characterisation of the passaged virus.
Welter, M.W. and Welter, M.J. (1990). Vet.Microbiology, 22, 179-186. Evaluation of killed and modified live porcine rotavirus vaccines in caesarian-derived colostrum-deprived pigs.
Woode, G.N., Bridger, J., Hale, G.A., Jones, J.M. and Jackson, G. (1976). J.Med.Microbiol. 9, 203-209. The isolation of reovirus-like agents (rotavirus) from acute gastroenteritis of piglets.

Caliciviruses in diarrhoea

Caliciviruses are RNA-containing viruses 37 nm in diameter with a petal-like arrangement of capsomeres and have been identified in cases of post-weaning diarrhoea in pigs in Britain and the US and Japan. Porcine isolates have a major structural and immunogenic proteinof 58 kDa and have been shown to be antigenically distinct from the calicivirus of vesicular exanthema. Porcine calicivirus has been grown in pig kidney cells in the presence of gnotobiotic intestinal content and alone eventually causes rounding and detachment of cells. Infection of gnotobiotic piglets caused diarrhoea lasting 3-7 days. Virus was present in the villous epithelial cells of the duodenum and jejunum and caused significant villous atrophy. It could be demonstrated in intestinal contents.

Calici-like viruses must be considered potential contributors to diarrhoea in piglets.

References

Bridger, J.C. (1980). Vet. Rec. 107, 532-533. Detection by electron microscopy of caliciviruses, astroviruses and rotavirus-like particles in the faeces of piglets with diarrhoea.
Flynn, W.T., Saif, L.J. (1988). J.Clin.Microbiol. 26, 206-212. Serial propagation of porcine enteric calici-like virus in primary porcine kidney cell cultures.
Flynn, W.T., Saif, L.J. and Moorhead, P.D. (1988). Am.J.Vet.Res. 49, 819-825. Pathogenesis of porcine enteric calici-like virus in four day old gnotobiotic pigs
Parwani, A., Saif, L.J., Kang, S.Y. (1990). Arch.Virol. 112, 41-53. Biochemical characterisation of porcine enteric calicivirus: analysis of structural and non-structural viral proteins.

Astroviruses in diarrhoea

Astroviruses are 29 nm in diameter and have a star-shaped pattern on their surfaces. They have been seen in the faeces of pigs with post-weaning diarrhoea with other viruses in the UK, and isolated from outbreaks of diarrhoea in Japan. The virus can replicate in primary calf kidney cells and has been grown in porcine embryonic kidney cells with added trypsin where CPE consisting of enlargement of cells and granularity of the cytoplasm occurs.

It is an RNA virus producing 13 kDa, 30 kDa, 31 kDa, 36 kDa and 39 kDa polypeptides. It is stable to lipid solvents and for 30 minutes at 50°C but is killed by acid at pH 3.0. The virus is antigenically distinct from calf astrovirus. Infected 4 day old hysterectomy-derived colostrum-deprived piglets developed mild diarrhoea. Seroconversion occurs and antibody was widespread in Japan in 50% of pigs tested, 0-83% in individual herds.

References

Bridger, J.C. (1980). Vet.Rec. 107, 532-533. Detection by electron microscopy of caliciviruses, astroviruses and rotavirus-like particles in the faeces of piglets with diarrhoea.
Shimizu, M., Shirai, J., Narita, M., Yamane, T. (1990). J.Clin.Microbiol. 28, 201-206. Cytopathic astrovirus isolated from porcine acute gastroenteritis in an established cell line derived from porcine embryonic kidney.

Toroviruses in Diarrhoea

Kidney-shaped torovirus-like particles l00 x 38nm and spherical particles 80 x 67nm were found in a 3 week-old piglet with diarrhoea.

Reference

Scott, A.C., Chaplin, M., Stack, M.J. and Lund, L. (1987). Vet.Rec. <u>120</u>, 583. Porcine torovirus

Picobirnavirus in Diarrhoea

Electron microscopy of faeces from pigs with and without diarrhoea has identified featureless virus particles 35nm in diameter, sometimes with a hexagonal profile and associated with bisegmented double stranded DNA in PAGE profiles in both the U.K. and Venezuela.

Their significance is currently unknown but 11% of samples from 15-35 day old pigs were positive on one farm.

References

Chasey, D. (1990). Vet.Rec. <u>126</u>, 465. Porcine picobirnavirus in U.K.?
Ludert, J.E., Hidalgo, M., Gil, F., Lipandi, F. (1991). Arch.Virol. <u>117</u>, 97-107. Identification in porcine faeces of a novel virus with a bisegmented double stranded RNA genome.

Orbiviruses in Diarrhoea

Orbivirus-like particles and RNA have been demonstrated in pig faeces. Their significance is not clear.

Bredaviruses in Diarrhoea

Particles resembling Breda virus have been demonstrated in diarrhoeic piglet faeces and have been associated with a sudden increase immortality in 6-8 week old piglets, reduction in appetite, weakness, tremor, recumbency and death.

Reference

Penrith, M.L., Gerdes, G.H. (1992). J.South African Vet.Ass. <u>63</u>, 102. Breda virus-like particles in pigs in South Africa.

Adenovirus Infection

Definition

Mild diarrhoea in pigs from 5 days to 24 weeks of age. Also involved in pneumonia and encephalitis.

Incidence

Adenovirus diarrhoea has been identified in the U.K., United States, Canada, Belgium, Japan and Hungary. Antibody to the virus has been identified in 70-80% slaughter pigs in the U.K. and the incidence of antibody increases with the age of the pigs. Similar findings are reported from Japan.

Aetiology

Adenoviruses are DNA viruses 75nm in diameter with 252 capsomeres arranged in cubic symmetry. Peripheral fibres exist. The virus can be cultivated in epithelial cell cultures eventually producing rounded cell cytopathic effects and intranuclear inclusions. They are resistant to ether, bile, detergents and acid and can persist for periods of up to 1 year at 4°C. They are susceptible to disinfectants. Five serological types have been identified in pigs.

Pathogenesis

Type 4 adenovirus has been shown to produce lesions repeatedly in experimental primary SPF piglets. Infection of week old piglets results in interstitial and proliferative pneumonia with thickened alveolar septa containing some intranuclear inclusions in septal cells. In the presence of *Mycoplasma hyopneumoniae* more severe lesions were produced. Encephalitis is also produced. Intestinal strains colonise the tonsil and intestine where they infect epithelial cells of the villi of the lower jejunum and ileum. Intranuclear Cowdry Type A inclusions (eosinophilic or amphophilic) develop in the epithelial goblet cells and are surrounded by a clear halo. Affected nuclei swell and often lie above the line of normal nuclei. Affected cells lose microvilli and their loss may be accelerated to cause villous shortening. Diarrhoea develops and affected cells are found progressively nearer the villus tips. Dehydration may result. Serum antibody can be demonstrated in recovered pigs.

Clinical signs

Infection can occur in pigs aged 5 days - 24 weeks but is commonest in piglets of less than 3 weeks of age. The incubation period is 3-5 days and diarrhoea lasts 3-6 days and is yellow, intermittent and of variable consistency. Diarrhoea has been associated with infection in 53% cases. Dehydration may occur in piglets but mortality is rare. Virus has been isolated from nasal discharge, abortions, and from stillborn piglets following transplacental infection. Severely dehydrated piglets unable to rise should be killed.

Pathology

Thinning of the intestinal wall with shortening of jejunal and ileal villi is described. Intranuclear inclusions are most commonly present in the epithelial cells of the short villi over Peyer's patches and in M cells but may occur more widely.

There may be an interstitial pneumonia or kidney tubule lesions.

Epidemiology

Rarely diagnosed at present but in one study 24% of piglets to 8 weeks, 60% of fat pigs and 90-93% sows had antibody to adenovirus group antigen. Infection is clearly widespread. Infection persists in herds for long periods.

Diagnosis

Based on histological finding of adenovirus intranuclear inclusions in histological sections or or the detection of viral particles in gut contents. A rise in serum precipitating antibody levels to adenovirus group antigen might also confirm. Cultivation in porcine thyroid cells has been described for Type 4 but blind passage in tissue culture is required isolation.

Treatment and control

Symptomatic treatment with fluid replacers and, possibly, feedback to sows.

References

Coussement, W., Ducatelle, R., Charlier, G. and Hoorens, J. (1981). Am.J.Vet.Res. 42, 1905-1911. Adenovirus enteritis in pigs.
Ducatelle, R., Coussement, W and Hoorens, J. (1982). Vet.Path. 19, 179-189. Sequential pathological study of porcine adenovirus enteritis.
Sanford, S.E., Hoover, D.M. (1983). Canadian J.Comp.Med. 47, 396-400. Enteric adenovirus infection in piglets.

Swine Influenza

Definition

A respiratory tract infection with Influenza A viruses resulting in coughing, dyspnoea and prostration which spreads rapidly through a herd and resolves within a week.

Incidence

Infection with classical swine influenza virus (HlN1) is a significant cause of respiratory disease in pigs in North America and since 1976 in most of Europe and Eastern Asia. Clinical disease was absent from Britain until 1986 when it occurred widely in England. Neither clinical disease nor serum antibody has yet been reported from Australia.

Antibody surveys in the U.S. suggest that classic disease is widespread in North Central States (51%) and that H3N2 infection is commonest in the South East (1.1%). Figures for some European countries may be even higher (East Germany 57%, Spain 60-78%).

Aetiology

Caused by Influenza A virus, an orthomyxovirus 80-120nm in diameter. These (and B and C viruses) have an RNA and protein core and surface spikes bearing haemagglutinating (H) and neuraminidase (N) antigens. They can be grown in embryonated eggs or on a number of porcine cell lines. Classical swine influenza is associated with influenza Virus A HlN1 in the U.S. but elsewhere in the world other strains are present in addition. A new strain, H1N1 A/swine/Eng/195852/92 was identified in UK in 1992. In many European countries, including Britain, Japan and other South East Asian countries H3N2 has also caused disease. Many H3N2 isolates from Europe are closely related antigenically to A/7/Port Chalmers/1/73, a human strain that appears to have persisted in pigs. In addition recombinants may occur and HlN2 has been reported from Japan. Recombination to give H1N2 has been demonstrated in Japan, and HlN1 and H3N2 have been reported in Italy, Japan, Hungary, Czechoslovakia and France and H1N7 (a horse/human recombinant) and H2N1 have been recorded in UK. Influenza viruses are sensitive to heat, drying, detergents and disinfectants. They are sensitive at high dilutions to modern disinfectants which contain oxidising agents and surfactants such as Virkon (Antec).

Influenza C infection has been reported in Japan and China.

Pathogenesis

In classic swine influenza, the virus enters the respiratory tract and multiplies rapidly from 2 hours in cells of the bronchial epithelium until at 24 hours post-infection most cells are infected and infected exudate is present in the bronchioles. Infection has largely disappeared by day 9. Infection of the alveolar septae and ducts occurs at the same time. The microscopic lesions develop as congestion followed by focal necrosis of bronchial epithelium. Small bronchi become blocked by neutrophil-rich exudate within 24 hours, alveolar necrosis and hyperplasia of the bronchial epithelium develop to give rise to the clinical signs and affected animals rapidly recover. The alveolar septae become thickened and cellular infiltrations of the alveolar septae and bronchial mucosa build up as recovery occurs. Serum antibody is produced. Viraemia can occur and transplacental infection has been recorded following infection up to 40 days before parturition and may result in failure of the lungs to develop. Antibody and antigen can be detected in foetuses. The severity of swine influenza infection may be much increased by the concurrent migration of Ascaris larvae through the lung and by infection with Aujeszky's disease virus, *A.pleuropneumoniae*, *H.parasuis* or *P.multocida*. Porcine respiratory coronavirus did not appear to exacerbate infection experimentally. In some cases "influenza-like" illness is not accompanied by the isolation of the swine influenza virus and other agents may also be responsible for the syndrome.

Clinical signs

In typical outbreaks, the incubation period is 1-2 days and there is rapid, virtually 100% involvement of all susceptible animals. Affected animals are apathetic, develop prostration, erythema of the skin, anorexia and fever (to 41.8°C, 107°F). Coughing occurs commonly and may be sufficiently severe for pigs to appear to vomit mucus exudate. Sneezing and dyspnoea are accompanied by reddened eyes and conjunctival discharge. Loss of condition rapidly becomes apparent. Recovery usually occurs suddenly at 5-7 days after the onset and mortality is low (usually less than 1%). Some pigs may remain depressed and growing pigs may reach slaughter up to 14 days later than expected. Piglets born to sows affected in pregnancy may develop disease at 2-5 days of age and adults kept in cold conditions may develop the clinical signs to a greater extent. In some herds infection may be completely subclinical and only be detected by seroconversion. Outbreaks may end at one time or continue in finishing pigs with new cases for periods up to 7 months. In atypical outbreaks only a few animals develop acute signs, others are scarcely affected and the disease spreads slowly. Influenza may be followed 3 days to 3 weeks later by abortions in sows in the second half of pregnancy. Conception to service during the outbreak may be reduced by up to 50% and litter sizes may be reduced.

Animals which remain prostrate or fevered for more than 7 days should be re-assessed and treated rather than killed.

Pathology

Animals with uncomplicated disease rarely die but sharply demarcated purple-red pneumonic lesions are present in the apical and cardiac lobes of the lung and may occur in the other lobes. Mucus and exudate are present in the bronchi and the mucosae are congested. Old lesions are depressed, greyish pink and firm on section. Microscopic lesions include thickened alveolar septae and bronchial epithelial changes. Bronchi are filled with neutrophils and later mononuclear cells. Finally, interstitial pneumonia and hyperplasia of the bronchial epithelium also occur. In some cases only congestion may be seen.

Recent reports of necrotising pneumonia from the U.K. and Canada may refer to the same condition. The U.K. H1 variant causes more pulmonary consolidation and congestion and the lesions are more severe with proliferative alveolitis, extensive necrosis of bronchioles and bronchi and peribronchial and peribronchiolar infiltration. The airways are filled with eosinophilic material.

Epidemiology

Virus spreads from pig to pig by snout to snout contact, by aerosol or droplet infection and does not persist for long in the environment. Disease may remain in large units for long periods, occurring particularly in newly-introduced susceptible breeding stock or feeder pigs. Maternal immunity may be demonstrable for up to 4 months. It may not prevent infection but may interfere with the production of active immunity. The disease is usually introduced to piggeries in carrier pigs. The virus survives best in the cold and disease is more common in cool conditions and in winter. Wind transmission to pigs kept partly outdoors may have occurred in France and some British outbreaks. Carrier pigs appear to have introduced the classical disease to Denmark, Japan, Italy and, possibly, the U.K. It appears that H1N1 occurs as a U.S. type (A/New Jersey/8/76/H1N1) and a European type in Europe. Oligonucleotide analysis has confirmed that some Swedish, Danish and Italian types, as well as those elsewhere in the world, are of U.S. origin.

The virus can persist on chilled meat for 8 days and in meat frozen at -20°C for 15 days, but this route of introduction to herds has not been documented.

Influenza may be carried by birds. turkeys have been shown to be capable of carrying and transmitting the disease to pigs. Influenza C in Japan occurs in dogs and influenzas in ducks are closely linked to pig disease in China.

Man may intorudce clinical infection with H3N2 which result in disease in pigs. Cases of influenza have been demonstrated in piggery workers in Europe and the U.S.. In one U.S. case, a human fatality was caused by H1N1 shown to be of pig origin by RNA fingerprinting. Others attending the same pig fair were infected and the disease spread to hospital staff.

Diagnosis

Clinical signs of a rapidly-spreading respiratory disease affecting all pigs in a herd and which does not respond to antimicrobial treatment is suggestive of influenza. The chronic disease is less easily identifiable on clinical grounds. Infection may be confirmed by a rise in serum antibody in paired serum samples taken 3-4 weeks apart. Antibodies to the virus can be detected using the haemagglutination inhibition (HI) test, single radial immunodiffusion or virus neutralisation tests. A four-fold rise in HI titre is considered diagnostic. HINI and H3N2 antigens should both be used. A blocking ELISA using a nucleoprotein monoclonal antibody has been described but still requires HI and N inhibition tests for typing. Virus isolation from nasal or tonsillar swabs and lung samples is possible if samples are taken within 2-5 days of the onset of clinical signs and submitted in virological transport medium. Fluorescent antibody to HINI and H3N2 can be used on lungs and nasal cells to demonstrate virus. Pathology is often complicated by the presence of other diseases. Influenza must be distinguished from porcine respiratory coronavirus infection and from Aujeszky's Disease in countries where these occur and in chronic disease or restricted outbreaks from pneumonic pasteurellosis, pleuropneumonia and chlamydial infection.

Treatment and Control

Vaccination with 2 doses of an oil adjuvanted vaccine e.g. (Suvaxyn Flu-3, Duphar) 3 weeks apart has been used widely in Europe (not yet U.K.) to protect against both clinical disease and loss of production. It contains A/Swine Ned/25/80 against European HINI viruses, A/Port Chalmers/1/73 against most H3N2 strains and A/Philippines/2/82 for protection against "Bangkok" H3N2 strains. Alum adjuvanted subunit and live virus vaccines have ben described. Control within herds consists of symptomatic treatment and antimicrobial treatment of secondary bacterial infection. Disinfectants can be used to prevent introduction on fomites. Sero-negative herds should only introduce pigs from similar herds. Total eradication from enzootically-infected herds must be by depopulation and restocking.

References

Abusugura, I.A., Linne,T., Klingeborn, B. (1989). J.Vet.Med. B. 36, 63-68. Analysis of some swine influenza H1N1 viruses by oligonucleotide fingerprinting.
Brown, I.H., Done, S., Hannam, D., Higgins, R.J., Machie, S.C., Courtenay, A. (1992). Vet.Rec. 130, 166. An outbreak of influenza in pigs.
Brown, I.H., Harris, P.A., Alexander, D.J. (1994). Proc.IPVS. 13, Studies of influenza virus in pigs in Great Britain 1992-1993.
Brown, I.H., Manvell, R.J., Alexander, D.J., Chakraverty, P., Hinshaw, V.S., Webster, R.G. (1993). Vet.Rec. 131, 461-462. Swine influenza outbreaks in E
Chambers, T.M., Hinshaw, V.S., Kawaoka, Y., Easterday, B.C., Webster, R.G. (1991). Arch.Virol. 116, 261-265. Influenza viral infection of swine in the U.S. 1988-89.
Kaufman, J., Hassan, M. and 13 others (1988). J.Am.Med.Ass. 260, 3116. Human infection with swine influenza virus - Wisconsin.
Madec, F., Kaiser, C., Gourreau, J.M., Martinat-Botte, F. (1989). Comp.Imm.Micro. and Inf.Dis. 12, 17-27. Consequences pathologiques d'un épisode grippal severe (virus swine A/H1/N1) dans les conditions naturelles chez la truie non immune en debut de gestation.
Nerome, K., Sakamoto, S. et al. (1983). J.Gen.Virol. 64, 2611-2620. The possible origin of H1N1 virus in the swine population of Japan and antigenic analysis of the isolates.

Onno, M., Jestin, A., Vannier, P. and Kaiser, C. (1990). Vet.Quarterly 12, 251-254. Diagnosis of swine influenza with an immunofluorescent technique using monoclonal antibodies.
Pritchard, G.C., Dick, I.G.C., Roberts, D.H., Wibberley, G. (1987). Vet.Rec. 121, 548. Porcine influenza outbreak in East Anglia due to influenza A virus (H3N2).
Roberts, D.H., Cartwright, S.F., Wibberley, G. (1987). Vet.Rec. 121, 53-55. Outbreaks of classical swine influenza in pigs in England in 1986.
Romijn, P.C., Swallow, C. and Edwards, S. (1989). Vet.Rec. 124, 224. Survival of influenza virus in pig tissue after slaughter
Sanford, S.E., Josephson, G.K.A. and Key, D.W. (1983). Canadian Vet.J. 24, 167-171. Pathology. An epizootic of swine influenza in Ontario.
Wells, D.L. and 6 authors (1991). J.Am.Med.Ass. 265, 478-481. Swine influenza virus infections: transmission from ill pigs to humans at a Wisconsin Agricultural Fair and subsequent probable person-to-person transmission.

Paramyxovirus infection

Paramyxoviruses have been recorded from pigs in many parts of the world. They include Sendai virus, Parainfluenza 3 and the virus of 'Blue Eye'. The best defined syndrome is 'Blue Eye'.

Paramyxovirus infection and 'Blue Eye'

Encephalomyelitis and corneal opacity associated with anterior uveitis have been recorded in young pigs 2-21 days of age in Mexico. The paramyxovirus has been found to cause stillbirths, mummified piglets and returns to oestrus. The causal agent in a paramyxovirus of 135-360nm and usually spherical, which is related most closely to SV5 and human mumps virus. Analysis of the genes for the Haemagglutinating and Matrix genes have been sequenced and code for proteins of 63;3 kDa, and 41; 6 kDa respectively. Other proteins, 59 kDa, 52 kDa, a nucleoprotein of 52 kDa and a large protein of 200 kDa have all been identified. The virus grows in Pig Kidney cells (PK15. CPE can be seen at 48 hours with cell rounding, death and syncytia. The virus haemagglutinates chicken, pig and human erythrocytes. Infectivity is destroyed by ether formalin, beta propiolactone and heat for 4 hours at $56^{o}C$. There is no cross neutralisation with other paramyxoviruses.

Infection is oronasal and spreads to brain, lung and reproductive tract in pregnant sows.

Affected piglets are usually 2-15 days old. Fever occurs suddenly and is accompanied by arching of the back, ataxia and rigidity. Conjunctivitis and corneal opacity may occur. Older piglets may develop listlessness and pneumonia and mummified piglets may be produced. Ataxic piglets should be killed.

Encephalomyelitis is the most obvious feature with some interstitial pneumonia, and corneal oedema occurs in 'Blue Eye'.

The disease appears to be confined to central Mexico. 'Blue Eye' has been reported from Northrn Ireland and, possibly, Czechoslovakia, but its relationship if any with the syndrome described here is unknown. Disease is maintained in continuous flow operations but is self-limiting in closed herds.

Diagnosis is based upon the clinical signs and the histological findings backed up by serology using HI and ELISA tests. The virus is most easily isolated from brain or tonsil on PK15 cells.

Control is based on isolation although a killed vaccine has been produced.

References

Moreno-Lopez, J., Correa-Giron, P., Martinez, A. and Ericsson, A. (1986). Arch.Virol. 91, 221-231. Characterisation of a paramyxovirus isolated from the brain of a piglet in Mexico.
Stephano, H.A., Gay, G.M., Ramirez, T.C. (1988). Vet.Rec. 122, 6-10. Encephalomyelitis, reproductive failure and corneal opacity in pigs associated with a new paramyxovirus infection ('Blue Eye').
Sundquist, A., Berg, M., Hernandez-Jauregui, P.

Pig Inclusion Body Rhinitis, Porcine Cytomegalovirus Infection (PCMV)

Definition

Infection with the porcine cytomegalovirus has been associated with rhinitis (Pig Inclusion Body Rhinitis, IBR, PIBR) and with lethal, generalised infection in very young pigs. It may cause disease in older animals in non-immune herds, crossing the placenta to cause an increase in embryonic and foetal mortality.

Incidence

Found worldwide and present in at least 9% of herds in Britain. The disease is usually identified when it enters a non-immune herd and may not be recognised in a given country until a clinical outbreak is investigated.

Aetiology

Porcine cytomegalovirus or porcine inclusion body rhinitis virus is a typical enveloped cytomegalo (herpes) virus approximately 150 nm in diameter which can only be cultured with difficulty and which is most easily isolated by the culture of lung macrophages from 3-5 week old pigs. . It can be cultivated *in vitro* in these or porcine tests or fallopian tube cell lines. In lung macrophage cultures C.P.E. does not occur although infected cells enlarge and form basophilic intranuclear inclusions which may be demonstrated by immunofluorescence or Giemsa stains.
The virus is inactivated by chloroform and ether but other physicochemical properties have not been reported. All isolates appear to belong to one antigenic type.

Pathogenesis

Primary replication appears to be in the nasal mucous glands in non-immune piglets infected by the oronasal route, in neutrophils in the viraemic stage 14-16 days p.i. and finally in epithelial sites such as nasal mucosa, seminiferous and kidney tubules at 3 weeks of age. Virus may cross the placenta and infect the foetus during the viraemic stage at 14-21 days after infection in non-immune sows. Viral isolation from the nose at 14-21 days post infection(dpi) is followed at 30-35 dpi by isolation from the cervix. Virus takes 14-20 days to multiply in the foetus and cervical virus may be of foetal origin. Multiplication occurs in foetal leptomeninges, hepatic sinusoidal cells, peritoneal macrophages and periosteal cells. Embryonic death occurs in early gestation. Foetuses exposed late in gestation are born seronegative. Boars can excrete virus in urine and nasal secretions. Serum antibody responses develop but low levels of antibody may not prevent infection of the products of conception. Serum antibody responses develop but low levels of antibody may not prevent infection of the products of conception.

Clinical signs

Few clinical signs other than anorexia and pyrexia occur in pigs of more than 3 weeks of age in herds where the infection is enzootic. Where individual sows or whole herds are non-immune, pigs may be infected *in utero* or within 2 weeks of birth and may develop rhinitis, sneezing and respiratory distress. Mortality in an affected litter may reach 25%. Piglets may be born dead, die without clinical signs or be pale anaemic and oedematous in the generalised form of the disease. A reduction in growth rate frequently occurs. Severe disease in adults has been recorded when infection enters non-immune herds. Anorexia, fever, coughing and serous, purulent and haemorrhagic nasal discharge have been recorded. Stillbirths and mummified foetuses may result and there may be an increase in returns to service and of small litters. Severely affected piglets should be assessed and killed as soon as they can no longer rise.

Pathology

Gross lesions are rarely visible in animals with localised upper respiratory tract infection but may appear as severe nasal congestion of the nasal septum with adherent tenacious mucus. Histological examination reveals cytomegaly with basophilic intranuclear inclusions in cells of the nasal mucus glands and other epithelial sites such as duodenum and renal tubules. Affected glands may be surrounded by macrophages and lymphocytes. Generalised lesions in young pigs and foetuses may be seen in the lung where pulmonary oedema occurs, and serous effusions and widespread haemorrhages may be seen, particularly in the kidneys. Inclusions may be seen in reticuloendothelial cells in lymphoid tissue, in the leptomeninges and hepatic sinusoidal cells, peritoneal macrophages, penosteal cells and, rarely in alveolar macrophages. Growth arrests may be present in the long bones. In field outbreaks, lesions may sometimes be complicated by other agents.

Epidemiology

Enzootic in many herds, virus can cross the placenta and therefore occur in hysterectomy-derived herds. There appear to be no vectors and infection appears to survive in carrier pigs, being spread to unaffected herds by the introduction of infected pigs. Infection can spread by direct contact with urine or respiratory secretions or by aerosol. Virus is shed in nasal secretions mostly between 3 and 8 weeks of age. Infection may occur even up to slaughter weight and may be reactivated by stress and mixing. There appears to be little persistence outside the host.

Diagnosis

Serum antibody can be detected by indirect immuno-fluorescence or ELISA tests. The clinical signs must be distinguished from those of Bordetella infection in piglets. The presence of the inclusions in sections or smears from nasal mucosa confirms the presence of infection. In sows and neonates the lack of abortion and the relatively low mortality distinguishes the disease from Aujeszky's disease. Viral isolation can be carried out but with difficulty.

Control and treatment

Secondary infection can be controlled and disease-free herds can be founded if pigs are screened serologically for 70 days after birth. Where severe infection occurs, neonatal piglets should not be exposed to it.

References

Edington, N., Plowright, W. and Watt, R.G. (1976). J.Comp.Path. 86, 191-202. Generalised cytomegalic inclusion disease: distribution of cytomegalic cells and virus.
Edington, N., Broad, S., Wrathall, A.E. and Done, J.T. (1988). Vet.Microbiol. 16, 189-193. Superinfection with PCMV initiating transplacental infection.
Edington, N., Wrathall, A.E. and Done, J.T. (1988). Vet.Microbiol. 17, 117-128. Porcine cytomegalovirus in early gestation.
Orr, J.P., Althouse, E., Dulac, G.C., Durham, P.J.K. (1988). Can.Vet.J. 29, 40-53. Epizootic infection of a minimal disease swine herd with a herpesvirus.

Reovirus

Reovirus has been isolated from a number of clinical syndromes including respiratory, enteric and nervous problems and from aborted foetuses in the U.K. (Type 1). Type 3 has been recovered from respiratory disease and untyped virus from outbreaks of abortion and foetal and early neonatal death. Mild microscopic lesions including infiltration of the interalveolar septae by macrophages, lymphocytes and fibroblasts have been described following experimental infection. Infection with the 75nm icosahedral double-stranded RNA virus may be demonstrated by culture in primary pig kidney cell lines where they eventually form intracytoplasmic eosinophilic inclusions or by serological methods such as the haemagglutination inhibition test. Paired sera are necessary to confirm a diagnosis. Antibodies to Type 1 and Type 2 were found in 30-40% of pig sera in Britain in 1971. Fifty-seven per cent of herds were found to be infected. Type 1 virus was most common in S.W. England and W. Scotland and Type 2 in the E. Midlands and N. Scotland. Higher prevalences have been detected in Japan and Brazil where the development of antibody occurred between 2 and 3 months of age.

Respiratory Syncytial Virus

Antibody to this virus has been found in the sera of Scottish slaughter pigs at levels which indicate that active infection has occurred. No clinical or pathological changes have yet been correlated with these. Virus established in the bronchi when hysterectomy-derived colostrum-deprived piglets were inoculated with human RSV, but lesions were confined to syncytia in the bronchiolar epithelium.

Swine Pox

Definition

A mild infectious disease caused by the swine pox virus in which red, circular pox lesions appear on the skin of the belly, axillae, face and head in young pigs. Rare congenital infections are fatal within 24 hours of birth.

Incidence

Widespread but rarely reported. Clinical case reports often represent a formal declaration of its presence in an area. In a 1990 survey of 150 sera from 69 herds in the U.K., 19.3% sows in 28.9% herds were antibody-positive.

Aetiology

Caused by the swine pox virus, a large ether-sensitive (300-400 x 176-200nm DNA virus of the swinepox group or in the past by Vaccinia virus. These viruses are extremely resistant to drying and may persist for years in exudates in which it can resist temperature of 100°C for 10 minutes. Swine pox virus grows in pig kidney cell lines or on the chorioallantoic membranes of eggs to cause C.P.E. and intracytoplasmic inclusions. Recent attempts to isolate the virus on the chorioallantoic membrane have been unsuccessful.

Pathogenesis

The virus enters locally via skin abrasions and multiplies there or attacks the skin after viraemia. The incubation period is 4-5 days from infection to the development of pustules and these last 10-14 days. All stages from vesicle, macule, pustule and ulcer may develop. Viraemia in sows results in the birth of congenitally-infected piglets. Serum neutralising antibody develops at 7 days, peaks at 20 days and has largely gone by 50 days, post infection. Cellular immunity peaks at 11-21 days post infection.

Clinical signs

The incubation period is 3-6 days but may be up to 14 days and the lesions persist for 1-3 weeks. Slight pyrexia (to 40°CF, 104°F) may accompany the appearance of the lesions. Red l cm. papules appear on the ventral abdomen and rapidly form circular red brown scabs, which rapidly blacken. In young piglets the bursting of the vesicular stage on the face may lead to wetting, scab formation and conjunctivitis. Slight inappetence may accompany the development of the lesions. Affected pigs appear hairy and growth may be depressed. A large percentage of successive litters of sucking and recently-weaned pigs may be affected but the disease is rare in adults. Mortality is rare although transplacental infection in newborn pigs can cause deaths. Lesions may be seen on the edge of the tongue, lips and all over the body. Badly affected neonates may have to be killed, but all other age groups normally recover.

Pathology

The skin lesions are those of a typical pox virus. Nuclear vacuolation and cytoplasmic inclusions may be seen at the papular stage in the cells of the epidermis. A mild vesicular stage occurs but the pustular and crusting stages are most prominent. Secondary bacterial infections may occur.

Epidemiology and Occurrence

The disease is widespread but is rarely reported, occurring in successive litters of sucking pigs, often becoming less common in the winter. Because good immunity is produced, adults are rarely affected. The virus may persist in a farm for years between outbreaks in dust and dried secretions in unused pens and fittings. The progeny of newly purchased pigs are often affected as are weaned pigs from non-immune farms when mixed with carriers. Lice and flies may transmit the disease within a farm.

Diagnosis

The size and colour of the lesions is characteristic. Flank biting, "spirochaetal granuloma" and local infections with *Staphylococcus hyicus* may also resemble pig pox but the agents of these are usually demonstrable. Electron microscopy or culture can confirm and differentiates from Orf.

Treatment and Control

Treatment or control are rarely attempted because of the mildness of the disease, but the use of insecticide to eliminate lice and the thorough cleaning and disinfection of pens in which outbreaks of the disease have occurred help to reduce the incidence. Vaccines have been produced experimentally but do not protect completely as fever may still occur on challenge.

References

Borst, G.H.A., Kimman, T.G., Gielkens, A.L.J., Kamp, J.S. vander (1990). Vet.Rec. 127, 61-63. Congenital swine pox.
Gorg, S.K., Chandra, R., Roo, V.D.P. (1989). Vet.Bull. 59, 441-448. Swine Pox.
Jubb, T.F., Ellis, T.M., Peet, R., Parkinson, J. (1992). Aust.Vet.J. 69, 99. Swine pox in Northern Western Australia.
Paton, D.J., Brown, I.H., Fitton, J., Wrathall, A.E. (1990). Vet.Rec. 127, 104. Congenital pig box: a case report.
Williams, P.P., Hall, M.R., McFarland, M.D. (1989). Vet.Immunol. Immunopath. 23, 149-159. Immunological responses of crossbred and inbred miniature pigs to swine pox virus.

The Porcine Reproductive and Respiratory Syndrome (PRRS)

(Porcine Epidemic Abortion and Respiratory Syndrome PEARS, Blue Ear)

Definition

A viral infection causing inappetance, laboured breathing, occasional fever, abortion and returns to service occurs in sows, accompanied by an increase in stillbirths and piglet mortality from birth to the early post-weaning stage. Respiratory distress, poor growth rates and increased mortality in weaned piglets are major features of the disease in chronically infected herds. Infection may be inapparent.

Incidence

The disease is widespread in the US where it was first seen in 1987, and in 1988 it was identified in Canada. In Europe it was seen first in Germany in 1990, and in 1991 was recorded in The Netherlands, Spain, Belgium and UK (May 1991, Humberside). It was identified in France in 1992 but has not yet been seen in Ireland. It has been recorded in Korea and Japan and must be regarded as occurring in most pig rearing countries. Most of these serological surveys suggest that over 50% of herds are infected. In all infected countries serologically negative herds exist.

Aetiology

PRRS is caused by an enveloped RNA virus 45-55 nm in diameter (50-60 nm negatively stained) with a 30-35 nm nucleocapsid. The genome has been cloned and sequenced and the virus has been found to be closely related to lactose dehydrogenase elevating virus of mice, equine arteritis virus and simian haemorrhagic virus (arteriviruses). Sequence and antigenic analysis suggest that European isolates are closely related to the Lelystad virus but that US (VR 2332) and Canadian isolates are more distantly related. Several different genomic and antigenic variants have been described from North America. Five viral proteins have been identified, 15 kDa (nucleo capsid protein common to all isolates), 16 (US)/15.5 kDa, 19 (US)/18 kDa, 22 kDa and 26 kDa glycosylated envelope proteins. Serum neutralisation tests can distinguish between strains.

The virus grows in the cytoplasm of cells, principally porcine alveolar macrophages but also in cell lines such as CL2621, budding into the smooth endoplasmic reticulum and accumulating within it. Infected cells such as macrophages may lyse within 12 hours but lysis and cytopathic effect do not occur in peripheral blood monocytes and some other permissive cells. Levels of $>10^7$ particles per ml can be produced by exocytosis. The virus has been shown to be stable at -70°C and -20°C, to persist for one month at +4°C, to be 93% inactivated and to be inactivated after 48 hours at 37°C and to persist less than 45 minutes at 56°C.

Pathogenesis

Infection is usually by the respiratory route or contact although infection has followed insemination. The virus multiplies in alveolar macrophages and other elements of the reticuloendothelial system including endothelial cells. The aleveolar macrophages are destroyed and multiplication of virus in the endothelial cells can give rise to vascular lesions including swelling of the endothelial cells of capillaries and small and large veins allowing plasma proteins to leak into the tissue. Secondary damage may result in thrombosis or complete occlusion. Many features of the disease and its development depend upon the ability of the virus to multiply in or destroy alveolar macrophages, endothelial and lymphoid cells.

Following infection viraemia rapidly develops and virus can be demonstrated in both serum and monocytes. There is a transient reduction in circulating white cells about four days' post-infection and this affects neutrophils and lymphocytes. CD4, CD8 and B cells are all affected in lymph nodes. Virus can be demonstrated in serum from the first day after infection and in the lung from them until day 7 post-infection but persists in spleen, tonsil, lymph nodes for longer. Viraemia may last for 1-9 days in sows but up to 3-8, or even 12 weeks in young pigs and continues in the presence of antibody. Throughout this period virus is shed in nasal secretions and faeces. The virus may penetrate the reproductive tract. In boars the virus may be shed in the semen and in the sow infection of the embryo can lead to resorption and in foetuses to mummification and stillbirths. Virus is present in lesions in both maternal and foetal placenta. Infection in young piglets leads to destruction of the alveolar macrophages rendering the lung susceptible to infection with bacteria such as *P.multocida*, *A.pleuropneumoniae*, *H.parasuis* and *Chlamydia sp.*. An interstitial pneumonia develops associated with capillary damage.

Antibody can be demonstrated from 7-9 days onwards and persists for more than 20 weeks in some animals.

Clinical signs

These are at their most severe when infection enters a non-immune herd, but infection may be inapparent.

In sows, there is usually an inappetance lasting 24-36 hours - 4 days in individuals and 7-10 days in the herd. Sows may be listless with laboured breathing but fever is not consistent, rarely exceeds 40°C and is transient, often lasting a single day. Abortion may occur at any stage of gestation, and is first apparent at 22 days, but most cases occur later. 2-3% of sows in a house may abort, many not even showing prior inappetance. There may be accompanying skin changes such as hyperaemia or congestion of the ears, nose and tail, but only 1-2% of animals develop these changes. Farrowing problems develop with a rise in stillbirths and increased mortality in piglets aged up to 1 week. This is partially due to premature farrowing (the herd gestation length may be reduced by two days). Lactation is affected in some sows and inappetance in lactation may lead to anoestrus. Returns to service may also occur although this may be partly attributed to boar fertility. A general rise in other diseases such as cystitis may be expected.

Boars may be listless and occasional animals develop blue ears. A drop in semen quality may occur but cannot be linked in every case to clinical signs.

In piglets, antenatal infection or effects on the sow may lead to an increase in stillbirths and antepartum deaths appearing as large mummified piglets. Many of the piglets born are weak, may have splayleg and do not survive. Affected piglets may have oedema of the eyelids which gives a spectacled appearance and there may be conjunctivitis. Bleeding from interference such as tail docking and tooth clipping is common and bruising may occur at iron injection and may be apparent as discolouration of the skin. Haemorrhage into the gut may lead to melaena and the appearance of a greyish diarrhoea. Laboured breathing may also be apparent. Occasional cases of meningitis have been reported.

In weaners and growers there is an increase in respiratory disease and skin changes may be seen in recovering pigs, 5-7 days after infection. An increase in any other disease endemic on the farm becomes apparent.

In the herd, the first 8 weeks of the disease are characterised by a rise in pre-weaning mortality (average 33%) and a dramatic rise in the number of stillbirths (average 18%). Later, mummified piglets appear and live births decrease (average reduction of 1.0 piglet/litter). Post-weaning mortality may increase (average 9%) and the number of treatments required increases markedly. In the second period of 6 weeks, there is an overall improvement but mummified piglets remain common and livebirths are still low. Returns to service increase (average 18%). Illness in piglets and weaned pigs remains common and numbers of treatments are still raised. In the third period, a drop in total births occurs as a result of continuing low numbers born and the increase in returns to service. A return to near normal levels of production can be expected 26 weeks after infection.

Annual levels of production may be affected as follows:

Returns to service	2.0% increase
Abortions	0.3% increase
Numbers born alive per littler	0.3% decrease
Stillbirths	2.7% increase
Piglet mortality	3.7% increase
Weaned pig mortality	1.1% increase

An overall loss of 2.54 pigs/sow/year may be expected and increases in the costs of feed medication may occur.

Once infection becomes enzootic, clinical disease is restricted to non-immune animals exposed to the disease for the first time. These are usually non-immune gilts introduced to n infected herd, weaners and growers. The disease in weaners and growers appears as fever (to 41°C), weakness and occasional cyanosis and raised respiratory rates. Diseases present on the farm may develop 5-7 days after infection. In gnotobiotic pigs or on SPF farms there may be no clinical signs and weight gains may be unaffected.

Humane destruction may be indicated in sows with blue-ear and severe and prolonged distress, particularly if they begin to lose condition or develop subnormal temperatures. Piglets with respiratory distress, weakness or severe splayleg may be destroyed. Weaners rarely require euthanasia in uncomplicated disease, but severe and prolonged respiratory distress which does not respond to treatment would be an indication.

Pathology

Affected piglets may have no gross lesions. There may be skin haemorrhages and bruising with bleeding into tissues, particularly where interference has occurred. The most consistent change noted is pulmonary congestion or anterior lobe pneumonia and excess pericardial or pleural fluid and type 2 pneumonocyte proliferation. There is perivascular cuffing, tracheal and nasal lesions are rare and there is vacuolation and surface blebbing of the bronchiolar epithelium which may not be functional. Alveolar macrophages are absent. Canadian cases have had a more severe proliferative necrotising pneumonia with lymphocytic rhinitis and perivascular cuffing. *Pneumocystis carinii* infection is commonly identified in these lesions. Necrotising pneumonia such as reported in Quebec is atypical and has not been reported in the UK. All post-mortem findings may be complicated by the presence of disease normally present in the herd. Influenza, porcine respiratory coronavirus, pleuropneumonia and *H.parasuis* infections are particularly important in the lungs and streptococcal meningitis and salmonellosis have also been recorded. Increases in enteric infections have also been reported.

<u>Epidemiology</u>

The disease spreads within a unit by aerosol or by direct contact between pigs. Nasal secretions are the main source of infection but faeces may also be infective. Serological studies have shown that infection may be confined to weaners and growers on a farm and that infection may be absent from sows and sucking pigs. Infection tends to appear as maternal antibody levels fall. Serology has also confirmed that spread amongst this age group is rapid and often complete within one or two weeks, and that antibody levels reach a peak at 6-12 weeks of age and are often declining by slaughter. Viraemia (and infectivity) may last for 8-12 weeks (and sometimes much less) in infected groups and pigs may be virus-free at slaughter.

Spread within groups of gilts, sows or boars varies in its speed and completeness. In some cases the introduction of an infected animal may not result in the infection of a farm and some infected farms spontaneously become seronegative and virus-free. Infection can be transmitted at service and virus has been isolated from semen from 13 to 43 days in one study. Natural service and artificial insemination with infected semen have both been shown to result in infection of the sow. Infection at day 1 of gestation (service) may not always result in reproductive failure but infection at 30 days may lead to 20% litters being affected.

The disease has been spread between farms by the introduction of carrier pigs which may remain infected for at least 12 weeks but it may also move locally by aerosol transmission. Spread between farms appears to occur over at least 3 km and occasionally up to 20 km, usually in low ambient temperatures, and high humidity on dull days. Semen produced by boars in the viraemic stage of infection is capable of introducing infection to non-immune herds.

Serological surveys suggest that inapparent infections are common and in a recent survey of 22 breeding herds and 10 feeding herds with no history of PRRS in Humberside, 50% were found to be seropositive. The development of clinical signs may depend upon the number of pigs present on the unit, their density and the hygienic conditions.

<u>Diagnosis</u>

Clinical signs such as an increase in stillbirths to 20%, in abortions to 8% and in pre-weaning mortality to 26% should lead to suspicion of PRRS. Lesser levels of these parameters and the other clinical signs described above may also lead to suspicion. The development of respiratory disease which is difficult to control in weaners or growers may also be associated with PRRS infection. The presence of the disease may also be suspected at post-mortem examination. Anterior lobe lung lesions and the presence of haemorrhages in the carcase may suggest the disease. Histological findings of the presence of an interstitial pneumonia and the absence of alveolar macrophages may also be noted. The presence of the virus may be confirmed by immunofluorescence or by immunoperoxidase using antibody to the p15 nucleocapsid protein (appears to react with all types) and a reverse polymerase chain reaction has been described.

Virus isolation may be carried out using porcine alveolar macrophages or one of the permissive cell lines such as CL2621. Cytopathogenic effects may be seen within 12 hours but not all isolates grow in both systems. Isolates should be further characterised as a number of other viruses may be isolated in this system. Lung tissue or serum may be used.

The detection of serum antibodies to the virus is the most commonly used way of confirming a diagnosis and may be used to construct serum profiles of infection in a herd and for disease monitoring. The most commonly used tests are:

ELISAs using cultures virus (Leleystad and US isolates may be required).

Immunoperoxidase monolayer assay (IPMA) is less frequently used now than the ELISA but detects antibody from 7-14 days.

Indirect fluorescent antibody test (IFA).

Serum neutralising test (SNT) which is strain specific. It can therefore be less useful in confirmation but very useful in identifying antibody to individual strains of virus.

Samples for serological testing can be taken from piglets 0-4 weeks of age (colostral antibody) and 10-12 weeks of age in enzootically-infected herds. Samples taken from slaughter pigs may be less satisfactory.

Other diseases which may need to be considered from a clinical point of view are Aujeszky's disease, African and Classical Swine Fever, Swine Influenza, Porcine Respiratory Coronavirus, Encephalomyocarditis, Porcine Parvovirus infection, Haemagglutinating Encephalomyelitis Virus infection, TGE, Porcine Epidemic Diarrhoea, Talfan, Chlamydia psittaci, erysipelas and leptospirosis. Serological testing will eliminate their involvement.

Treatment and control

There is no specific treatment but a series of measures have been recommended to reduce the economic and welfare impact of the disease:

1. Proved electrolytes for all weak/diarrhoeic pigs.
2. Delay iron injection to 3 days and tail docking to 3-5 days. Do not clip teeth.
3. Stop induced farrowings.
4. Give artificial colostrum to piglets at birth and 4 hours of age.
5. Treat sows with acetyl salicylic acid (aspirin) daily for 7 days prior to farrowing at 8g/sow/day by top dressing of feed for first 4-6 weeks of outbreak.
6. Do not serve sows until 21 days after farrowing regardless of the fate of the litter. Do not restore depleted litters to full size.
7. Sows weaned during the acute phase of the disease should be given high energy diets to reduce the effects of inappetance on reproductive performance.
8. Allow minimum of 21 days before re-service following abortion of litters of 70 days' gestation.
9. Re-serve immediately sows aborting earlier litters.

10. Check all sows for pregnancy weekly from 4-5 weeks' gestation onwards.
11. Supplement all services with A1 for 6 weeks from appearance of acute disease due to effects on semen quality.
12. Be prepared for the onset of disease in the feeding herd and treat as appropriate.
13. Maintain normal health procedures if possible.

Eradication has been achieved successfully by preparing antibody profiles in herds. Where there is no infection in sows or sucking piglets, and disease is confined to weaners and growers, depopulation, cleaning, removal of slurry, disinfection and three weeks' rest of the accommodation, followed by restocking, can lead to elimination of the infection.

The use of separate site weaning and growing and finishing accommodation (Isowean, P.I.C.) may also eliminate infection. Continuous medication with antibacterials over the period of risk may reduce the economic effects.

References

Albina, E., Baron, T. and Leforban, Y. Vet.Rec. (1992). 130, 58-59. Blue eared pig disease in Brittany.

Albina, E., Leforban, Y., Baron, T. and Duran, J.P. Vet.Rec. (1992). 130, 83-84. Blue eared pig disease in Brittany: a new test.

Albina, E., Leforban, Y., Baron, T., Duran, J.P., Vannier, P. (1992). Annales de Recherche Veterinaires 23, 167-176. An ELISA for the detection of antibody to the PRRS virus.

Albina, E., Madec, F., Cariolet, R., Torrison, J. (1994). Vet.Rec. 134, 567-573. Immune response and persistence of the PRRS virus in infected pigs and farm units.

Anon (1992). Vet.Rec. 130, 87-89. (Review) Porcine reproductive and respiratory syndrome (PRRS or blue-eared pig disease).

Benfield, D.A. Nelson, E., Collins, J.E., Harris, L., Goyal, S.M., Robison, D., Christianson, W.T., Morrison, R.B., Gorcyca, D. and Chladek, D. (1992). J.Vet.Diagn.Invest. 4, 127-133. Characterisation of swine infertility and respiratory syndrome (SIRS) virus (isolate ATCC VR2332).

Christianson, W.T., Collins, J.E., Pijoan, C., Joo, H.S., Benfield, D.A., McCullough, S.J. (1991). Pig Vet.J. 27, 9-12. Swine Infertility and Respiratory Syndrome.

Dee, S.A., Joo, H.S. (1994). Vet.Rec. 135, 6-9. Prevention of the spread of PRCV in endemically infected herds by nursery depopulation.

Gordon, S.C. (1992). Vet.Rec. 130, 513-514. Effects of blue-eared pig disease on a breeding and fattening unit.

Morin, M. and Robinson, Y. (1991). Vet.Rec. 129, 367-368. Porcine reproductive and respiratory syndrome in Quebec.

Paton, D.J., Brown, I.H., Scott, A.C., Done, S.H., Edwards, S. (1992). Vet.Microbiol. 33, 195-201. Isolation of a Lelystad virus-like agent from British pigs and scanning electron microscopy of infected macrophages.

Robertson, I.B. (1992). Vet.Rec. 130, 478-479. Transmission of blue-eared pig disease.

Rossow, K.D., Bautista, E.M., Goyal, S.M., Molitor, T.W., Murtaugh, M.P., Morrison, R.B., Benfield, D.A., Collins, J.E. (1994). J.Vet.Diagn. Invest. 6, 3-12. Experimental PRRS virus infection in 1, 4 and 10 week-old pigs.

Stevenson, G.W., Alsine, W.G. van, Kanitz, C.L. (1994). J.Am.Vet.Med.Assn. 204, 1938-1942. Characterisation of infection with endemic PRRS virus in a swine herd.
Swenson, S.L. and 10 other authors (1994). J.Am.Vet.Med.Assn. 204, 1943-1948. Excretion of PRRSV in semen after experimentally-induced infection in boars.
Wensvoort, G., Terpstra, C., Pol, J.M.A. (1991). Vet.Quarterly. 13, 121-130. Mystery Swine Disease in the Netherlands: the isolation of Lelystad virus.
Woensel, P. van., Wouw, J. van der, Visser, N. (1994). J.Virol.Methods 47, 273-278. Detection of PRRSV by the polymerase chain reaction.
Yoon, I.J., Joo, H.S., Christianson, W.T., Kim, H., Collins, J.E., Morrison, R.B., Dial, G.D. (1992). J.Vet.Diagn.Invest. 4, 144-147. An indirect fluorescent antibody test for the detection of antibody to SIRS virus in swine sera.

Aujeszky's Disease (Pseudorabies)

Definition

Aujeszky's disease is a herpes virus infection of pigs characterised by nervous and respiratory signs associated with a rise of temperature and often leading to death in young pigs. Infection in adults may be inapparent or associated with stillbirths or abortion.

Incidence

Widespread in the United States, Europe, South America and South East Asia. Aujeszky's disease occurred sporadically in Britain; only 3 outbreaks were confirmed in 1970, but from then onwards, numbers of outbreaks rose to 12-20 p.a. and in 1982 43 outbreaks were recorded. A rise in confirmations to 470 was recorded in 1983-84 when an eradication campaign began in Great Britain and by 1988 only 6 infected herds were recorded, some as serological reactors. Five were recorded in 1989 and eradication was then complete. The disease is still present in Ireland.

The disease has been eradicated from Denmark, is absent from Switzerland and is the subject of eradication campaigns in other parts of the world.

Aetiology

The causal agent of Aujeszky's disease is a herpes virus, Suid herpesvirus I (SHVI), the complete enveloped particle of which has a diameter of 180nm. It may be cultivated in tissue cultures of porcine origin or in embryonated hens' eggs. Cowdry Type A intranuclear inclusion bodies are produced in tissue culture and *in vivo* and the C.P.E. produced in tissue culture is characterised by the formation of syncytia. The virus is 150-180nm in diameter and consists of a DNA core of 75nm in diameter, a nucleocapsid of 105-110nm consisting of 162 capsomeres and an envelope bearing glycoproteins. These glycoproteins include gI, gII, gIII, gVI (gp50) and gp63. Other important viral proteins include the thymidine kinase (TK) and nucleocapsid proteins. The genes for these proteins have been identified, sequenced, cloned and used to produce recombinant proteins, primers for the polymerase chain reaction (PCR) and probes. Cell penetration appears to be associated with gI, gII and gp50, cell fusion with gI and gp50 and central nervous system spread with gI. Monoclonal antibodies have been used to study epitopes on the proteins and for diagnostic tests. Restriction endonuclease fragment analysis has been used on the whole genome to sub-divide Aujeszky's Disease Virus into RF types. Molecular biology has been vital in the development of new vaccines, diagnostic tests, control measures and epidemiology and additional information appears below.

Only one major antigenic type of the virus is recognised, but strains of virus producing predominantly nervous lesions and others producing predominantly pneumonic lesions have been described. Other biological differences include a few entirely genital strains and some isolates which do not produce syncytia in tissue culture. The virus is ether sensitive and is readily inactivated by heat (30 minutes exposure to 57°C). It is stable between pH 6 and 11 at 23°C when suspended in tissue culture fluid. Low concentrations of disinfectant e.g. 2% lysol and 5.25% sodium hypochlorite will inactivate it as will formaldehyde and detergents. Disinfectants combining surfactants and other agents are particularly useful.

Pathogenesis

Infection with Aujeszky's disease virus occurs via the epithelium of the upper respiratory tract and multiplication of the virus in this site is followed by invasion of the central nervous system and by passage of the virus along the course of the olfactory, trigeminal and glossopharyngeal nerves to the medulla and pons. A non-suppurative meningo-encephalitis and myelitis is produced. Strains of the virus found in Northern Ireland and Central Europe also produce pneumonia. Local multiplication in the upper respiratory tract also occurs. Viraemia may accompany the invasion of the C.N.S. or lungs and give rise to lesions elsewhere in the body, but viraemia is not essential to the production of the clinical signs of the disease. Virus is shed in nasal and respiratory tract secretions. 10^{10} tissue culture infectious doses may be present per ml of nasal secretion. Infected alveolar macrophages are less effective and lymphocyte lysis and focal necrosis in lymph nodes depress the immune response. Invasion of the uterus, maternal and foetal placentas and foetuses occurs and can cause abortion, foetal death, mummification and foetal resorption if it occurs in the first half of gestation, and mummification in some cases in the last third. The virus can be adsorbed onto embryonated eggs and can infect recipient sows in embryo transfer. Infection of the genital tract may occur in boars and virus may be shed in the semen for up to 10 days. Virus shedding from animals infected by any route may occur between 2 days post-infection and continue until 10-14 days post-infection in most cases and exceptionally until 19-20 days. Latent infections commonly develop. Virus can be demonstrated by co-cultivation, PCR and labelled DNA probe in trigeminal ganglia and other areas of the brain for up to 7 months after infection and, following immunosuppression using corticosteroids for up to 18-19 months. Immunosuppression, whether artificial or natural by means of stress can be followed by a period of virus shedding for 4-11 days after the event. Latent virus may be present in nervous tissue only as viral DNA sequences. Up to 30 copies of viral genome may be present in infected cells. Restriction endonuclease techniques confirm its identity and that of re-isolated virus with initial infecting virus. Recovered animals develop both humoral and cellular immunity. The humoral response can be demonstrated by day 8 post exposure at titres of 1:2-1:4 and rises to 1:128 or 1:512 at which level it remains for some weeks. IgM, IgG1 and IgG2 antibodies are most important in quantity and for protection but an IgA response has been demonstrated in the nasal mucosa. Cellular immunity develops by day 7-14 post infection and persists for up to 170 days post infection. Colostral antibody levels may be double or treble those in maternal serum and piglet serum levels are the same as those in colostrum by 1 day post partum. Antibody cannot be demonstrated by 14 weeks post partum. The presence of neutralising antibody may not prevent colonisation of the nasopharynx, the development of viraemia on challenge or the development of microscopic lesions and cellular immunity may not prevent colonisation of the nasal epithelium.

Clinical signs

The clinical signs of Aujeszky's disease differ according to the infectious dose and the age of the animals affected. They are most severe in pigs aged 0-4 weeks in which morbidity and mortality may reach 100% in newborn animals declining to 40-60% in 4 week-old animals. Animals aged between 1 and 5 months are less severely affected (mortality up to 15%) and in adults the disease may produce few clinical signs.

Piglets newborn - 4 weeks of age

Clinical signs begin 3-7 days after infection in natural outbreaks and affected piglets may vomit or show diarrhoea and then become depressed, with trembling, incoordination (including circling), the adoption of a dog-sitting position, spasms of opisthotonus and prostration followed by death after at least 12 hours. Body temperature rarely exceeds 41.5°C, 107°F. The course of the disease is longer in older piglets and it may be accompanied by constipation. Mortality is less common in older piglets and death takes longer from the onset of clinical signs. Skin lesions resembling those of human cold sores may be present on the snout, lips and face.

Weaned pigs 4 weeks - 5 months of age

Clinical signs begin 5-7 days after infection with a rise in temperature to 40.6-41.7°C, 105-107°F, which may continue for 4-8 days. Anorexia with occasional vomiting occurs within 3 days of the onset of fever and is accompanied from the 4th day by nervous signs which begin with tremor and incoordination, in particular of the hind limbs, and progress to tonoclonic spasms of various muscle groups and to convulsions which may last only 45 seconds. These nervous signs are usually followed by prostration and death. The course of the disease usually takes 4-8 days from the onset of clinical signs. Finishing periods may be extended by 10-14 days. In outbreaks in Northern Ireland, and in growing and finishing pigs elsewhere, severe pneumonia has been recorded in addition to the nervous signs described above.

Adults

Infection may be asymptomatic or consist only of anorexia but is usually followed by a rise in temperature accompanied by coughing, salivation and other upper respiratory signs, anorexia, constipation and depression which may lead to recovery after 4-5 days or rarely to central nervous involvement and death (2%). Up to 50% of affected pregnant animals abort or give birth to mummified or macerated foetuses. Reproductive failure may follow these abortions or the early weaning consequent upon death of a litter. Boars may be affected and semen quality may decline from 10-14 days post-infection for a period of 1-2 weeks. Some sperm abnormalities may occur.

Humane endpoint: Animals which are ataxic or undergoing convulsions should be killed as should those with acute respiratory distress.

Pathological findings

Gross changes

Few gross changes are seen. There may be small haemorrhages and congestion of lymph nodes and petechiation of the kidney cortex. Where nervous involvement has occurred, there may be congestion of the meninges and excess cerebrospinal fluid may be present. Congestion of the nasal mucosa with necrotic foci and pulmonary oedema are common. Necrotic foci on the tonsil are a common finding and give it a "speckled" or white appearance. In the pneumonic form, large areas of the apical and cardiac lobes of the lung were consolidated and dark red with oedema of the interlobular septa. Necrotic foci in liver and small intestine may also occur. Lesions in boars include changes in the seminiferous tubules of the testis and local lesions in the prepuce and penis. Aborted foetuses may have scattered 2-3 mm yellow-white necrotic foci in liver, spleen and lung. The placenta is often grossly normal, but necrotic lesions may be present. There may be mild endometritis and the wall of the uterus may be thickened and oedematous..

Histological findings

The major histological lesions occur in the C.N.S. and consist of a diffuse, non-suppurative meningoencephalitis which is most intense in the cerebral and cerebellar cortices. Neuronal necrosis, glial cell degeneration and lymphocytic accumulation occur about the blood vessels. Intranuclear inclusion bodies of the Cowdry Type A variety are rarely found in nervous tissue, but may be present in necrotic areas in tongue, muscle, adrenal or tonsil. Widespread necrosis with necrotising bronchitis, bronchiolitis and alveolitis and the exudation of fibrin were found in the pneumonic variant. In one study, infected cells in pulmonary necrotic foci were characterised by a thickened nuclear membrane and an amphophilic ground-glass appearance to the nucleus. Lymphoid hyperplasia, haemorrhages and intranuclear inclusions may be found in lymph nodes. In aborted foetuses, foci of coagulation necrosis may be seen in the liver and spleen. Inclusion bodies may be present in cells at the edges of the lesion. Necrotic lesions may also be found in the placenta and inclusion bodies may be seen.

Epidemiology

The disease is important in densely-stocked areas, particularly where rapid expansion of the pig population and unrestricted movement occurs between herds. Such conditions have occurred in Belgium, France, the Netherlands, Singapore and parts of the United States. The widespread use of vaccination in many countries has made the epidemiology of the disease difficult to monitor by conventional means and the presence of infection with wild type virus can only be followed where the vaccine types used can be complemented by an appropriate ELISA system e.g., Gi, TK deleted vaccine and gl ELISA.

Spread within a herd occurs by direct oronasal contact with affected animals, carriers or those shedding virus from reactivated latent infections, at service or during artificial insemination and by vertical transmission. Infected pigs produce large quantities of virus in nasal secretions and where these exceed 10^3 TCD50/100mg mucus, aerosols are generated and spread the virus within the unit. Indirect spread within the unit may be by aerosol, by survival on concrete, clothing, soil, in slurry, in flies and other animal species such as birds (pigeons) mice, rats and sheep.

Spread within a unit depends upon its immune status and the nature of the introduction. Single serological reactors may not spread the virus, but those with latent infections often do (3/4 in one study). Widespread clinical disease may be followed by little or no disease for 2-3 years. Active disease may be restricted to a particular house or age group (e.g. finishers) and infection may die out in herds with fewer than 200 sows. Risk factor analysis suggests that high herd sizes, breeder-finisher units, indoor housing and density of the pig population all predispose to transmission and that low age at weaning, all-in-all-out housing reduce it.

Spread between units or areas, or after depopulation may, in order of importance, be by -

1) the introduction of carrier pigs - shedding virus for 7-14 days after clinical recovery or latently-infected for up to 170 days (exceptionally to 19 months)

2) in travelling boars and semen from affected animals. Unwashed embryos have caused seroconversion in recipient sows.

3) aerosol for short distances of up to 2 km. Distances of 17 km overland and 60-70 km over water have been recorded (maximum halflife of 43 minutes at 4^oC and 55% relative humidity).

4) rapidly lose infectivity at 25^oC (but in fomites which infection persists on clothing, feed, straw and in faeces for 2-4 days at 25^oC, longer at 4^oC, long enough to allow transmission between units.

5) in vectors such as rodents (rats and mice) carnivores such as cats, dogs and foxes, sheep and cattle which cannot infect others of their species but may infect pigs, birds such as pigeons and flies which may carry the virus for up to 6 hours at 20^oC.

6) in buildings which may remain infective for 4-7 weeks. Infection persists in animals (see above) on soil, fixtures and fittings, feed, straw, in slurry for 3-4 weeks and, potentially in the carcases of dead animals in cold conditions.

7) in meat products. This is unlikely as the virus dies out within 35 days even when frozen at -18^oC and does not survive processing for swill or meat and bone meal.

Risk to man. Transient seroconversions have been recorded but virus has not been re-isolated.

Diagnosis

Abortion, neonatal deaths, nervous signs in piglets and coughing and listlessness in finishing pigs spreading through a non-immune herd should suggest Aujeszky's Disease. Clinical signs may be slight or undetectable in vaccinated, partially immune herds or those with breeding herds or finishers only. Pruritis and death may occur in other species in contact may be of value. Pruritis in other species in contact may be of value in reaching a diagnosis in pigs and death in farm cats and dogs is a common early sign. Gross pathological findings may be of little use in diagnosis but the presence of necrotic tonsils or a necrotic nasal septum and turbinates may indicate

Aujeszky's disease. The presence of the characteristic intranuclear inclusion bodies is diagnostic, but they may be found in histological sections of less than half the field cases examined. Laboratory confirmation may be obtained using a fluorescent antibody test to detect the presence of virus in the tonsil, olfactory bulb or pons. Tissue should be frozen. Virus can be demonstrated in tissue using immunoperoxidase with monoclonal antibodies directed against antigens present in wild type and/or vaccine viruses. DNA probes directed against individual genes may also be used in fixed tissue or tissue samples such as nasal swabs, brain or tonsil.

Virus can be isolated from the brain, spleen and lung of acutely-affected pigs. Material should be refrigerated or frozen at -70°C. Virus isolates may be subjected to gene probes or restriction endonuclease fragment analysis and this information may be used to confirm whether an isolate is wild or vaccine type and may be of value in deciding its origin.

Serological testing is the most widely used method of identifying infected herds or recovered animals. Virus neutralisation, complement fixation and gel diffusion tests may be used from antibody from vaccination with gl deletion mutants. Commercial ELISA kits are available for use with most recombinant or deletion vaccines. Significant levels of antibody are determined for each test using positive and negative control sera.

Control

No treatment is possible at present. In some countries, prophylactic administration of hyper-immune serum may be given to piglets less than 4 weeks old.

Vaccination

Killed whole virus vaccines

A number of adjuvanted killed virus vaccines have been produced and are widely available in many parts of the world. They may be prepared from wild type virus or from gene-deleted virus. Oil adjuvanted vaccines are intended for sows and may give protection for a year to the sow and to her litters for up to 9-10 weeks. A double infection 4 weeks apart may be necessary for initial immunisation. Finishing pigs may be vaccinated using alum adjuvanted vaccines.

Subunit vaccines

Subunit vaccines have been shown to be effective experimentally and in the field. They have been prepared from viral envelopes from both wild type and gl-deleted virus. Recombinant gl, gll, glll and gp50 subunit vaccines have all been prepared. New adjuvants such as ISCOMS have been used.

Live vaccines

The original live vaccines were produced by attenuation in tissue culture or other host species and have been widely used (by Bartha K61). Some of these had the gene deletions subsequently engineered into wild type virus. More recently, a series of gene-deleted mutants have been produced. Thymidine kinase (TK) and glycoprotein 1 (gl) deletion mutants have been used and a number of other combinations (TK⁻gIII⁻, TK⁻, gI, gIII) have been described. Some live vaccines have been found to be more effective if emulsified in oil. Live vaccines may be given parenterally or intranasally.

Recombinant vectored vaccines

Vaccinia virus recombinants expressing gp50, gII and gIII alone or together have been prepared and shown to be effective in pigs. Adenoviruses incorporating gp50 have also been prepared. Neither type of vaccine is yet available commercially.

Vaccination is an effective means of protecting a herd against the economic consequences of Aujeszky's Disease infection. All vaccines are considered to be effective if they prevent reduction in weight gain in the face of challenge with wild type virus. Few, if any, vaccines prevent the colonisation of the nasal mucosa and the development of latent infections by wild type virus, but they reduce the period of viral shedding and its level, and have a similar effect on reactivated latent infections.

All vaccines and natural infection in the sow give rise to maternal immunity in the piglet. This maternal immunity lasts for a variable length of time, from 9-10 weeks and sometimes longer. Its presence in neonates, sucking piglets and weaners may interfere with vaccination and live vaccines may have to be given in 3 successive occasions in order to ensure that protective immunity of weaned animals lasts until slaughter. Killed adjuvanted vaccines can often overcome this.

Serum profiling

Serum antibody levels can be plotted against age in a farm or within a single building in order to identify the most economic point for administering vaccine. A single dose of live vaccine administered when maternal antibody has disappeared and prior to the rise in active antibody, may be sufficient for control. Serum profiling should be repeated annually.

Recombination

Live virus vaccines may recombine with others or with wild type virus and revert. Genes from other herpesviruses may be incorporated.

Distinction between vaccinal virus infection and wild type virus infection

ELISAs prepared with antigens missing from the vaccine in use can detect antibody to wild type virus and the two types of virus may be distinguished in tissue or in culture by the use of probes, PCR or restriction endonuclease fragment length polymorphism (RFLP). Reagents may be chosen with regard to the deletions present in the vaccine used in a herd or region.

(a) The Slaughter of positive herds and repopulation. This expensive option was used in Great Britain and, subsequently in Denmark. In Great Britain, the disease the disease was made notifiable under the Aujeszky's Disease Order 1979 and the movement of affected pigs controlled under the Aujeszky's Disease of Swine Order 1982. A producer funded eradication campaign began in March 1983 and was substantially complete by September 1983 with 447 herds slaughtered and compensation paid. The campaign was carried out in stages: Phase 1, herds positive between May 1982 and March 1983, Phase 2, those positive between August 1979 and May 1982 and, finally, Phase 3, those prior to August 1979. Infected herds were slaughtered and normal animals sent for human consumption. Movement and neighbourhood tracing and 2 km (or later, 5 km) patrols examined nearby farms. A national serum survey and a survey of culled sow sera has continued and was extended to boars in 1988. 470 herds were slaughtered in the first year (to March 1984). Subsequently herds with 10+ reactors or active infection were slaughtered, but where less than 10 reactors were found with no subsequent transmission only the reactors were slaughtered.

Seven infected herds were identified in 1989 and slaughter or partial slaughter was carried out. Since that time Great Britain has remained free from Aujszky's Disease. A total of 523 herds was found to be infected, of which 82 were treated by removal of reactors and the remainder slaughtered completely. 440,190 pigs were slaughtered and the whole exercise cost £37,490,000 at contemporary prices.

In Denmark the disease has reappeared as a result of aerosol spread from Schleswig Holstein. The risk of further recrudescence has been reduced by vaccination in the border zone.

b)   Test and removal.   On a limited basis, the removal of all pigs which are seropositive from a herd has been shown to reduce the incidence of seroconversion and clinical disease and some serologically negative herds have resulted.

Danish, British and US results suggest that this approach may work.

c)   Isolation.   Isolation of herds appears to be a satisfactory method of control although spread by aerosol or vectors may occur. In infected small herds (50 sows or less) the disease may die out once isolation is practised. It is unlikely to be successful in herds of 200 sows.

d)   All-in, all-out husbandry. This technique may prevent infection if piglets are weaned at 10-20 days and reared in isolation (contrary to legal commitments to UK welfare codes). This is particularly useful for the reduction of disease in finishing pigs.

e)   Early weaning to different sites. An elaborate form of d) has been introduced to supplement early weaning.

f)   Vaccination alone. Northern Ireland, US, French and Belgian experience suggests that herds may become seronegative after continued vaccination. This does not occur in every case and does not appear to apply to herds with more than 200 sows. U.S. experience suggests that vaccination in the early stages of an outbreak, coupled with the removal of clinically-affected pigs, may succeed.

g)   Vaccination with serological testing and removal of pigs infected by wild virus can eliminate infection and is in use in a number of European countries and the US. This policy depends upon the widespread use of a single gene deleted vaccine in an area and the use of complementary

ELISAs for wild type antigens such as gl when gl deleted vaccines are in use. Pigs with wild type virus are removed.

h) Vaccination and hysterectomy. Successful eradication from infected herds has been reported following the production of piglets by caesarian, hysterectomy or even snatching from vaccinated sows and rearing on separate premises.

i) Washing embryos. Genetic transfer may be carried out from infected herds by washing harvested embryos to remove any adsorbed virus.

Supportive measures

The success of all these measures presupposes a supply of clean breeding stock for repopulation (such as the nucleus herds of the UK breeding companies in the 1980s) and the removal of infection by disinfecting buildings and slurry (by adding lime at 30 kg per m^3 of slurry to give a pH of 11.5). The entry of pigs should be controlled and quarantine practised. Entry of potentially infected personnel of vehicles should be prevented and clean units should be sited outside the range of aerosol transmission of the virus if at all possible.
Some killed virus vaccines are made from gene deleted vaccines.

References

'Aujeszky's Disease' A seminar in the Animal Pathology Series of the E.E.C. Programme of Co-ordination of Agricultural Research held at Tubingen, Federal Republic of Germany, June 9-10, 1981. Eds. Wittman, G. and Hall, S.A., Martinus Nijhoff the Hague Netherlands (1982).

Banks, M. and Cartwright, S. (1983). Vet. Rec. 113, 38-41. Comparison and evaluation of four serological tests for detection of antibodies to Aujeszky's Disease virus.

Banks, M. (1993). Br.Vet.J. 149, 155-163. DNA restriction fragment length polymorphism among British isolates of Aujeszky's Disease Virus: use of the PCR to discriminate amongst strains.

Basinger, D. (1990). Pig Vet J. 24, 102-121. The politico-economic aspects of Aujeszky's Disease control in Great Britain from 1955-1989.

Beran, G.W. (1993). Vet.Med. 88, 70-79. Understanding the transmission of pseudorabies virus (Aujeszky's virus).

Botner, A. (1991). Vet.Microbiol. 29, 225-235. Survival of Aujeszky's Disease virus in slurry at various temperatures.

Bourgueil, E. et al. (1992). Res.Vet.Sci. 52, 182-186. Air sampling procedures for evaluation of viral excetion level by vaccinated pigs infected with Aujeszky's Disease (pseudorabies) virus.

Brown, T.T. (1981). Am.J.Vet.Res. 41, 1033. Laboratory evaluation of selected disinfectants as virucidal agents against porcine parvovirus, pseudorabies virus and transmissible gastroenteritis virus.

Christensen, L.S. et al. (1990) Vet. Rec. 127, 471-474. Evidence of long-distance airborne transmission of Aujeszky's Disease (pseudorabies) virus.

Christensen, L.S. (1988). Arch.Virol. 102, 39-47. Comparison by restriction fragment pattern analysis and molecular characterisation of some European isolates of Suid herpesvirus I : a contribution to strain differentiation of European isolates.

73

Donaldson, A.I., Wardley, R.C., Martin, S. and Harkeness, J.W. (1984). Vet. Rec. 115, 121-124. Influence of vaccination on Aujeszkys Disease: virus and disease transmission. in Yorkshire 1981-82: the possibility of airborne disease spread.

Gloster, J., Donaldson, A.I. and Hough, M.N. (1984). Veterinary Record 114, 234-239. Analysis of a series of outbreaks of Aujeszky's Disease.

Harris, D.L. (1992). Veterinary Medicine 87, 166-170. Producing pseudorabies-free swine breeding stock from an infected herd.

Henderson, L.M., Levings, R.L., Davis, A.J., Sturtz, D.R. (1991). Am.J.Vet.Res. 52, 820-825. Recombination of pseudorabies virus vaccine strains.

Hoblet, K.H., Millr, G.Y., Barkter, N.G. (1987). J.Am.Vet.Med.Assn. 190, 405-409. Economic assessment of a pseudorabies epizootic breeding herd removal/repopulation and downtime in a commercial swine herd.

Kit, S. (1990). Vaccine 8, 420-424. Genetically engineered vaccines for the control of Aujeszky's Disease (Pseudorabies).

McCullough, S.J. and Todd, D. (1988). Vet.Rec. 122, 77-81. Subclinical Aujeszky's disease virus infection a a pig herd and characterisation of the strain of virus isolated.

Maes, R.K., Kanits, C.L., Gustafson, D. (1983). Am.J.Vet.Res. 44, 2083-2086. Shedding patterns in swine of virulent and attenuated pseudorabies virus.

Martin, S., Wardley, R.C. (1987). Res.Vet.Sci. 42, 170-174. Local humoral and cellular responses in Aujeszky's disease virus infections in pigs

Mengeling, W.L. (1989). Am.J.Vet.Res. 50, 1658-1664. Latent infection and subsequent activation of pseudorabies virus in swine exposed to pseudorabies virus while nursing immune dams.

Mellencamp, M.W., Pfeiffer, N.E., Sutter, B.T., Harness, J.R., Beckenhauter, W.H. (1989). J.Clin.Micro. 27, 2208-2213. Identification of pseudorabies virus-exposed swine with a gl glycoprotein enzyme-linked immunosorbent assay.

Miry, C., Pensaert, M.B. (1989). Am.J.Vet.Res. 50, 345-348. Sites of virus replication in the genital organs of boars inoculated in the vacum vaginale with pseudorabies virus.

Oirschot, J.T. van. (Ed.) (1988). Vaccination and Control of Aujeszky's Disease, Dordrecht Netherlands, Kleaver Academic Publishers.

Oirschot, J.T. van., Waal, C.A.H. de., (1987). Vet.Rec. 121, 305-306. An ELISA to distinguish between Aujeszky's disease vaccinated and infected pigs.

Oirschot, J.T. van, Wismuller, J.M., Waal, C.A.H. de., Lith, P.M. van. (1990). Vet.Rec. 126, 159-163. A novel concept for the control of Aujeszky's Disease: experiences in two vaccinated pig herds.

Paul, S., Mengeling, W.L., and Pirtle, E.E. (1982). Arch.Virol. 73, 193-198. Differentiation of pseudorabies (Aujeszky's disease) virus by restriction endonuclease analysis.

Riviere, M.et al., 1992). J.Virol. 66, 3424-3434. Protection of mice and swine from pseudorabies virus conferred by vaccinia virus based recombinants.

Rziha, H.J., Mittenleiter, T.C., Ohlinger, V., Wittmann, G. (1986). Virology 155, 600-613. Herpesvirus (pseudorabies virus) latency in swine: occurrence and physical state of viral DNA in neural tissues.

Schoenbaum, M.A., Beran, G.W., Murphy, D.P. (1990). Am.J.Vet.Res. 51, 334-338. Pseudorabies virus latency and reactivation in vaccinated swine.

Wittmann, G., Ohlinger, V. and Rziha, H.J. (1983). Arch.Virol. 75, 29-41. Occurrence and reactivation of latent Aujeszky's disease virus following challenge in previously vaccinated pigs.

Zimmerman, J.J., Hallam, J.A., Beran, G.W. (1989). Preventive Vet.Med. 7, 187-189. The cost of eradicating pseudorabies from swine herds in Iowa.

Classical Swine Fever (Hog Cholera)

Definition

Classical Swine Fever (CSF) or Hog Cholera (HC) is a highly contagious viral disease of pigs characterised clinically by rapid spread, fever, high morbidity and mortality in a susceptible herd and by characteristic haemorrhagic lesions at post mortem.

Incidence

Swine fever is a notifiable disease in the EC, US, Canada, Australia and many other areas of the world. It was eradicated from Britain in 1966. Three outbreaks of swine fever occurred in Britain in 1971 on farms near Hull on which pig swill was fed and 3 primary outbreaks in 1986 led to a total of 10 infected herds and 7 with antibodies. A further outbreak occurred in 1987. The United States, Canada, Australia and Scandinavian countries such as Norway, Sweden and Finland are free from the disease. The EC countries are officially free from the disease but outbreaks have occurred in several countries in recent years. Denmark, Ireland, Portugal, Greece and UK, but Germany has suffered many outbreaks, 99 (1993) 87 (9/1994) and Belgium 7, (1993), 45 (9/1994), France 1 (1993 0 (9/1994), Italy 12 (1993), 12 (9/1994), The Netherlands 5 (1992) and Spain have all suffered small numbers of outbreaks.

Aetiology

Swine fever is caused by an ether-sensitive RNA virus belonging to the Pestivirus subgroup of the Flavoviridae. The virus varies in size but is mostly 40-50 nm in diameter with a 29 nm cubic nucleocapsid and spikes 8-9 nm in length on the envelope. The RNA genome is 12 kilobases in size and has been partially sequenced. Genes for a number of proteins have been identified and cloned. Important protein constituents of the virus include envelope glycoproteins of 55 kDa (E1), 44-48 kDa and 33 kDa and a number of core proteins of 36 kDa, 23 kDa and 14 kDa. The genome can now be distinguished from those of related pestiviruses, Bovine Viral Diarrhoea Virus (BVDV) and Border Disease Virus (BDV). It multiplies in cell cultures prepared from pig tissues (including leucocyte cultures) but the vast majority of strains do so without producing C.P.E. It can persist in cell cultures.

Swine fever virus is acid resistant (pH 5) and relatively heat stable. One hour at 66°C is required for total inactivation of the virus in blood, but it survives in frozen pork for at least 1,500 days and in chilled meat and in carcases preserved by pickling, salting or smoking for 3-6 months or more. It can survive in Parma ham for 313 days.

Exposure of hams to 70°C for 1 minute and 65°C for 90 minutes eliminates virus. The bone marrow is frequently the site of persistence. In conditions where putrefaction occurs, the virus is rapidly destroyed and rarely survives for more than 2 days in faeces or infected pens at 37-65°C but may survive for 4 weeks in winter. It is rapidly destroyed by 2% sodium hydroxide, ether, chloroform or bile and at pH 3.

Swine fever virus occurs as a single major antigenic type although minor differences in antigens have been recorded. Isolates have been shown to differ in pathogenicity for pigs and to share a soluble antigen with BVDV to a varying extent. Swine fever virus can replicate in sheep and cattle although it does not produce clinical signs and BVDV can infect pregnant sows and may initiate antibody response. Swine fever virus isolates of high pig pathogenicity seem to be less closely related to BVDV than those of low pathogenicity. Border disease virus may also infect pigs.

Pathogenesis

The virus enters the body through the upper digestive tract or through the upper respiratory tract. It appears to be taken up by macrophages and reaches local lymph nodes, e.g. the tonsils and the pharyngeal and submandibular lymph nodes in which it multiplies. Twenty four hours after the initial multiplication, a transient viraemia occurs during which the virus becomes localised in the endothelial cells of the blood vessels and lymphatics. It reaches parenchymatous organs after 3-4 days. A secondary viraemia follows 5-6 days after infection as the clinical signs develop and the virus reaches its peak titre in the blood on the 7th day after infection. The pathological findings are related to the fact that the virus primarily attacks (1) the endothelial cells of small blood vessels and (2) reticuloendothelial cells. The blood vessels become occluded by proliferation of the vascular endothelium.

Virus spreads to epithelial surfaces such as salivary gland and bladder where it is shed. Infection is followed by a rise in antibody levels but may also be accompanied by widespread depletion of the lymphoid system and effects on body defences such as those of the lung and intestine. Virus may cross the placenta in pregnant sows and lead to abortion, the birth of pigs with persistent viraemia (up to 90 days) and no antibody. Foetuses infected after 65-67 days' gestation may develop antibody, be aborted or born with haemorrhagic lesions or become mummified.

Clinical signs

Acute, chronic and mild forms of swine fever occur in countries where the disease is enzootic, and, although it is thought outbreaks in swine-fever-free countries may be of the classic, acute type, outbreaks in susceptible pigs in Australia and the US have been caused by low virulence virus which has produced less striking clinical signs. The disease has an incubation period of 5-10 days (range 2-30 days) after which the following signs may be observed.

Hyperacute disease. One or two young pigs may be found dead and others may show signs of the acute type when examined.

Acute disease. Affected animals are dull, lethargic, anorexic and show fever of 40.5-41.5°C, 105-107°F at first. These signs are followed by conjunctivitis, in which the eyelids may be stuck together by exudate, and constipation followed by diarrhoea with occasional vomiting. The animals often huddle in piles in the bedding, walk reluctantly with a swaying movement of the hindquarters and may seek the support of walls or posts. Erythema and blotching of the skin and dyspnoea occur and may be present until death. Nervous signs, in particular, convulsions, occur early in the disease and are followed by circling, incoordination and ataxia. Death normally occurs within 4-8 days of infection in hyperacute cases, 9-19 days in acute cases and in some cases a chronic disease may occur in which death occurs between 30 and 95 days after onset. Emaciation, with blotching and necrosis of the ears may occur. Adult sows may abort in the acute stage of the disease, foetal resorption may occur, or weak and trembling piglets may be born.

Leucopaenia is a prominent finding and levels as low as 3-9,000/µl may be found (normal >18,000) within 2-6 days of infection.

Chronic disease. Few clinical signs may be observed. Fever may appear within 4-5 days of infection and persist accompanied by leucopaenia. Temporary recovery may be followed by death in 30-95 days. In some infected herds individual affected litters may be the only clinical signs of infection.

Low virulence virus. Infections often resemble chronic disease but may be less severe. Transient pyrexia and inappetence with no clinical signs other than leucopaenia may occur. Posterior ataxia has been recorded 4 months after birth in pigs born to sows infected with low virulence virus. There may be reproductive signs such as abortion and the birth of mummified or stillborn piglets.

Humane slaughter of affected animals should be carried out.

Pathological findings

Gross lesions

In hyperacute cases there may be no gross lesions, but in acute cases the skin may be redden may be widespread. Enlarged haemorrhagic "strawberry" lymph nodes are commonly found, in particular in those of the pharyngeal, submandibular and abdominal regions. The haemorrhage is distributed peripherally. Petechiation and ecchymoses are found in the kidney (80% of cases) as the "turkey egg" kidney (also seen in other septicaemic conditions), in the skin (50%) and in the bladder and lung (30%).

Infarction of the spleen occurs in 20% of cases and is due to thrombosis of small end-arteries in the spleen and ischaemia of the areas supplied. "Button ulcers", circular ulcers 1-2 cm in diameter with a necrotic centre are commonly found in the proximal portion of the colon but can occur elsewhere in the intestine. They result from damage to mucosal arteries with infarction distal to the occluded, damaged part and occur later in the disease.

In chronic or persistent infections, atrophy of the thymus and general lymphoid atrophy are common. Adrenal cortical hyperplasia and chronic rib lesions with a band of calcification proximal to the costochondral junction are present.

Cerebellar hypoplasia may be present in newborn trembling pigs (see Congenital Tremor Type AI).

The basic lesions are the hydropic degeneration and proliferation of the vascular endothelial cells leading to occlusion of blood vessels. A marked non-suppurative encephalitis is present in most cases.

Epidemiology

Infection takes place as a result of the ingestion of virus-contaminated feed or litter or through abrasions. Virus is present in all body secretions, especially in the urine, and close contact between infected and susceptible pigs is necessary for transmission to occur. It is present in all tissues of affected pigs and ingestion of meat or other tissues frequently results in infection. Virus may be present in semen. Animals housed in pens separated by pig-proof partitions may remain uninfected during outbreaks of the disease on a farm.

Transmission between farms is normally by:-

1. The purchase of infected pigs direct from an infected farm. A number of recent European outbreaks have resulted from the purchase of such animals.
2. Direct contact between infected and susceptible pigs at markets or in transport
3. Feeding improperly boiled swill containing infected pork products (1971 and 1986 UK outbreaks). In some cases infected meat has been fed to pigs, particularly in the 1993 outbreaks in Germany. The survival time of the virus in some meat products is given above. Recent studies with silage suggests that virus may survive for up to 5 months in meat fragments in silage and that such material is not safe until 9 months after production.
4. The purchase of infected pregnant sows. These may show low clinical signs of the disease after recovery, but the virus may cross the placenta and the resulting litter may show "trembling" or myoclonia congenita and may excrete virulent virus for up to 56 days after birth. Horizontal transmission amongst the offspring appears to result in seroconversion but not clinical disease. Low virulence virus may persist a a viraemia but does not appear to be shed under these circumstances.
5. Indirect transfer. This mechanism of spread is relatively unimportant and includes the use of contaminated vaccines, sera, semen or embryos. One recent outbreak in Belgium was traced to a veterinarian and spread in this way is always possible.
6. Spread from wild boar. Although wild pigs in Australia and the US are not infected, eradication of the disease from domesticated pig populations in Europe has revealed that wild boar are an important reservoir of infection. Infection has spread from wild boar in Germany, France and Italy. Disease has been identified in wild boar in Sardinia and Tuscany. Recent studies with monoclonal antibodies to envelope proteins have confirmed that wild boar and domestic pig isolates are similar.

Diagnosis

The clinical signs accompanied by the findings of a high fever in large numbers of pigs, and some deaths should lead to suspicion of swine fever, particularly if the herd affected is swill-fed or if animals have been recently bought it. Trembling piglets with cerebellar hypolasia must also be considered possible cases of congenital infection. If the disease is suspected, the Ministry of Agriculture should be notified immediately. Diagnosis is confirmed by:

1. Post mortem findings - the haemorrhagic lymph nodes and petechial haemorrhages in the acute form, splenic infarcts and button ulcers in more chronic cases.

2. Clinical Pathology - A white blood cell count of less than 10,000 cells/μl in affected pigs more than 5 weeks of age and affected for less than 6 days indicates swine fever. Leucopaenia is a prominent clinical pathological finding in early cases.

3. Demonstration of virus

(a)   Fluorescent antibody test.   Frozen sections of tonsil, kidney, spleen or ileum, mandibular, maxillary and mesenteric lymph nodes from animals which have been affected for between 5 and 10 days may be used for the highly specific fluorescent antibody test for the virus. Specific cytoplasmic fluorescence is considered diagnostic.

(b)   Peroxidase-linked antibo has been used in similar circumstances. Peroxidase-linked monoclonal antibodies are more sensitive and can be more specific than polyclonals.

(c)   Virus isolation may be attempted in pig kidney cells (PK 15) using spleen or leucocytes as a source of infectious material. Infected cells are identified by immunofluorescence or peroxidase-linked monoclonal antibodies at 22-72 hours post-inoculation.   The tissues listed above, and the blood in EDTA should be submitted.
Panels of monoclonal antibodies have been developed to distinguish isolates of swine fever virus from other pestiviruses isolated from pigs..

(d)   Immunoassay for antigen.   An antigen-capture ELISA for virus antigen in peripheral blood, leucocytes and spleen cells has been described.

(e)   Polymerase chain reaction. Reverse transcriptase - coupled PCR using primers for pestivirus in general and classical swine fever in particular has been described.

Monoclonal antibodies capable of distinguishing between BVDV and swine fever virus have been used for (a) and (b).

4.   Serology

Serum antibody may be detected by:

(a)   Serum neutralisation tests.   Cytopathogenic virus or non-cytopathogenic virus detected by immunofluorescence of immunoperoxidase neutralisation peroxidase-linked assay (NPLA) or the fluorescent antibody virus neutralisation test. The presence of higher titres to CSFV than to BVDV or BDV confirms that the antibody is to CSFV.

(b)   Complement fixation tests may also be used.

(c)   ELISAs. Whole virus may be used to identify antibody to CSF presumptively but monoclonal antibody blocking ELISAs or BDV ELISAs are necessary to confirm the antibody as being CSF.
A specific ELISA based on gp54 and a complex trapping blocking ELISA have also been described.

5.   Animal transmission - The final definitive test for swine fever in newly affected areas. The use of controls immunised against swine fever is of value in separating the disease from African Swine Fever.

The disease may be differentiated from acute African Swine Fever in countries where both are present by the persistent high temperature in Swine Fever (it falls prior to the clinical signs in African Swine Fever), the appearance of the disease in pigs vaccinated against swine fever and the lack of button ulcers, laryngeal haemorrhages and turkey-egg kidney in African Swine Fever. Lesions occurring in the latter but not in Swine Fever include oedema of the lung and gall bladder and massive infarction of the hepatic lymph node. Haemorrhages on the heart are more common. Laboratory tests confirm.

BVDV and BDV infections may be distinguished from classical swine fever using the tests described above.

Acute erysipelas, salmonellosis, congenital tremor and some types of abortion and foetal mummification may all lead to suspicion of swine fever.

Control

Swine fever is controlled in the EC at present by a slaughter policy in which all pigs in contact with confirmed cases are slaughtered and buried or burned on the affected farms. These are disinfected and left depopulated for a period. All markets in the affected area are closed until danger of further infection has passed and pig movements in the affected areas are strictly controlled. As a precautionary measure, all swill fed to pigs in Britain is heat treated in an attempt to prevent the re-entry of swine fever. Legislation dealing with swine fever includes the Swine Fever Order 1963 made under the Diseases of Animals Act 1950. Other orders such as the Diseases of Animals (Waste Foods) Order 1974 and the Movement and Sale of Pigs Order 1975 act to prevent the introduction and spread of Swine Fever. EC regulations to control swine fever within the Community include agreement on the diagnostic criteria to be used in the Community.

Vaccination

In countries in which the disease is enzootic, live attenuated (lapinised) virus vaccine (LPC - China virus) or the cell culture attenuated Japanese GP strain can be given either before colostrum is taken by newborn piglets or at 30-60 days of age. Vaccination should be repeated at 9 month intervals and does not eliminate infection but reduces multiplication of virus in the tonsil. Vaccine virus may be present in the semen of recently-vaccinated boars and cross the placenta. Maternal vaccinal titres may be differentiated from swine fever antibody. Antibody titres of 1:32 or less allow LPC vaccine to provide protection, those greater than 1:32 do not and animals with that level of passive immunity at vaccination later become susceptible. At 5-6 weeks 11% piglets respond to vaccine, 42% at 7-8 weeks and 77% at 10 weeks in vaccinated herds.

A vector vaccine, using vaccinia virus expressing core protein p23 and envelope proteins gp55 and gp33, has been shown to be protective.

Disinfection

An important part of the control of swine fever is disinfection between farms in enzootic areas, disinfection of implements and vehicles and disinfection of infected premises. Infected areas should be disinfected, cleaned and finally disinfected once more. The concentrations appropriate for use are given in the UK in the lists of approved disinfectants under the Diseases of Animals

(Approved Disinfectants) Order 1978 updated at intervals. Sample dilutions include phenols at 1:50-80 and Antec Farm Fluid S 1:160.

References

Dahle, J., Liess, B. (1992). Comp.Immunol.Microbiol. and Infectious Disease 15, 203-211. A review of classical swine fever infection in pigs: epizootiology, clinical disease and pathology.

Edwards, S., Moennig, V. , Wensvoort, G. (1991). Vet.Micro. 29, 101-108. The development of an international reference panel of monoclonal antibodies for the differentiation of hog cholera virus from other pestiviruses.
Harkness, J.W. (1985). Vet.Rec. 116, 288-293. Review: Classical swine fever and its diagnosis.
Le Forban, Y., Cariolet, R. (1992). Annales de Recherche Veterinaire 23, 93-100. Characterisation and pathogenicity for pigs of a hog cholera virus strain isolated from wild boars.
Liess, B. Ed. (1988). Classical Swine Fever and related viral infections. Martinus Nijhoff in the series 'Developments in Veterinary Virology.
Meyers, G., Rumenapf, T., Thiel, H.J. (1989). Virology 171, 555-567. Molecular cloning and nucleotide sequence of the genome of hog cholera.
Moennig, V. (1992). Comp.Immunol.Microbiol. and Infectious Disease 15, 189-201. The Hog Cholera Virus.
Pearson, J.E. (1992). Comp.Immunol.Microbiol. and Infectious Disease 15, 213-219. Hog cholera diagnostic techniques.
Robertson, I., Owen, J. (1994). In Practice 16, 110-128. Notifiable Diseases of Pigs.
Rumenapf, T., Stark, R., Meyers, G., Thiel, H.J. (1991). J.Virol. 65, 589-597. Structural proteins of hog cholera virus expressed by vaccinia virus: further characterisation and induction of protective immunity.
Shannon, A.D., Morrisy, C., Mackintosh, S.G., Westbury, H.A. (1993). Vet.Microbiol. 34, 232-248. Detection of hog cholera virus antigens in experimentally-infected pigs using an antigen capture ELISA.
Terpstra, C., Wensvoort, G. (1988). Res.Vet.Sci. 45, 137-142. Natural infections of pigs with Bovine Viral Diarrhoea Virus associated with signs resembling swine fever.
Wirz, B., Tratschin, J.D., Muller, H.K., Mitchell, D.B. (1993). J.Clin.Microbiol. 31, 1148-1154. Detection of hog cholera virus and differentiation from other pestiviruses by polymerase chain reaction.
Wood, L., Brockman, S., Harkness, J.W., Edwards, S. (1988). Vet.Rec. 122, 391-394. Virulence and tissue distribution of UK 1986 viruses.
Williams, D.R., Matthews, D. (1988). Vet.Rec. 122, 479-483. 1986 UK outbreak and its control.

African Swine Fever

Definition

African Swine Fever is a highly contagious often highly fatal viral disease of pigs characterised by clinical signs and gross lesions which may be difficult to distinguish from European Swine Fever. It is caused by an unrelated virus.

Incidence

African Swine Fever has never occurred in Britain and was confined to Africa until 1957 when infection spread through Portugal, Spain, Southern France and Italy. Infection persists in Spain, Portugal and Sardinia but has been eradicated from the Italian mainland, France, Belgium, Malta, Cuba, the Dominican Republic, Brazil and The Netherlands in all of which countries small numbers of outbreaks have occurred. Eighteen outbreaks were recorded in Sardinia in 1992, 83 in Spain and 2 in Portugal.

Aetiology

The African Swine Fever virus is a large ether-sensitive DNA iridovirus which is icosahedral in form, enveloped and 175-215nm in diameter. Restriction endonuclease analysis can distinguish between different field isolates and between these and tissue-culture adapted stains. Up to 37 viral proteins have been described, one of which, Vp73, may be useful as an antigen in ELISA tests but is unrelated to protection. Protein P12 is associated with adsorption to cells and antibody to it can prevent adsorption *in vitro*. The genome of the virus has been largely characterised and several genes have been sequenced, their proteins cloned and expressed in *E.coli*. There is molecular biological evidence of a relationship to pox viruses. Isolates of African swine fever virus from Africa are very variable. The variation in the DNA is reflected in antigenic differences between strains and primers for PCR have to be chosen from non-variable regions of the genome.

The virus grows in cultures of porcine bone marrow and buffy coat with the production of syncytia. In kidney cell cultures some strains produce C.P.E. preceded by haemadsorption. It has been grown in some arthropod cell lines. In the field the virus is found in pigs, multiplies in ticks and pig lice and is found in the blood of wild pigs in Africa, in particular in wart hogs. The virus is very resistant and survives conditions of putrefaction and sunlight which would destroy swine fever virus.. It can survive 2 hours at $56^{o}C$, survive for 6 months in carcases held at $4^{o}C$, for 2 years when dried at room temperature and almost indefinitely when frozen in meat at $-20^{o}C$. It is stable between pH 3 and pH 10 but is inactivated by 1% formaldehyde in 6 days and by 2% NaOH in 24 hours.

Pathogenesis

The main route of infection is via the upper respiratory tract and initial virus replication occurs within 24 hours of infection in the lymphoid tissue draining the nasal mucosa and in the pharyngeal tonsil. Viraemia follows and the virus affects the vascular endothelium and causes lymphopaenia. Thrombin clotting times increase from day 4 post-infection and thrombocytopaenia occurs from day 6 post-infection. After 4-5 days the sub-endothelial lesions involve basement membranes and death ensues due to pulmonary oedema.

Virus multiplies in monocyttes, macrophages, hepatocytes, endothelial cells and some epithelial cells throughout the body. Virus may be shed within 24 hours of the onset of fever. Surviving animals are persistently infected and viraemia persists in spite of the presence of high levels of circulating antibody. This may result in immune glomerulonephritis. Antibody may be detected first at 11 days post-infection and from that time virus levels in the plasma fall to disappear by day 46 post-infection. Haemadsorption of red cells to infected cells occurs *in vivo* and virus in the blood is adsorbed onto erythrocytes and 95% infectivity is associated with them. Reduction in levels of virus is related to the presence of antibody. Protection against re-infection appears to be related to cellular immunity which may develop within 7-10 days of infection and be antibody-dependent cell-mediated cytotoxicity (ADCC).

Clinical signs

The incubation period averages 1 week (5-15 days) and is followed by pyrexia (40-42°C, 104-108°F) for a period of 48 hours during which affected animals remain bright and continue eating. Clinical signs begin as the temperature drops and consist of dullness, anorexia, huddling together, incoordination, dyspnoea and coughing (30% of cases), skin cyanosis and occasional vomiting or diarrhoea, sometimes with serous mucopurulent or bloody ocular and nasal discharges. Death occurs within 7-10 days of the onset of clinical signs and in classic outbreaks the mortality rate is 95-100%. Chronic cases appear emaciated with lameness, swollen joints and skin ulceration. Mild forms may occur in herds or areas in which the disease is enzootic. Abortion may occur in sows in all stages of pregnancy 5-8 days after infection or 1-3 days after fever develops. A high proportion of such mildly affected animals may recover.
Affected pigs should be slaughtered humanely.

Pathological findings

Severe haemorrhages are widespread throughout the body. The lymph nodes are so haemorrhagic that they resemble pieces of spleen, the ecchymoses on serous membranes are severe and those on the epicardium may lead to haemopericardium and those on the pleura and peritoneum may stain the peritoneal and pleural effusions with blood. Haemorrhages may also be found in the myocardium, lung, liver, kidney and bladder. The gall bladder is oedematous and the hepatic lymph node is haemorrhagic even in cases of mild disease. There may be oedema of the lung. Haemorrhagic ulceration may develop in the large intestine, but button ulcers are rare and the laryngeal haemorrhages and turkey egg kidney found in swine fever are uncommon. In chronic cases, pericarditis, pleuritis, pneumonia, arthritis and cutaneous ulcers are seen. Some African isolates may only cause petechiation of the kidney and visceral lymph nodes with an increase in abdominal fluid. Aborted foetuses have ecchymotic placental and petechial cutaneous haemorrhages.
Histological findings include congestion, lymphoid infiltration of the letptomeninges of the brain and nuclear changes in lymphocytes in all tissues. There is thickening of blood vessels and severe damage to vascular endothelium with perivascular haemorrhages. A fall in the number of lymphocytes is common. The use of peroxidase-linked monoclonal antibodies to the virus or its subunits can demonstrate virus in phagocytes, hepatocytes, endothelial cells and some epithelia throughout the body.

Epizootiology

Infected pigs have a persistent viraemia and the virus is present in all body fluids, secretions and excretions. Virus is shed for 7-10 days after the onset of fever, can form aerosols but is present in greatest amounts in faeces. It persists in blood for up to 8 weeks and in lymphoid tissues for 12 weeks or more and has been recorded for up to 21 weeks. Animals which have recovered are immune to challenge with homologous virus but can succumb to other strains of virus. Maternal immunity may protect for up to 7 weeks.

Transmission in Europe is by the following routes in order of importance:

a)   direct contact with pigs excreting virus
b)   the ingestion of infected meat products (often improperly cooked swill)
c)   the bites of biological vectors such as *Ornithodoros erraticus* (Iberia) and *O.moubata* (Africa). Ticks may remain infective in disused piggeries for 5 years
d)   the bites of mechanical vectors such as biting flies, lice etc.
e)   parenteral inoculation which allows infection from low titres of virus.

In Africa the infection is derived from carrier wart hogs which are the source of infection for ticks. The disease persists on infected premised for long periods of time. Where the disease has become enzootic in Southern Europe, the clinical signs are less dramatic and chronic infection may occur so that carrier pigs are important in the spread of the disease. Onward transmission from recovered animals is not inevitable as many antibody-positive animals are virus-negative. Wild boar are infected in Sardinia, and in 1990 1.5% of wild boar sampled were seropositive. The relationship between infected ticks, boar and domestic pigs is not clear in some areas. In the Caribbean outbreaks, spread within a farm was slow and from pen to pen. Adjacent buildings were unaffected for a long period. The virus is introduced to countries in pig products and then spread by the methods noted above. In Belgium (1985) spread by fomites was particularly important.

Diagnosis

African Swine Fever should be suspected where a highly infectious syndrome causes 95-100% mortality in pigs of all ages with clinical signs resembling those of swine fever. A point of difference is the fall in temperature before the onset of clinical signs. Mild forms of the disease may be more difficult to diagnose. At post-mortem findings of multiple haemorrhages, petechiated kidneys, haemorrhagic lymph nodes (especially the hepatic, in chronic or wild cases) and splenic infarcts also suggest one of the swine fevers. Laboratory confirmation should always be sought. The actual techniques used are to be found in the current O.I.E. handbook, but material for investigation should include clotted blood and blood in EDTA, lymph node, kidney, spleen and lung. In abortion from African Swine Fever, infection is more easily demonstrable in the sow rather than the foetus. Placenta is best in the products of abortion for diagnosis.

The tests used are as follows:

a)   Demonstration of antibody in tissue or body fluids. Classically by indirect immunofluorescence on infected tissue culture monolayers, immunoperoxidase can improve results. ELISAs have been described using whole virus or p73 (recombinant or tissue-culture-derived) as antigen. Other tests such as complement fixation, immunoblotting, radioimmunoassay, radio-immune-precipitation have all been used.

b)   Demonstration of virus in tissue. Classically by immunofluorescence on frozen tissue sections, immunoperoxidase may be of equal value. ELISA using monoclonal antibody may also be used but may be of reduced value where antibody complexes mask antigen. Electron microscopy may reveal virus on red cells or macrophages The polymerase chain reaction (PCR) has been used with primers from non-variable regions on extracts from tissue and body fluids and can detect 10 pg of virus. It does not require live virus.

c)　Virus isolation in cultures of buffy coat leucocytes or macrophages. Cytopathic effects may be seen, but the presence of virus is usually demonstrated primarily by the haemadsorption test in which infected cells are ringed by erythrocytes. The presence of virus can be confirmed by ELISA, neutralisation, PCR, immunofluorescence, immunoperoxidase or gel diffusion, immunoblot etc.

d)　Animal transmission. The ultimate confirmation, especially of new introductions and to distinguish it from classical swine fever.

Carrier pigs may be identified by serological tests. these include a commercial ELISA or indirect tests using infected monolayers and fluorescent antibody to pig immunoglobulins. Monoclonal antibodies can be used to detect IgM or IgG antibody. Immunoelectrophoresis and immunoradial diffusion can also be used

Control

African Swine Fever is currently controlled by restrictions on movement of pigs or meat from infected areas. In all EC countries and most American countries it is a notifiable disease (1980, UK). Measures such as the boiling of swill and the prohibition of the import of infected pigs or meat have safeguarded the UK but infected meat has caused outbreaks in Belgium and The Netherlands. The recent (1989) EC decision to allow the export of meat from areas of Spain other than Estremadura, has confirmed that country's claims to general freedom from disease. Outbreaks of the disease outside the enzootic areas have been controlled by slaughter of all pigs on the infected farm and any farms in direct contact. Affected farms have been disinfected and sentinel pigs introduced prior to restocking depopulated farms. Movement has been prohibited in the surrounding areas.

Disinfectants with specific claims for use in ASF outbreaks include Farm Fluid S (1:160) and Virkon S (1:100); Antec International. In enzootic areas, education, restriction of animal movement and prompt and generous compensation have reduced the levels of disease to low levels.

References

Beeker, Y. (Ed.) (1987) . African Swine Fever, Martinus Nyhoff Publishers. Developments in Veterinary Virology series.

Biront, P., Castryck, F., Leunen, J. (1987). Vet.Rec. 120, 432-434. An epizootic of African Swine Fever in Belgium and its eradication.

Galo, A. (1993). Agriculture: Coordination of Agricultural Research, African Swine Fever: Proceedings of a workshop of agricultural research, Lisbon, Portugal 7, 8, 9 October 1991. Luxembourg, Commission of the EC.

McVicar, J.W. (1984). Am.J.Vet.Res. 45, 1535-1541. Quantitative aspects of transmission of African swine fever virus.

Oleaga-Perez, A., Perez-Sanchez, R., Encinas-Grandes, A. (1990). Vet.Rec. 126, 32-37. Distribution and biology of *Ornithodoros erraticus* in parts of Spain affected by African swine fever.

Pastor, M.J., Arias, M., Escribiano, J.M. (1990). Am.J.Vet.Res. 51, 1540-1543. Comparison of two antigens for use in an ELISA to detect African swine fever antibodies.

Petit, F., Boucraut-Baralon, C., Py, R., Benazet, F., Picavet, D.P., Chantal, J. (1991). Annales de Recherche Veterinaire 22, 201-209. Detection of African swine fever virus by a biotinylated DNA probe: assay on cell cultures and field samples.

Schlafer, D.H., McVicar, J.W., Mebus, C.A. (1984). Am.J.Vet.Res. 45, 1361-1366. African swine fever convalescent sows: subsequent pregnancy and the effect of colostral antibody on challenge inoculation of their pigs.

Schlafer, D.H., Mebus, C.A. (1984). Am.J.Vet.Res. 45, 1353-1360. Abortion in sows experimentally-infected with African swine fever virus: clinical features.

Schlafer, D.H., Mebus, C.A. (1987). Am.J.Vet.Res. 48, 246-254. Abortion in sows experimentally-infected with African swine fever virus: pathogenesis studies.

Schlafer, D.H., Mebus, C.A., McVicar, J.W. (1984). Am.J.Vet.Res. 45, 1367-1372. African swine fever in neonatal pigs: passively acquired protection from colostrum or serum of recovered pigs.

Steiger, Y., Ackerman, M., Mettraux, C., Kihm, M. (1992). J.Clin.Microbiol. 30, 1-8. Rapid and biologically safe diagnosis of African swine fever using polymerase chain reaction.

Robertson, I., Owen, J. (1994). In Practice 16, 110-128. Notifiable Diseases of Pigs.

Wardley, R.C., Norley, S.G., Wilkinson, P.J., Williams, S. (1985). Vet.Immunology and Immunopathology 9, 201-212. The role of antibody in protection against African swine fever virus.

Wilkinson, P.J. (1980). Pig News and Information 1, 17-20.

Wilkinson, P.J. (Ed.) (1983). African Swine Fever: Proceedings of an EC Seminar, Sardinia 1981. Eur 8466.

Swine Vesicular Disease

Definition

Swine vesicular disease is an infectious disease of pigs clinically indistinguishable from foot and mouth disease and is caused by an enterovirus.

Incidence

A vesicular disease of pigs was first observed in Italy in 1966 and then in Hong Kong in 1971. In December 1972, an outbreak occurred in swill-fed pigs in Staffordshire and was thought to be Foot-and-Mouth disease. Similar outbreaks also occurred in Poland, Austria, France and Italy within a few weeks of each other. The disease in Britain was shown to be caused by a virus distinct from that of foot and mouth disease and related to those previously identified from Hong Kong, Italy and elsewhere in Europe on the basis of serum neutralisation tests. It is distinct from the viruses of vesicular stomatitis and vesicular exanthema. It occurred sporadically in Britain, particularly in Humberside, from

1979-82. It has recently occurred in several EC countries. In 1992 outbreaks were identified in Belgium (1), Italy (31) and The Netherlands (6), the source of some pigs affected in Italy. In 1993 it was present in Belgium (1), Italy (8) and Spain (3).

Aetiology

The disease is caused by a picornavirus 30-32 nm in size (as opposed to 24-25 nm for that of Foot-and-Mouth Disease. The virus is fatal to newborn mice, a character of the Coxsackie group of enteroviruses and it appears to be related to the human strain Coxsackie B5 on the basis of virus neutralisation tests and the nucleotide sequences of the 3 capsid genes. Its genome is closely (90%) related to that of coxsackie viruses B1, B3, B4, B5, A9 and A16 and it is regarded by some as a porcine coxsackie virus.

The virus has been named Porcine Enterovirus England/72. Swine vesicular disease virus is stable at pH 5 and more resistant to acid and alkaline conditions than F.M.D. virus. A pH below 2.5 or above 12.5 is necessary to destroy the virus. It is destroyed by moist heat at 60°C within 30 minutes, of 9°C for 15 minutes, but in cool, humid conditions it can persist for more than 4 months and it survives indefinitely in infected refrigerated pig tissues. A number of antigenic types (5 at present) have been identified using polyacrylamide gel electrophoresis. The 1979 strain, UK 1/79, differed from those found here previously and from those present at that time in Europe.

Pathogenesis

The exposure of susceptible pigs to infected animals results in infection through the tonsil in 90% of cases. Virus may also enter through the skin of the head, tongue and especially the foot, and also through the gut. It then multiplies in the draining lymph node and subsequently gives rise to a viraemia which results in the clinical signs. The gastrointestinal tract may be exposed to $10^{7.5}$ particles without the occurrence of infection but the dose required to infect the coronary band is only $10^{3.6}$ viable virus particles. Infections from swill may, therefore, take place through the skin. There is field but little experimental evidence for transplacental infection. Neutralising antibody can be detected 7 days after infection and peaks at 28 days post-infection.

Clinical signs

The disease in the field is indistinguishable from foot and mouth disease in pigs but does not affect sheep or cattle although the virus may be present in these animals.

The development of lesions is accompanied by fever (40-41°C, 104-106°F) and by 1 or 2 days' inappetence. Lameness or tenderness of the feet is apparent and affected pigs may be disinclined to move and may arch their backs or group their feet beneath themselves. In severe cases, they may scream or walk on their knees, although the lesions are said to be less painful than those of F.M.D.

The lesions first appear as blanched areas of skin or epithelium which develop into vesicles within 2-4 hours and then rupture a few hours later to leave clean ulcers with, at first, a ragged periphery. Healing by granulation may be complete within 4 days. The incubation period varies with the weight of infection but is usually 2-4 days for local, primary lesions, 56 days after viraemia and 7-11 days after ingestion.

The lesions are most commonly found on the coronary band of the feet and the supernumerary digits but also extend into the inter-digital space. Under-running of the horn and sloughing of the claw may occur. Vesicles also occur on the skin of the limbs, the mammary glands and in about 5% of animals, on the snout and in the mouth, especially on the dorsum of the tongue. In many cases, especially in sows, the lesions may be mild and may pass unnoticed until later cases have been traced.

In some outbreaks, nervous signs have been recorded. They include head-pressing and disturbances of gait and may result in death following convulsions. From 25-70% of pigs may be affected, mainly those over 3 months of age. Mild cases occur and there is little mortality except when CNS involvement occurs. Some animals show no clinical signs but develop neutralising antibody.

The humane endpoint is when severe lameness is accompanied by loss of digital horn and when nervous signs lead to paralysis or convulsion.

Epidemiology

The incubation period is 3-7 days and virus may be shed as early as the second day after infection and shedding usually ceases 8-15 days after the appearance of the lesions. Subclinically-infected pigs can transmit the disease to others after mixing; virus is excreted in the faeces. No carrier state has yet been identified. Virus is shed in vesicular fluid and spread on the farm appears to be largely by pig-pig contact.

The ability of the virus to survive in pig faeces (138 days in moist faeces stored between 12 and 17°C) means that environmental contamination may be a significant cause of the persistence of disease on premises and is important in the spread of the disease by lorries and by human carriage (on clothing, footwear, etc.). The 5 primary outbreaks appeared in pigs fed swill containing pork products of foreign origin and the secondary outbreaks appear to have resulted from direct movement of pigs from infecting premises, movement through markets (including contact infections) and infection through lorries. Swill-fed pigs have proved to be responsible for many outbreaks. At first, disinfection measures were inadequate and some recrudescence of infection occurred.

Examination of sera from slaughter pigs for antibodies to S.V.D. in 1974 showed that there was no widespread undisclosed disease in the most heavily infected areas, Lancashire and Yorkshire, although one farm was found to have evidence of active infection and significant antibody levels were found on 3 others out of 369 surveyed. Serological surveys in EC countries such as The Netherlands show that antibody is not present in the general pig population although the situation in Italy is less clear.

Diagnosis

The clinical signs only allow a diagnosis of a vesicular condition to be made unless the case is linked to a confirmed outbreak of S.V.D. Laboratory tests carried out at Pirbright in confirmation include complement fixation tests, virus isolation and, in long-standing cases, serum virus neutralisation tests and double immunodiffusion tests. Recent studies suggest that, although the serum neutralisation test is most accurate, counter-immunoelectrophoresis tests can used and ELISA tests are most useful for widespread screening and distinction between Foot-and-Mouth and S.V.D. A liquid phase blocking sandwich ELISA has recently shown to be comparable to viral neutralisation. False positives in some ELISAs may result from antibody to other enteroviruses and neutralisation tests may be necessary to confirm their identity.

Control

Swine Vesicular Disease is controlled under the Swine Vesicular Disease Order 1972 which resembles the F.M.D. Orders, but only apply to pigs. The Diseases of Animals (Waste Foods) Order 1974 made the installation of adequate swill treatment mandatory for swill feeders. In consequence, the number of licensed swill feeders dropped from 4,300 to fewer than 1,000, a major step in the control of the disease. Movement of pigs is controlled under the Movement and Sale of Pigs Order 1975. This order slows down pig movement which can only be made under local authority licence except for pigs going direct to slaughter from premises where no swill is fed. Swill-fed pigs must be licensed and can only move to a slaughter house.

Pigs going to market or other farms must be licensed and come from farms on to which no pigs have been moved within the preceding 21 days and be free from notifiable disease. Markets for pigs of 21 day status and those for slaughter pigs cannot be held on the same premises. Strict rules for disinfection of lorries and premises are in force.

Clinically affected pigs must be reported and are slaughtered under the S.V.D. Order 1972. Disinfection with 1% sodium hydroxide and flame guns is carried out, although certain other disinfectants, e.g. iodophors may be used. A full list is given in the Disease of Animals (approved disinfectants) Order 1978.

In spite of apparent eradication, the disease reappeared in Autumn 1976, Winter 1977 in 5 swill-fed herds and a reservoir of infection may have existed in frozen pork. The origin of the 1979 outbreak was not clear, particularly in view of the different antigenic nature of the virus. There were only 14 outbreaks of swine vesicular disease in 1982 and no evidence of infection has been found since in spite of widespread serum surveys. Recent studies of Group III enteroviruses which are epitheliotropic suggest that they could cause vesicular diseases.

References

Anon., Vet. Rec. (1973) 92 , 234-235.
Armstrong, R.M., Barnett, J.T.R. (1989). J.Virol.Methods 25, 71-79. An ELISA for the detection and quantitation of antibody against swine vesicular disease virus.
Ferris, N.P., Dawson, M. (1988). Vet.Microbiol. 16, 201-209. Routine application of ELISA in comparison with complement fixation for the diagnosis of foot-an-mouth and swine vesicular diseases.
Herniman, K.A., Medhurst, P.M., Wilson, J.N. and Sellers, R.F. (1974) Vet. Rec. 93, 620-625.
Lowes, E. Vet. Annual 1973 pp, 51-54.
Mann, J.A. and Hitchings, G.H. (1980) J.Hygiene 84, 355-363. Swine vesicular disease: pathways of infection.
Mowat, G.N. (1972) Vet.Rec. 90, 618-621.
Robertson, I., Owen, J. (1994). In Practice 16, 110-128. Notifiable Diseases of Pigs.
Seechum, P., Knowles, N.J., McCauley, J.W. (1990). Virus Research 16, 255-274. The complete nucleotide sequence of a pathogenic swine vesicular disease virus.

Sellers, R.F. (1982) Pig News and Information, 3, 21-24. Swine vesicular disease.

Zhang, A., Wilsden, G., Knowles, N.J., McCauley, J.W. (1993). J.Gen.Virol. 74, 845-853. Complete nucleotide sequence of Coxsackie B5 virus and its relationship to SVDV.

Foot and Mouth Disease

Foot-and-Mouth Disease in pigs is an acute and very contagious viral disease characterised by fever, the formation of vesicles on the coronary band and less frequently, on the lips and tongue. Morbidity is high but mortality is low, except amongst young pigs in which sudden death commonly occurs.

Incidence

Foot-and-Mouth Disease is absent from Britain, Ireland and several other countries in Northern Europe. It occurs from time to time in most of Europe as isolated outbreaks or as epizootics, the last of which in Britain occurred in 1967-68 when 113, 800 pigs were slaughtered. The disease is present in South America, in some parts of Southern Europe (Italy 1985 onwards), in Africa, in many parts of Asia, but is not present in Australia and North America. Fifty-seven outbreaks occurred in Italy in 1993.

Aetiology

Foot-and-Mouth Disease virus is an aphthovirus with a particle size of 23 nm and a cubical capsid containing 32 capsomeres. Four polypeptide chains and occasionally a fifth are present in the virion. The virus may be cultivated in bovine or pig kidney cells, calf thyroid cells or bovine lingual epithelium. Baby hamster kidney cells are widely used. The virus is highly cytopathic for porcine cell lines and, unlike swine vesicular disease virus, for bovine thyroid cultures. It is inactivated below pH 6 and above pH 8. 0 and is rapidly destroyed by sunlight.

Infectivity is lost within a few days at 37°C but remains for many months at 4-7°C and for years when frozen, particularly at temperatures as low as -30 to -70°C. Under natural conditions, the virus can remain infective for years in tongue epithelium stored at +4°C, in blood or vesicular fluid, for 4 weeks on hair, 15 weeks on leather and 20 weeks on hay or straw at room temperature, and for up to 6 days in milk. Pasteurisation by the flash process (72°C for 15 seconds) may not inactivate the virus completely and it may be present in milk powder for years. Survival in meat products varies. The virus is rapidly destroyed by lactic acid formation in muscle but may persist for up to 6 months in bone marrow and 4-5 months in parenchymatous organs and lymph nodes. In pickled meats, the virus may survive for 1-2 months and in Parma ham for 3-5 months.

Seven serotypes exist. They are: 3 European (A, 32 subtypes; O, 11 subtypes and C, 5 subtypes), 3 South African Territories (S.A.T. 1, 7 subtypes - S.A.T. 2, 3 subtypes - S.A.T. 3, 4 subtypes) and Asian (Asia 1 , 3 subtypes) . Only types A, O and C have been recorded in Europe. There is no cross-immunity between types and only partial immunity between subtypes within a type. All 3 were identified in the recent Italian outbreak. Recent studies suggest that the RNA polymerase genes of all types are high conserved.

Pathogenesis

Infection takes place by inhalation and ingestion and can also result from the infection of abrasions on the skin and other body surfaces. Initial virus multiplication takes place in the pharyngeal region or at the point of inoculation and viraemia then results. Local spread to the tongue may occur. Secondary vesicles appear on the coronary band, back of the snout and on the udder of suckling sows, often within 24 hours of the appearance of lesions in the mouth. Maximum shedding of virus by aerosol occurs at this time, much of it from early replication in the upper respiratory tract and the lungs and trachea. Vesicles rupture and if uncontaminated, heal rapidly. Those on the feet may result in destruction of growing horn and loss of the hoof. Immunity to the type and subtype of the infecting virus develops within 3-7 days of the clinical signs but may last for only 6 months. Piglets can be protected by colostral antibody.

Clinical signs

The sudden onset of severe lameness is the commonest finding in affected pigs, the feet of which are obviously painful. The back may be arched, reluctance to move is common and movement may be accompanied by squealing. Vesicles appear as raised white areas 0.5-1 cm in diameter on the dorsum of the tongue and on the snout and may rupture readily to leave small ulcers. Frothy saliva may be present and vesicles develop on the coronet in the interdigital space, and on the supernumerary digits. When they rupture, the cause "thimbling" as the damaged horn is shed. Fever (up to 41°C-106°F) accompanies the earliest stages of the disease. Affected animals are depressed, anorexic and lose condition. Mortality rarely exceeds 5%, but it may reach 50% in piglets in which sudden death may occur before vesicles develop in either piglets or the sows. Animals with loss of horn or acute lameness should be killed humanely.

Pathology

Apart from the presence of vesicles and the appearance of a fevered carcase, patchy necrosis of the heart muscle may be seen in young pigs which have died suddenly. The latter may not have vesicles.

Epidemiology

The incubation period is 2-7 days and virus is shed even before the appearance of the lesions, particularly from the upper respiratory tract. As there is no carrier state and the ability of the virus to survive under various conditions is important and has been listed above. Foot-and-Mouth disease in pigs is a major source of virus for other species. The high concentration of virus produced in early stages of the disease, coupled with the large numbers of pigs in an airspace and forced ventilation, can give rise to virus aerosol plumes which can travel long distances. Infection results from direct or indirect contact with affected animals, carcases or animal products. Transmission may be by the aerosol route, by contact with other species of affected livestock, by fomites and from infected material of animal origin in incompletely cooked swill. Milk, either skim or whole, may be a source during outbreaks. Following infection, pigs do not remain carriers.

Diagnosis

The clinical signs only allow a diagnosis of a vesicular condition to be made but Foot-and-Mouth disease may be suspected if the case is linked to a confirmed outbreak of F.M.D. Laboratory diagnosis is based on the examination of fresh lesion material taken from suspected clinical cases. Material for examination should be transported in 50/50 glycerol/phosphate buffer kept at 4°C or lower. The complement fixation test is performed using lesion material as antigen against all 7 serotypes. A polymerase chain reaction has been described using a primer for the RNA polymerase gene and a reverse transcriptase ELISA and radioimmunoassay tests are also used. Passage through baby mice or in tissue culture may be used. Acid sensitivity distinguishes the virus from S.V.D. virus. Serum from recovered cases and populations may also be tested by ELISA, especially the liquid phase blocking ELISA and virus neutralisation. Blood dried in paper discs may be used.

Prophylaxis and control

Control in the EC is based on early recognition, followed by slaughter, disinfection and strict control of movement which is cheaper to operate than the alternative of annual vaccination Foot and Mouth Disease Order, 1983. The disease is kept out of the EC by control over the import of animals and animal products and by the UK policy, under the Diseases of Animals (Waste Foods) Order and Movement and Sale of Pigs Order 1975, of ensuring that swill is properly cooked and that swill-fed pigs go only to slaughter (introduced for the control of S.V.D.).

In future outbreaks, the use of vaccination may be used strategically in areas surrounding an outbreak in combination with the existing slaughter policy Foot and Mouth Disease (Infected Areas) (Vaccination) Order 1972. This combination of using vaccination and slaughter has been used with success elsewhere. In countries where the disease is enzootic, annual vaccination is practised.

Both live, attenuated and inactivated vaccines are available.

Inactivated vaccines are made from virus growth in bovine tongue epithelium or other suitable cells, inactivated with formalin, acetylethyleneimine (AEI) and other ethyleneimines and incorporated with oil, saponin or aluminium hydroxide adjuvants. Pigs are not readily immunised and require high concentrations of virus, although immunity has been demonstrated for up to 9 months using oil-adjuvanted vaccines. These cause granulomatous reactions and should be given into the pinna of the ear or intraperitoneally. One or more different serotypes may be included. Protection may take 7-20 days to develop and re-vaccination is required every 6-8 months. IgG appears to be the important protective antibody.

Attenuated vaccines are not widely used in pigs but are continuously under review.

Subunit vaccines are being developed by genetic engineering and direct synthesis from viral polypeptides but are not commercially available. Subunits as small as 3 amino acids have been shown to provide some protection.

Reference

Armstrong, R.M., Crowther, J.R., Denyer M.S. (1991). J.Virol.Methods. 34, 181-192. The detection of antibodies against FMDV in filter paper eluates from pig sera or whole blood by ELISA.

Barteling, S.J., Vreeswick, J. (1991). Vaccine. 9, 75-88. Developments in Foot-and-Mouth vaccines.

Donaldson, A.I., Ferris, N.P. and Wells, G.A.H. (1984). Vet.Rec. 115, 509-512. Experimental foot-and-mouth disease in fattening pigs, sows and piglets in relation to outbreaks in the field.

Ferris, N.P., Dawson, M. (1988). Vet.Microbiol. 16, 201-209. Routine application of ELISA in comparison with complement fixation for the diagnosis of FMD and SVD.

Meyer, R.F., Brown, C.C., House, C., House, J.A., Molitor, T.W. (1991). J.Virol.Methods. 34, 161-172. Rapid and sensitive detection of FMDV in tissues by enzymatic RNA amplification of the polymerase gene.

Morgan, D.O., Moore, D.A. (1990). Am.J.Vet.Res. 51, 40-45. Protection of cattle and swine against FMD using biosynthetic peptide vaccines.

Robertson, I., Owen, J. (1994). In Practice 16, 110-128. Notifiable Disease of Pigs.

Vesicular exanthema

A calicivirus disease which caused vesicular lesions resembling those of foot-and-mouth disease and S.V.D. in California. Not seen since 1959, the virus is present in fish and sea lions and these might at any time form a source for pigs. The virus is spread by contact and fomites, but primary cases followed the feeding of contaminated uncooked swill.

Reference

Berry C.S., Skilling, D.E., Barlough, J.C., Vedros N.A., Gage, L.J., Smith, A.W. (1990). Am.J.Vet.Res. 51, 1184-1187. New marine calicivirus serotype infective for swine.

Vesicular stomatitis

Another vesicular disease of the Western Hemisphere caused by two RNA vesiculoviruses (members of the rhabdoviridae) and rarely found in pigs. The virus also affects cattle, horses and man, possibly from a wild life or insect reservoir and probably transmitted by the sand fly *Lutzomyia shannoni* associated with maritime live oaks. It is enzootic in Mexico and other parts of Central America and occasionally occurs in the Southern US e.g. 1985. It is seasonal, occurring in the summer. Antibody levels in the South Eastern US. can vary from 12-60%. Once in pig populations the virus may be transmitted by contact and fomites.

Control should include disinfection and protection from insects.

Rabies

A rare, fatal viral disease of pigs in rabies-infected areas characterised by sudden onset, nervous signs and death.

Incidence

Less than 0.05% of rabies cases notified in Europe occur in the pig. It is equally rarely diagnosed in pigs in other parts of the world in which rabies is present.

Aetiology and pathogenesis

Caused by an R.N.A. by lyssavirus (rhabdoviridae), 75 x 180 nm with a characteristic shape. Exposure from bites or aerosol infection results in passage of the virus up nerves to central nervous system.

Clinical signs

Sudden onset, loss of coordination, twitching of the nose, excessive salivation and muscular spasm followed by prostration and death within 72-96 hours. Incubation period 50-120 days. Affected pigs should be killed.

Pathological findings

No gross changes; central nervous system changes may include the presence of Negri bodies. Other changes are very variable but may include diffuse meningitis

Diagnosis

Clinical signs and history of exposure to rabies. Presence of rabies antigen in brain using specific immunofluorescence or animal inoculation.

Control

General control of other rabid animals. Successful vaccination has been reported from China.

Not Present in UK or Eire, notifiable (Rabies (Control Order) 1974) and transmissible to man as a fatal disease.

Reference

Hazlett, J. and Koller, M.A. (1986). Canadian Vet.J. 27, 116-118. Small outbreak in housed pigs exposed to a rabid cat.

Japanese B. Encephalitis

Definition

A viral infection of pigs in Eastern Asia transmitted by mosquitoes responsible for reproductive failure.

Aetiology

A flavi virus (RNA) 40 nm in diameter. It has been defined antigenically and by restriction endonuclease techniques. It is extremely labile and rapidly inactivated by disinfectants, heat and extremes of pH. It grows well in most cell types.

Pathogenesis

Infection results from mosquito bites and viraemia results. The central nervous system may be affected but the major effects result from infection of the testis and the development or orchitis and multiplication in the foetus between 40 and 60 days' gestation to cause foetal death.

Clinical signs

Clinical signs may follow infection in piglets but it is normally asymptomatic. The major effects are on numbers born alive which are reduced. Mummified foetuses, stillborn and weak pigs are produced Boars lose libido, develop abnormal semen and azoospermia.

Pathology

Largely restricted to affected foetuses or stillborn pigs where there may be oedematous changes and neuronal changes.

Epidemiology

Transmitted by mosquitoes, principally *Culex tritaenorhynchus* but other mosquito species may be involved. Wild birds may be a reservoir and infection can be transmitted to man. Infection may be transmitted in semen.

Diagnosis

Antibody can be detected by haemagglutination inhibition tests and by ELISA (especially an IgM capture ELISA).

Control

Live attenuated virus vaccines should be given to breeding stock twice 2-3 weeks before the start of the mosquito season. Semen from affected boars should not be used.

Reference

Habu, A. (1991). Bull.Nippon Veterinary and Animal Science University 40, 107-108. Studies on the disorders of spermatogenic function in boars infected with Japanese Encephalitis Virus and its prevention.

Getah Virus Infection

A haemagglutinating virus causing viraemia and foetal death in sows one week after infection. Described from Japan and confirmed serologically by ELISA and haemagglutination Inhibition tests.

Reference

Izumida, A., Takuma, H., Inaga, S., Kubota, M., Hirahawa, T., Kodama, K., Sasaki, N. (1988). Japanese J.Vet.Si. 50, 679-684. Experimental infection of Getah virus in swine.

Other Arthropod-Transmitted Viruses

Other arthropod-transmitted viruses have been identified in pigs.

In Asia these include Apoi, Akabane, Ibaraki Batai (Japan), Dengue, West Nile and Chikungunya (India and in Europe, West Nile virus and tickborne encephalitis (Rumania) and Louping III (Scotland).

Louping III

Louping III is transmitted by ingestion and by the tick *Ixodes ricinus* and has caused nervous signs including hydrophobia. A non-suppurative meningo-encephalitis with neuronal necrosis, neuronophagia and lymphoid perivascular cuffing has been described in the brain stem. Virus has been demonstrated in, and is isolated from, the brain.

Prevention by the use of the oil-adjuvanted killed vaccine would be possible subject to local reaction.

Louping III is a zoonosis.

Reference

Ross, H.M., Evans, C.C., Spence, J.A., Reid, H.W., Krueger, N. (1994). Vet.Rec. 134, 99-100. Louping III in free ranging pigs.

Hepatitis E

Experimental infection of pigs with faeces from an affected human case resulted in jaundice 3-4 weeks post-infection, histological evidence of hepaitis and is of particular relevance to human health in areas with street pigs and poor sanitation.

Retrovirus

Retroviruses have been identified in porcine cell lines but clinical disease has not been reported.

Reference

Phanh Thanh, L., Kaeffer, B., Bottreau, E. (1992). Arch.Virol. 123, 255-265. Porcine retrovirus: optimal conditions for its biochemical detection.

Porcine Spongiform Encephalopathy

Bovine spongiform encephalopathy has been experimentally-transmitted to a pig by inoculation of bovine brain. Depression, inappetence, aimless biting and ataxia developed after 69 weeks. Spongiform lesions of the mid-brain were identified.

Reference

Dawson, M., Wells, G.A.H., Parker, B.N.J., Scott, A.C. (1990). Vet.Rec. 127, 338. Primary parenteral transmission of bovine spongiform encephalopathy to the pig.

Porcine Circovirus

Infection with circovirus, a small circular single-stranded DNA virus is widespread in pig populations where it has been sought (South Africa, New Zealand, UK). No clinical syndrome has yet been associated with it but its ability to multiply in bone marrow suggests the possibility of anaemia as in chicks.

BACTERIAL DISEASES

Diseases caused by bacteria, mycoplasmas, rickettsiae, chlamydia and eperythrozoon are all considered in this section. The identification of bacterial cause to an infectious syndrome is subject to the same criteria that have already been outlined for viral diseases with two important differences:

1) Many bacterial diseases respond to appropriate antimicrobial treatment.

2) A few bacteria may produce toxins in the feed which can be ingested to cause disease.

Bacterial diseases may be recognised by the identification of clinical signs, post-mortem findings or epidemiological features with those of the diseases described below and under Differential Diagnosis at the end of the book. These diseases can then be confirmed by the demonstration of the agent, its products or antibody to it. Some bacterial diseases are enzootic in pig herds (enzootic pneumonia, *Mycoplasma hypopneumoniae* and *E.coli* post-weaning diarrhoea) and it should be realised that the disease may behave very differently in a herd with enzootic infection anidentify where more than one agent may be present in a lesion and because bacteria are capable of colonising lesions caused by other agents. This problem is particularly acute when considering enteric lesions which may be initiated by viruses, parasites or bacteria and then colonised by other bacterial pathogens. In these complicated syndromes associated with bacteria, a decision has to be made about the most significant agent or agents present and these can then be controlled. Successful identification of the initiating agent can only be confirmed by a favourable response to a specific vaccine, a particular control measure or therapy in a controlled split herd study or laboratory confirmation..

Minor pathogens or opportunists are described here in order to provide some ideas about possible causes or contribution to bacterial disease.

When disease fails to respond to control measure expected to be effective, consider that:

a) antimicrobial may be ineffective because it is given too late, in too low levels (inactivated in water, by pelleting, by settlement in feed) or may be given by a route inappropriate to the body system affected. It may also fail because the wrong antimicrobial was chosen for the organism concerned due to innate or acquired resistance.

b) Vaccine may be inappropriate because a different serotype of the organism is involved in disease or antibody/cellular immune levels are too low.

c) Re-infection is taking place because of mixing of stock or survival of the agent in the environment.

If none of these factors account for the problem, reconsider the diagnosis.

Leptospirosis

Definition

Infection with *Leptospira interrogans* serotypes and serovars may be inapparent, or may cause fever, meningitis, icterus and death in piglets and abortion and stillbirth in sows. *Leptospira canicola, L. icterohaemorrhagiae* and members of the *L.australis* serogroup are the most important causes of the syndrome in Britain. *L.pomona* is most important worldwide, perhaps followed by *L.tarassovi* and *L.bratislava*

Incidence

Leptospirosis occurs in pigs worldwide. The range of serotypes and serovars reported from each country varies. Reporting depends upon a) those actually present and b) those sought for which can vary according to the strains used as antigens and the ability of laboratories to isolate and identify them. It is more common in animals kept outside, but infection with *L.bratislava* occurs and *L.canicola*, and *L.icterohaemorrhagiae* occurred in Britain in housed pigs in the past. In a serological survey of pig herds in Britain, antibody to the following serotypes of *L.interrogans* was found: *australis* 23%, *cynopteri* 12%, *icterohaemorrhagiae* 4%, ballum 3% and others 3%. Studies in Northern Ireland have shown that *australis* (*bratislava* and *muenchen*) was present in 71% of aborted piglets and on 68% farms examined. Infection with *australis* serovars has been identified in the US. and Canada as well as many European countries, Australia and South America. Infection rates vary. In many countries *pomona* and *tarassovi* infections may be present in up to 30% of herds and outbreaks of *L.canicola* and *L.icterohaemorrhagiae* may occur from time to time.

Aetiology

Leptospira are fine spiral bacterial (spirochaetes) (10 μm in length and 0.2 μm in diameter) with a central body which is hooked at the end and surrounded by an envelope. Within this lies a single axial filament arising from each end and overlapping centrally. They may be grown in complex media such as EMJH and E medium, and are aerobic. Primary isolation from tissue takes 2-6 weeks and 5 fluorouracil, rifampicin, amphotericin B or cycloserine are included in isolation media. The bacteria are divided into serogroups by the production of antisera which are then absorbed with organisms of other groups. The groups have been shown to be associated with the possession of particular combinations of envelope antigens. Each serogroup consists of a number of serovars which are distinguished using monoclonal antibodies. Serovars have been sub-divided in their turn by the use of factor analysis with monoclonal antibodies and more easily by restriction endonuclease analysis. Particular subdivisions of serovars have been associated with particular syndromes such as *L.australis* serovar *bratislava* genotype B2b and serovar *muenchen* M2 in abortion and serovar *bratislava* B2a in meningitis.

Leptospirae are sensitive *in vitro* to many antimicrobials such as penicillin and streptomycin and are sensitive to most disinfectants, to soaps, detergents and are rapidly destroyed by drying. They may, however, persist for weeks or months in water.

Antibodies to *L.pomona, canicola, hyos/tarassovi, icterohaemorrhagiae, sejroe, hardjo, ballum, bratislava* and *autumnalis* have all been found in pigs.

Infections with *L.pomona* and *L.tarassovi* are an important cause of morbidity in the United States, Australia and Europe, but in Britain *L.canicola*, *L.icterohaemorrhagiae* and *L.australis* are the most important serotypes. *L.muenchen* and *L.bratislava* are the two most common australis serovars found. *L.pomona* serovar *mozdok* has been identified in Dorset but *L.pomona*, *kennewiki*, the classic pig adapted *pomona* has never been found.

Pathogenesis

Infection is by ingestion, direct contact and entry through abrasions, transplacental transmission or by the venereal route. The organisms multiply to produce a septicaemia which may produce clinical signs. They may cause damage in the liver and elsewhere in the body and penetrate basement membranes into sites protected from circulating antibody which normally limits leptospiraemia within 7-10 days of infection. In pomona infections, organisms penetrate from the blood vessels through the interstitial tissue of the kidney to the basement membrane within 3-5 days of infection and cause swelling of the tubular epithelial cells. By 7 days post-infection they are present within the tubular epithelial cells and macrophages are prominent in the interstitial tissue and by 14 days after infection are restricted to the microvilli of the lumenal surface. Plasma cells and lymphocytes are prominent in the interstitial tissue. Leptospirae are shed in the urine from time to time during a period of months after clinical recovery. Localisation may also occur in the pregnant uterus, cause foetal invasion and abortion 10 days to 4 weeks after infection and may also occur in the fallopian tubes and seminal vesicles. Penetration into the central nervous system may result in meningitis and damage to the liver in the acute stage may result in jaundice. The pathogenesis of muenchen infections in sows appears to be similar with few detectable clinical signs and a shorter period of leptospiruria (30 days). Leptospirae may enter the genital tract from systemic infection or from venereal infection. Embryos and foetuses must be infected prior to 50 days of gestation for death to result. The organisms may persist in the genital tract of both sows and boars.

Clinical signs

Three main clinical syndromes are associated with leptospira infection in pigs.

1. Subclinical infection

    Serological evidence of infection (see above) is widespread in pig populations in Britain, especially in finishing pigs and gilts reared extensively in which clinical signs of disease are rarely seen. Leptospirae may be isolated from the kidneys and genital tracts of these animals

2. Acute or subacute infection

    Fever to 40°C (105.8°F) for 3-5 days has been recorded in *L.canicola* and *L.icterohaemorrhagiae* infection in piglets and in *pomona* and *tarassovi* infections. Affected pigs become dull, anorexic, show diarrhoea and rarely develop icterus with or without haemoglobinuria. Heavy mortality may occur. Nervous signs may be seen, e.g. weakness of the hindquarters, meningitis or tremor if leptospirae enter nervous tissue.

Animals with severe jaundice, haemorrhagic disease or nervous signs such that prostration occurs, should be killed humanely if treatment is ineffective.

3.   Reproductive disorders

Abortion, stillbirth and neonatal mortality accompanied by fever, loss of milk and jaundice in the sows are common consequences of leptospiral infection in breeding herds. *L.muenchen*, *L.bratislava* and *canicola* are often implicated in Britain, but *L.pomona* is an important cause abroad. In experimental infections, abortion occurred 4-7 days after infection with *L.canicola* in sows less than 4-5 weeks pregnant. In sows which were infected later, weak piglets were born.   Mummified and macerated foetuses also occur commonly amongst the litters of sows with leptospirosis. Abortion in the last trimester of pregnancy is common. Infertility associated with venereal spread in non-immune herds may be responsible for returns to service, particularly with the *australis* serovars *bratislava* and *muenchen.*

Pathology

Death from leptospirosis only occurs infrequently in Britain, so post-mortem findings are mainly incidental, e.g. at slaughter, or as a result of the examination of aborted foetuses.   In acute cases, signs of generalised septicaemia occur, often coupled with jaundice and signs of liver damage. Kidney lesions may be present.   In leptospiral abortions, associated with *L.pomona* and *L.icterohaemorrhagiae,* affected foetuses may be mummified, or have uniformly pale organs with or without jaundice. Freshly aborted foetuses often have petechiae on the skin and haemorrhages in kidney, lungs and liver. Excess straw-coloured fluid is often present in the serous cavities. In other cases few distinctive changes may be present.   In *australis* abortions mummification is not a feature and abortions take place in the last third of gestation or litters of stillborn piglets are produced at full term. Renal lesions are the most common finding, and often occur in clinically-normal pigs. The basic lesion is a greyish-white focus 1-3 mm in diameter in the cortex. This lesion may be surrounded by an area of congestion, may be seen when the capsule is stripped. Petechiation may be present. Histological findings in the early stages include the presence of the organism in silver-stained sections, especially in the kidney tubules. Tubular damage and mononuclear cell infiltration may be seen in sections of affected kidneys. Leptospirae may also be demonstrated by immunofluorescence and immunoperoxidase in tissue. Antigen demonstrated by these means remains detectable after whole organisms have disintegrated and can no longer be cultured or recognised in silver-stained sections. DNA probes have also been used and may detect 10^2 organisms/g tissue.

Epidemiology

Infection with *Leptospira* may arise from the organisms shed in the urine of carrier animals, from organisms shed by carrier rodents or by venereal spread.   Rat infestation is a common source of infection due to *L.icterohaemorrhagiae* and in Europe and other countries, *L.pomona* infections may be associated with infections in field mice. Pigs infected with leptospira may act as sources of infection for dogs and for man. The organisms may persist in clean water for periods up to 30 days and infections may be water borne from a source upstream or from drinking water contaminated with rodent urine. *L.pomona* infections due to *L.pomona kennewiki* may be enzootic in herds. In such a herd, the prevalence of serum antibody in young piglets is high, falls to a low point by 6-10 weeks of age and rises rapidly thereafter to a high prevalence. In herds with sporadic infection, such as *australis* infections in Britain in which infection is contracted from rodents or by venereal spread, the prevalence of specific antibody rises gradually with age. Many animals with localised infections may not have serum antibody levels and thus escape detection.

Diagnosis

Clinical signs such as abortion in the last trimester of pregnancy, reduced conception, vulval discharge, the birth of weak piglets, and fever with icterus and mortality in older piglets and weaners may suggest leptospirosis. The post-mortem findings, especially the kidney lesions, may also be suggestive. Diagnosis is usually confirmed by demonstration of the organism or by antibody to it.

The organism may be demonstrated by dark ground microscopy of the urine of aborting sows or in urine, semen, aborted foetuses and the organs of slaughtered pigs by culture. Culture requires specialist media and is most reliable when the tissue concerned is fresh and uncontaminated.

Contamination may be reduced by using fresh urine, kidneys with the capsule intact, or the anterior chamber of the eye in aborted foetuses. Liver, lung, brain, the blood, exudates and reproductive organs and secretions may all be examined. Samples should be submitted in a transport medium similar to the isolation medium and isolation can be carried out by a specialist laboratory but may take 6-12 weeks. Isolation is one of the most sensitive methods of confirmation of diagnosis.

The organism, its antigens or products may also be demonstrated in tissue by silver staining of fixed tissue, by immunofluorescence or immunoperoxidase, and by DNA probes.

Serological tests are widely used. Antibodies to leptospira appear in the serum with 1-2 weeks of infection and reach titres of 1:10,000-1:30,000 (Microscopic Agglutination Lysis Test, MAT) which may persist for some weeks. The MAT, using live organisms, is the most sensitive test and detects rising titres which follow infection particularly well. Microscopic agglutination tests can be carried out using killed antigen but are less sensitive (94.%). An IgM Enzyme Immunoassay (EIA) with 82% sensitivity and whole cell ELISA and axial filament ELISAs with 97% sensitivity have also been described.

Serum antibody can only be used as a herd test. Antibody levels suggestive of chronic infection are 1:100 (MAT) but infected animals may be seronegative. Antibody occurring in thoracic exudates in stillborn foetuses is diagnostic. Cross reaction between serogroups and serovars may occur and accurate serology is best carried out using local serovars.

Treatment

The parenteral administration of a number of antibiotics such as penicillin, semisynthetic penicillins, streptomycin and tiamulin is of value in acutely ill animals. Abortions may be prevented and renal carriers eliminated by parenteral treatment with streptomycin (25 mg/kg) as a single dose or for 3-5 days. Treatment 1 week before service and 2 weeks before farrowing has been found to be most satisfactory in preventing reproductive losses. Feed or water medication with tetracyclines may be of value. Re-infection should be prevented by hygiene and isolation.

Control

Vaccination of sows with killed vaccines containing the appropriate serotype or serotypes before service may prevent abortion. Piglets should be vaccinated before the period of risk (6-10 weeks of age). Only *L.icterohaemorrhagiae*, *L.canicola* and *L.hardjo* vaccines are available in the UK. but elsewhere *L.pomona*, *L.tarassovi*, *L.hardjo*, *L.bratislava* and *L.grippotyphosa* have been used either alone or in various combinations. Vaccination may not prevent renal colonisation. *L.bratislava* vaccine has been known to produce significant improvements in numbers born in the face of *L.bratislava* infection.

The disease may be eliminated by hygiene, vaccination, treatment or slaughter of carriers or a total slaughter policy combined with disinfection, elimination of rodents and restocking. As leptospirae can survive freezing, the practice of feedback for parvovirus control may predispose to leptospiral infection.

References

Baker, T.F., McEwen, S.A., Prescott, J.F. and Meek, A.H. (1989). Can.J.Vet.Res. 53, 290-294. The prevalence of leptospirosis and its association with multifocal interstitial nephritis in swine at slaughter.
Chappel, R.J., Prince, R.W., Mullar, B.D., Mead, L.J., Jones, R.T. and Adler, B. (1992). Vet.Micro. 30, 151-163. Comparison of diagnostic procedures for porcine leptospires.
Ellis, W.A. (1989). Pig Vet.J. 22, 83-92. *L.australis* infection in pigs.
Ellis, W.A., McParland, P.J., Bryson, D.G. and Cassells, J.A. (1986). Vet.Rec. 118, 63-65. Prevalence of leptospira infection in aborted pigs in Northern Ireland.
Ellis, W.A., McParland, P.J., Bryson, D.G. and Cassells, J.A. (1986). Vet.Rec. 118, 563. Boars as carriers of leptospires of the Australis serogroup on farms with an abortion problem.
Ellis, W.A., McParland, P.J., Bryson, D.G., Thiermann, A.B. and Montgomery, J. (1986). Vet.Rec. 118, 294-295. Isolation of leptospires from genital tract and kidneys of aborted sows.
Ellis, W.A., Montgomery, J.M. and McParland, P.J. (1989). Vet.Rec. 125, 319-321. An experimental study with an *L.interrogans* serovar *bratislava* vaccine.
Ellis, W.A., Montgomery, J.M. and Thiermann, A.B. (1991). J.Clin.Microbiol. 29, 957-961. Restriction endonuclease analysis as a taxonomic tool in the study of pig isolates belonging to the Australis serogroup of *L.interrogans*.
Franz, J.C., Hanson, L.E. and Brown, A.L. (1989). Am.J.Vet.Res. 50, 1044-1047. Effect of vaccination with a bacteria containing *L.interrogans* serovar bratislava on the breeding performance of swineherds.
Hathaway, S.C., Little, T.W.A. and Stevens, A.E. (1981) Res. in Vet. Sci. 31, 169-173. Leptospira hardjo in pigs. A new host - parasite relationship in the UK.
Kingscote, W.F. (1986). Can.Vet.J. 77, 188-197 Leptospirosis outbreak in a piggery in Southern Alberta.
Michna, S.W. and Campbell, R.S.F. (1969) Vet.Rec. 84, 135-138. Leptospirosis in pigs: Epidemiology, microbiology and pathology.

Actinobacillosis

Definition

Actinobacillus suis and *A.equuli* may cause fatal septicaemia, endocarditis and arthritis in pigs 1-6 weeks of age. In older animals, skin lesions may be seen and a focal necrotising pneumonia may occur.

Incidence

Present in many countries but reported from few. First identified in UK in 1971, it is not uncommon. It has been studied most extensively in Canada in recent years.

Aetiology

Actinobacillus suis and *A.equuli* have both been reported. Both produce 2 mm translucent regular colonies on blood agar and small pink colonies on MacConkey agar after 24 hours' incubation. *A.suis* produces alpha-haemolysis on horse blood agar and B-haemolysis on sheep blood agar. *A.suis* also hydrolyses aesculin, produces acid from arabinose, cellobiose and salicin and is pathogenic for mice. *A. suis* has been shown to produce the 104 kDa cytolysin also found in *A.pleuropneumoniae*, although the genes are arranged differently.

Pathogenesis

Infection appears to occur via the upper respiratory tract in young pigs and results in septicaemia. The animal may die at this stage or the infection may localise to give vegetative endocarditis or arthritis. It is sometimes considered that the actinobacilli are opportunist pathogens. In older pigs infection may be by the respiratory route.

Clinical signs

Sudden death may occur in piglets and in some cases the cause of death in neonates is assumed to be crushing or still birth. Others may be found to be febrile (39-40.5°C, 102.5-105°F) with multiple haemorrhages on the skin, particularly of the ears and abdomen. Swollen joints and septic or necrotic lesions of the skin may also be seen. Recovering animals remain unthrifty. Adults may have round or rhomboid subcutaneous abscesses, particularly on the neck, withers and flanks which may resemble those of erysipelas. Adults are rarely affected but deaths have been reported following the introduction of the disease to high health herds.

Death is often sudden and mild cases respond to antimicrobial treatment, but animals with chronic arthritis or vegetative endocarditis should be killed humanely.

Pathology

Animals which have died from actinobacillus infections may have discoloured areas, purpura or necrosis of the skin. The carcases may appear normal apart from the presence of petechiae on lung, the kidney and an excess of pleural fluid. Histological lesions in the lung are characteristic as they consist of a microcolony of bacteria surrounded by necrosis and inflammatory cells. The skin lesions contain thromboemboli in both superficial and deep vessels surrounded by infarcted dermal and epidermal tissue. Chronic cases may have vegetative endocarditis, fibrinous pericarditis, pneumonia or polyarthritis. Lesions resembling those of pleuropneumonia in fattening pigs have yielded *Actinobacillus spp. A.equuli* or, more commonly, *A.suis*, may be isolated in pure culture from the kidney, liver, or heart blood and from localised lesions.

Epidemiology

There are some reports of contact with horses in *A.equuli* cases and outbreaks may occur following the introduction of carrier animals to the farm. Studies of enzootically-infected herds show that antibody to the 104 kDa toxin are present in colostrum and that active antibody appears at 6-8 weeks of age. *A.suis* can be recovered from the tonsils of sucking pigs and from sow vaginas.

Diagnosis

The clinical signs and post-mortem lesions are not specific, although the skin lesions are suggestive of this disease, particularly when fever and purpura are found erysipelas should be ruled out. Isolation of the organism will confirm. *Pasteurella haemolytica* septicaemia usually follows contact with sheep. Serological cross reactions with *(A) pleuropneumoniae* occur in the C.F. test for the latter and tests using the 104 kDa toxin will also cross-react.

Treatment

Tetracyclines, ampicillin or other antibiotics may be given parenterally or orally if necessary in small pigs. Recovery is normally complete after 2-5 days' treatment.

References

Jones, J.E.T. and Simmons, J.R. (1971). Brit.Vet.J. 127, 25-29. Endocarditis in the pig caused by *Actinobacillus equuli*. A field and experimental case.
Miniats, O.P., Spinato, M.T. and Sanford, S.E. (1989). Can.Vet.J. 30, 943-947. *Actinobacillus suis* septicaemia in mature swine. Two outbreaks resembling erysipelas.
Sanford, S.E., Josephson, G.K.A., Rehmtulla, A.J., Tilker, A.M.E. (1990). Can.Vet.J. 31, 443-447. *Actinobacillus suis* infection in pigs in south western Ontario.

Actinobacillus ureae

This organism, formerly *Pasteurella ureae* has been recorded in placentitis and abortion. There is no experimental evidence for its causal role.

Reference

Orr, J., Chirino-Trejo, M., Saunders, B., Kumor, L., Sawatsky, J. (1990). Can.Vet.J. 31, 42. Association of *A.ureae* with porcine abortion.

Brucellosis

Definition

Brucella suis infection may be inapparent or may result in stillbirths, abortions and infertility in both sexes. In the boar, infection of the testicles and accessory sex glands is common.

Incidence

Brucellosis does not occur in pigs in Britain or Ireland but still occurs in many countries in Europe and in half the states of the US. It appears to be absent from Canada. In most countries with developed pig industries the incidence is declining.

Aetiology

B.suis biotype 1 (worldwide), biotype 2 (West Central Europe), biotype 3 (US., S. America, S.E. Asia) is the causal agent. It is a small, slender, aerobic gram-negative bacillus and forms 1-2 mm domed colonies on blood agar after 2-4 days' aerobic incubation.

Pathogenesis

B.abortus and B.melitensis have been found to infect pigs. Infection by the oral or venereal route is followed by multiplication in local lymph nodes. After 1-2 weeks a bacteraemia develops and persists for at least 5 weeks. The organisms remain in lymph nodes, joints and the genital tract. Invasion of the foetus may lead to abortion. Infection may persist for at least 64 months and, in boars, for life.

Clinical signs

Early abortion (returns to oestrus 5-8 weeks after service) results from infection at service, but infection later in pregnancy gives rise to litters with mummified, stillborn or weak pigs. Copious bloody vulval discharge and endometritis occur. Testicular swelling, orchitis and epididymitis may occur in boars within 7 weeks of infection and testicular atrophy may be present within 19 weeks. Bones and joints may be involved in both sexes and posterior paralysis and lameness may occur. Lame animals and those with paralysis should be destroyed on humane grounds.

Pathology

Necrotic or abscessed testicles may be seen in boars and there may be marked enlargement or atrophy of these organs. In the sow there may be oedema, haemorrhage and necrosis in the uterine lining. There may be a purulent arthritis in both sexes. Granulomatous lesions may be present in the liver, kidney and spleen.

Epidemiology

Infection is introduced to a herd by live infected pigs or contact with infected hares or, less commonly, by contaminated meat products and semen or ova. Infection is often oral. Infected boars form a major source of infection within a herd and transmit the disease by natural service or artificial insemination. Sows may remain carriers and up to 10% of their progeny may contract infection which they retain until adulthood. Lateral spread may also occur amongst weaners. Infection may persist in dried secretions in cold conditions for up to 2 years and reservoirs of infection in the European brown hare and Wild Boar are important in Europe while infected feral pigs are important in Australia and the South Eastern US. The organism infects man to cause brucellosis.

Diagnosis

Clinical signs may suggest brucellosis but diagnosis is often made by isolating the organism by culture of the mandibular, gastrohepatic and external iliac lymph nodes on a regular basis and from other organs affected in the particular outbreak. Serological tests are also important but may be misleading. Some infected animals are antibody-negative. *B.abortus* standard antigen is used for tests as the same antigens are present in *B.suis*. Tube and plate agglutination tests can be used but the brucellosis card test and the Rose Bengal Plate Test are widely used for large scale surveillance. ELISA tests have been tested. Antibody to *Yersinia enterocolitica* type IX may cause cross reaction and false positives.

Control

Vaccination with attenuated strains such as the Chinese S2 strain and treatment are not 100% effective and slaughter followed by restocking is the most successful method of control. Disinfection is a vital part of control. International trade is safeguarded by the export of seronegative pigs and the testing of boars upon entry to AI stations.

References

Cornell, W.D., Chengappa, M.M., Stuart, L.A., Maddux, R.L., Hail, R.I. (1989). J.Vet. Diagnostic Investigation 1, 20-21. *Brucella suis* biovar 3 infection in a Kentucky swine herd.
Rogers, R.J., Cook, D.R., Ketterer, P.J., Baldock, F.C., Blackale, P.J., Stewart, R.W. (1989). Aust.Vet.J. 66, 77-80. An evaluation of three serological tests for antibody to *B.suis* in pigs.
Wrathall, A.E., Broughton, A.E., Gill, K.P.W., Goldsmith, G.P. (1993). Vet.Rec. 132, 449-454. Serological reactions to Brucella species in British pigs.

Listeriosis

Infection with *Listeria sp.* is common in pigs. Studies in Denmark, Japan and Yugoslavia suggest that about 10% of slaughter pigs may be contaminated in life and that the organisms, principally *L.monocytogenes* and *L.innocua* are present in tonsils and in faeces. Carriage rate increases when silage is fed.

L.monocytogenes is a Gram-positive bacillus 1.2 µm by 0.5 µm which grows from $4^{\circ}C$ to $37^{\circ}C$. Colonies on blood agar are beta-haemolytic, greyish and opaque with a narrow zone of haemolysis.

Infection rarely causes disease, but sudden death in piglets, septicaemia and nervous signs have all been recorded. Abortion, stillbirths and the birth of weak piglets may all occur in sows. Lesions in piglets may include necrotic lesions in the liver, patchy lesions in the lung and hydrothorax. Histological lesions include meningitis, perivascular cuffing and microabscess formation in the brain. The bacteria may be seen in these.

Listeria infection in pigs is a potential source of infection for man. Up to 30% of minced pork products may be infected and preservatives such as sodium chloride 3%, dextrose 1% and phosphate 0.04% have been shown to enhance resistance to heating. Diagnosis is based on isolation of the organism but serum antibody may be present in infected pigs, especially in sows after abortion.

The organism is sensitive to a number of antimicrobials and may be treated in piglets if caught in time. Paralysed pigs should be destroyed.

Reference

Lopez, A. and Bildfell, R. (1989). Can.Vet.J. 30, 828-829. Neonatal porcine listeriosis.

Eperythrozoonosis

Definition

Infection results in anaemia fever and icterus in pigs of 0-5 days of age. Growing pigs and sows may also be affected.

Incidence

Present in the US, Germany, Taiwan and many other pig-rearing countries. Recently reported in the UK, the earlier reports of *E.parvum* may have been erroneous. The use of tetracyclines may reduce the incidence of disease.

Aetiology

Clinical disease is associated with *E.suis*. Another organism, *E.parvum*, was originally described but differed only in size and lack of clinical disease. *E.suis* is coccoid, disc-like or ring-like, 0.8-1 µm in diameter and is located on the erythrocyte membrane.

Pathogenesis

After infection by parenteral or oral transmission the organisms begin to multiply and to cause disease in as little as 5-6 days. Most studies have been carried out in splenectomised pigs which are sensitive indicators. At the onset of clinical signs, up to 80% of erythrocytes are infected. They cause increased fragility of the red cell membranes leading to breakdown, anaemia and icterus. Hypoglycaemia occurs because the consumption of blood glucose exceeds gluconeogenesis. Liver enzymes and bilirubin levels rise and intravascular coagulation occurs.

Antibody levels rise to a peak lasting 2 months and cold (IgM) agglutinins may also affect red cell integrity. PRRS may be a predisposing factor.

Clinical signs

Pallor and icterus has been described in neonatal pigs 0-5 days of age and then resolves leaving the animals uneven in size. In weaned pigs, varying degrees of unthriftiness, jaundice (bilirubin values 46-68 μ.mole/l.) and anaemia. In sows these signs are accompanied by fever (40-41.5°C, 104-107°F) and oedema. Secondary infections and effects on reproduction are common.

Pathology

Anaemia, watery blood, icterus of the carcase, enlargement of liver and spleen and fluid in all cavities with reddening of the bone marrow may be seen.

Epidemiology

Related at present to PRRS, infection can be transmitted to non-immune pigs by bites from lice (*Haematopinus suis*), infected needles, rough handling (nasal snares) and the ingestion of blood or secretions containing it. *In utero* transmission has been described but not venereal transmission.

Diagnosis

Based on clinical signs and confirmed by demonstrating the organisms on erythrocytes in blood smears stained by Giemsa or acridine orange. DNA probes and PCR have recently been described. Antibody can be detected by Indirect Haemagglutination but recently ELISAs, using whole organisms, have been described.

Treatment

Tetracyclines given by injection or orally for 14 days will eliminate all organisms. Symptomatic treatment may also be required.

Control

Reduction in exposure to susceptible pigs to blood of infected animals.

References

Gresham, A., Rogers, J., Tribe, H., Phipps, L.P. (1994). Vet.Rec. 134, 71-72. *Eperythrozoon suis* in weaned pigs.
Gwaltney, S.M., Hays, M.P., Oberst, R.D. (1993). J.Vet.Diagnostic Investigation 5, 40-46. Detection of *Eperythrozoon suis* using the polymerase chain reaction.
Hsu, F.S., Liu, M.C., Chou, S.M., Zachary, J.F., Smith, A.R. (1992). Am.J.Vet.Res. 53, 352-354. Evaluation of an ELISA for the detection of *Eperythrozoon suis* antibodies in swine.
Oberst, R.D., Hall, S.M., Jasso, R.A., Arndt, T., Wen, L. (1990). Am.J.Vet.Res. 51, 1760-1764. Recombinant DNA probe detecting *Eperythrozoon suis* in swine blood.
Smith, J.E., Cipriano, J.E., Hall, S.M. (1990). J.Vet.Med. Series B. 37, 587-592. *In vitro* glucose consumption in swine eperythrozoonosis.

Clostridium perfringens Type C

Clostridium perfringens type C produces a fatal necrotic and haemorrhagic enteritis in piglets less than 7 days of age and may cause chronic infection in older piglets.

Incidence

The disease occurs in most pig keeping countries. In Britain, 3-4 litters or part of a litter in a herd may be affected by severe disease. In other countries up to 50 litters have been reported to be affected in outbreaks.

Aetiology

Clostridium perfringens type C is a large Gram-positive rod which only occasionally forms spores. It bears attachment factors and produces toxins the most important of which is the protease/trypsin-sensitive beta toxin. The organism grows readily on blood agar on which it forms 3 mm greyish colonies with an irregular edge and varying degrees of B-haemolysis after 24 hours. It is capable of forming spores and in this form is very resistant to heat although it can be killed by formalin. Varying amounts of alpha, beta and delta toxin are produced by porcine type C.

Pathogenesis

C.perfringens type C colonises the neonatal bowel within 12-24 hours of birth on contaminated farms, and, in the absence of specific colostral immunity multiplies to cause damage to the cells of the epithelial cells of the villi of the jejunum and ileum by means of the beta toxin. Toxic damage is rapidly followed by penetration of the damaged epithelium by organisms which then adhere to the basement membrane of the villi. Necrotic damage to the core of the villus follows and the villi are shortened and covered in necrotic debris. The sensitivity of the toxin to trypsin means that disease is most likely when antitryptic factors such as those in colostrum are being ingested i.e. in the neonatal period and in the piglets of non-immune sows. Systemic absorption of the toxin occurs.

Clinical signs

Affected pigs are normal at birth and may sicken on the first or second day of life and usually die within 12-24 hours of the onset of clinical signs. A dramatic, profuse diarrhoea occurs and rapidly becomes claret-coloured. The hindquarters may be soiled with bloody faeces. Affected piglets become weak, collapse and die. Some may be found dead. In more chronic cases, shreds of necrotic material may appear in the reddish-brown watery faeces. Affected animals become very thin and pale before death. Depression of growth rate may be a feature in chronically-infected piglets.

Piglets with abdominal discolouration, subnormal temperatures or severe blood-stained diarrhoea do not recover and should be killed.

Post-mortem findings

The jejunum of affected piglets is a swollen, angry purplish-red colour and if death has been sudden, is usually full of pasty, blood-stained contents. In

110

more chronic cases, a diptheritic layer forms and the contents are more watery. Shedding of the villi of the jejunum and the presence of Gram-positive rods at the bases of the crypts may be seen in histological sections.

Epidemiology

Outbreaks often follow the introduction of infected breeding stock and disease persists in herds for up to 2 months in most cases. In some cases where new stock is constantly introduced, outbreaks may continue for up to 15 months. Farrowing houses or areas may become heavily contaminated and some organisms may sporulate. Transmission of vegetative organisms occurs in faeces. Other animal species may be infected but may theoretically represent a source of infection for pigs. Organisms of pig origin have caused disease in man.

Diagnosis

The clinical signs and the post-mortem findings of haemorrhagic enteritis in the jejunum of piglets of this age are suggestive. Mouse protection tests may confirm the presence of *C.perfringens* type C toxin in filtrates of intestinal contents and the organism may be demonstrated in smears of the small intestinal contents. Beta toxin may be demonstrated by ELISA in intestinal contents and in culture filtrates. Clostridia may be isolated in profuse culture from the lesions in anaerobic conditions but culture filtrates must be shown to contain type C toxin before the organism can be said to be involved. The organism may be present in lesions of other diseases such as T.G.E. in older pigs and may occur when antitryptic factors are present in the diet of weaned pigs.

Treatment and control

Affected animals die, but prophylactic injection of 2 ml hyperimmune antiserum to type C toxins gives complete protection to animals protected at birth, and usually protects animals which have not yet developed clinical signs. Oral ampicillin can be used to treat the survivors of an affected litter and, when given at birth may reduce the mortality in litters at risk or prevent the occurrence of the disease completely. It may be necessary to give more than one daily dose.

These measures, coupled with improved hygiene, may stop an outbreak but more permanent control is obtained by vaccination. Alum adjuvanted vaccines containing the toxoids of *C.perfringens* type C, or killed cultures of the organism, may be used alone or in combination with other vaccines such as *E.coli*. Sheep vaccines may also be used. Sows should be vaccinated 6 and 2 weeks prior to farrowing and piglets will be protected provided they ingest colostrum. Levels of antibody in colostrum may vary considerably. Very low levels of protection may allow the development of chronic disease.

References

Arbuckle, J.B.R. (1972). J.Pathology 106, 65. The attachment of *Clostridium welchii* (*Cl.perfringens*) type C to intestinal villi of pigs.
Bergeland, M.E. (1972). J.Am.Vet.Med.Ass. 160, 658. Pathogenesis and immunity of *C.perfringens* type C enteritis in swine.

111

Mackinnon, J.D. (1989). Pig Vet.J. 22, 119-125. Enterotoxaemia caused by
C.perfringens type C.
Ripley, P.H. and Gush, A.F. (1983). Vet.Rec. 112, 201-202. Immunisation
schedule for the prevention of infectious necrotic enteritis caused by
C.perfringens type C in piglets.

Clostridium perfringens Type A

Definition

Causes a syndrome in piglets resembling that caused by *C.perfringens*
type C but less severe. Involved in and able to cause diarrhoea in weaned pigs.

Incidence

Syndromes of the type described here appear to be present in many
countries and to be fairly common in Britain. They have been identified in the
Netherlands, Belgium, France, Germany, Rumania and Japan.

Aetiology

C.perfringens type A resembles type C but vegetative cells produce
alpha toxin as the major toxin. This, with the theta toxin, enables colonies to be
identified by the double zone of haemolysis on blood agar and by its lecithinase
effect on egg yolk agar. Sporulation is rare in *C.perfringens* type A but
sporulating strains have been isolated from weaned pig and piglet diarrhoeas
and enterotoxin, produced during sporulation, has been demonstrated in
intestinal contents and faeces.

Pathogenesis

Oral infection leads to multiplication in the small intestine but attachment
to the villi has not been demonstrated. In neonatal piglets the same factors
appear to operate as in *C.perfringens* type C disease with colostrum from
immune sows protecting against clinical signs but not colonisation. Organisms
multiply in the gut lumen of the unprotected piglet and reach high numbers in
the ileum, caecum and colon. Lesions of mild villous atrophy, mucosal
hyperaemia and mild necrosis develop. The reason for the enteritis is not clear
as pure alpha toxin protects piglets against infection with vegetative forms.
Infection with sporulating strains producing enterotoxin appear capable of
causing diarrhoea within 24-72 hours of infection and enterotoxin can be
demonstrated in terminal ileum, large intestine and faeces. It can be
demonstrated adsorbed to colonic epithelial cells and its action may persist in
this site. Enterotoxin from pig strains of *C.perfringens* type A can cause fluid
production and transient diarrhoea when introduced into the small intestine.
Serum antibody to alpha toxin can be demonstrated in some older pigs.
Antibody to enterotoxin is passed in the colostrum and falls to levels of 1:4
(counter immunoelectrophoresis) at 4-6 weeks of age to rise again thereafter to
adult levels. Many sows and finishing pigs in the UK have demonstrable
antibody to enterotoxin. Other agents are frequently present.

Clinical signs

Vegetative strains may cause sudden death within 48 hours of infection or birth in non-immune piglets or may cause diarrhoea. Affected diarrhoeic sucking piglets appear dull with sunken flanks and evidence of loss of condition. The perineal area is heavily pasted with yellowish faeces. The faeces present on the pen floor frequently contains some mucus but is often creamy or pasty containing flecks of fresh blood or of a pinkish tinge. Marked depression of growth occurs. Sporulating strains may produce a transient watery diarrhoea with no mortality. In weaned pigs immunity is common but non-sporulating strains can induce transient nervous signs and minor faecal changes, sometimes accompanied by loss of condition in experimental infection. Sporulating strains cause a greyish, sometimes mucoid diarrhoea lasting 3-7 days or more after the onset of clinical signs. Inappetence and reduction in weight gain occur. Loss of condition and faecal staining of the perineum and coat are common.

Affected pigs rarely die, but piglets with low rectal temperatures and discoloured abdomens will not survive and should be killed.

Pathology

The small intestine of dead piglets is often congested and its contents creamy or watery but not blood filled as in type C infections. Necrotic areas may be seen on the mucosal surface of the jejunal and ileal mucosa with a dissecting microscope and villous atrophy is obvious. Few changes apart from congestion and darkening of the carcase are seen outside the gut. Similar findings may be seen in chronically infected piglets and *C.perfringens* may contribute these changes to syndromes initiated by other agents. Histological changes include widespread shedding of villous epithelial cells and destruction of the villi.

C.perfringens type A may be seen in direct smears and isolated in profuse culture from the small intestine, its contents and from the faeces of live affected piglets. Spores may be identified in direct smears where enterotoxigenic strains are involved. In weaned pigs it is present in the small intestines which are flaccid and often contain mucopus and bubbles of gas. The histological changes described above are present to a lesser extent. *C.perfringens* type A may be isolated in profuse culture from the small intestines of animals with enteritis caused by a number of agents such as T.G.E. virus, rotavirus and cryptosporidial infections. Lesions are those of the most important contributor to the syndrome present.

Epidemiology

The organism is ubiquitous, being present in soil, intestinal contents and faeces. Nothing is known about the existence of pig-specific strains of the organism or transfer between species. *C.perfringens* type A sporulating strains have been identified in meat and may cause food poisoning in man Antibody to both alpha toxin and enterotoxin is widespread in pig populations and levels often rise with age.

Diagnosis

Requires the demonstration of *C.perfringens* type A by direct culture or immunofluorescence and the elimination of other causes of similar disease of piglets such as type C disease and coccidial infections. A marked response to penicillin therapy may be suggestive of a clostridial condition. Diagnosis of uncomplicated *C.perfringens* type A disease in older pigs relies on the clinical signs of greyish diarrhoea or soft motions, and loss of condition in pigs aged from 5-6 weeks onwards. The presence of enterotoxin in faecal filtrates can be confirmed using commercial Reversed Passive Latex Agglutination tests, counter immunoelectrophoresis, ELISA and Vero cells. Sporulating strains may be isolated by dilution of faeces in ethanol for 1 hour or by heating at 80°C for 10 minutes and then culturing anaerobically.

Treatment

Penicillin, ampicillin or antibiotics other than neomycin or other aminoglycosides given orally may be used to treat the disease in neonates. Avoparcin included in the feed at 40 ppm will prevent the development of the disease, reduce the numbers of organisms dramatically and prevent enterotoxin production. A vaccine has been described in combination with *C.perfringens* type C but is not available in the UK. Some protection may be afforded by other clostridial vaccines.

References
Estrada Correa, A., Taylor D.J. (1986). Proc.IPVS. 9, 171. Enterotoxigenic *C.perfringens* type A as a cause of diarrhoea in pigs.
Estrada Correa, A., Taylor, D.J. (1988). Proc.IPVS. 10, 138. Enterotoxigenic *C.perfringens* type A as a cause of diarrhoea in weaned pigs.
Jestin, A., Popoff, M.R., Mahe, S. (1985). Am.J.Vet.Res. 46, 2149-2151. Epizootiological investigations of a diarrhoeic syndrome in fattening pigs.
Nabuurs, M.J.A., Haagsma, J., Molen, E.J. van der. and Heijden, P.J. van der (1983). Annales de Recherches Veterinaire 14, 408-411. Diarrhoea in 1-3 week-old piglets associated with *C.perfringens* type A.
Taylor, D.J., Estrada Correa, A. (1988). Proc.IPVS. 10, 139. Avoparcin in the prevention of enterotoxigenic *C.perfringens* type A infections and diarrhoea in pigs.
Taylor, D.J., Olubunmi, P.A. (1982). Proc.IPVS. 7, 66. Enteric disease in sucking and weaned pigs initiated by and associated with *C.perfringens* type A.

Tetanus

Definition

Infection with *Clostridium tetani* causes stiffness and abnormal gait leading to tetanic spasms and death. The condition occurs sporadically in young pigs and may be associated with umbilical infections or with castration, especially when a contaminated knife has been used or where sheep have been lambed in the same accommodation.

Aetiology

C.tetani is a slender rod-shaped Gram-positive anaerobic bacillus 0.4 by 3-8 µ with terminal spherical spores and forming weakly haemolytic colonies with fibrils of growth extending over the medium from their edges. The clinical signs result from the peptide toxin tetanospasmin.

Pathogenesis

Following inoculation into penetrating wounds or the umbilicus, spores germinate in the anaerobic, often contaminated tissue debris and form toxin. This diffuses from the site of multiplication to affect the central nervous system mostly by travel in the axoplasm and sheaths of peripheral nerves. Recovery is associated with the development of circulating antibody to the toxin.

Clinical signs

Clinical signs appear a few days to weeks after wound infection and affected animals show abnormalities of gait and can be identified in this way in affected batches. Within 1-2 days the muscles stiffen, the ears are held erect and the tail straight and affected pigs finally lie on their sides in opisthotonus with fore and hind limbs rigidly extended and pointing backwards. Stimuli, e.g. noise, result in tetanic spasm of the muscles. Death normally results. Affected sucking pigs should be killed but affected weaners may recover with treatment. If severely affected and unable to stand they should be killed.

Diagnosis

Diagnosis is based on the characteristic clinical signs. Dead pigs may be rigid in the characteristic attitude, but no specific gross lesions are seen at post-mortem examination. A wound abscess or umbilical lesion may be present and a smear may be made from this and the diagnosis may be confirmed if the characteristic "drum-stick" bacilli and spores are seen.

Treatment and control

Severely affected animals rarely recover after treatment. Tetanus antitoxin may be given intramuscularly or intrathecally to mildly affected animals or intramuscularly to those at risk and antibiotic injections should also be given. Affected animals may also be given barbiturate as a relaxant, (in EU may not be appropriate for food animals) and should be given an antibiotic such as penicillin. The disease is normally controlled by hygiene, particularly at castration, although vaccination either of sows or piglets may be carried out using tetanus toxoid alone given in divided doses of 1 or 2 ml subcutaneously with an interval of 4 weeks. Tetanus toxoid is included in many sheep vaccines for protection against *C.perfringens* type C and other clostridia.

Clostridium novyi (*C. oedematiens* infection)

Definition

Clostridium novyi type B infection causes sudden death in large fattening pigs and sows.

Incidence

Sporadic, particularly in swill fed pigs and sows. Worldwide.

Aetiology

C.novyi (oedematiens) type B a large clostridium 5-10 µm or more in length with oval, central or subterminal spores is a fastidious anaerobe and is difficult to isolate.

Pathogenesis

Unknown at present, but these organisms produce powerful toxins and multiplication in the liver appears to follow or be associated with decrease in liver oxygenation resulting from chronic pneumonia or enteritis.

Clinical signs

Often found dead.

Pathology

Findings include submandibular swelling, pulmonary oedema and tracheal froth, sero-fibrinous or bloody exudates in the pericardial and peritoneal cavities, and most frequently, the presence of excess gas in the liver which appears light in colour and resembles "Aero" chocolate or foam rubber.

Diagnosis

Other causes of death should be excluded and C.novyi type B identified in the liver by fluorescent antibody staining. The organisms are large Gram-positive rods with oval subterminal spores. They may be post-mortem invaders and for that reason, culture may be unreliable. 10^3-10^6 organisms per g of liver can be demonstrated in affected livers. The diagnosis is complicated by post-mortem change, but is probable if the above changes are seen in freshly dead animals.

Treatment and control

Treatment of predisposing conditions such as pneumonia or enteritis with appropriate antimicrobials reduces the mortality and protection with a vaccine containing C.novyi (oedematiens) type B antigens may prevent the disease if given before the period of risk, e.g. in weaners or store pigs. Vaccines intended for sheep have been used.

Botulism

A rare, sometimes fatal flaccid paralysis of pigs resulting from ingestion of preformed toxin of Clostridium botulinum in food.

Incidence

Worldwide but rarely described.

Aetiology

C.botulinum is capable of multiplying in decaying animal and plant material at temperatures of 25-30°C and producing toxin. Six toxin types (A-F) exist.

Pathogenesis

Preformed toxin is ingested with contaminated food and is absorbed, probably via the lymphatics, to fix to the myoneural junction and prevent muscular contraction.

Clinical signs

Flaccid paralysis may occur 8 hours to 3 days after exposure and begins with the forelegs, progresses to the hindlegs and results in lateral recumbency and death. Anorexia, blindness and inability to control salivation and micturition may occur.

Animals which have collapsed should be killed.

Pathology

No gross lesions.

Epidemiology

The organism is widespread and the pig is relatively resistant. Ingestion of sufficient toxin to cause clinical signs depends upon consumption of sufficient contaminated feedstuff such as fish, meat or possibly vegetation such as spoiled silage. There is a risk to man from the ingestion of meat from affected pigs.

Other clostridia

C.difficile has been isolated from the small intestine of a pig with chronic diarrhoea and toxin has been demonstrated in faeces.

C.septicum and *C.chauvoei* may be isolated from cellulitis and gangrene as may *C.perfringens* type A or other clostridia.

Escherichia coli infections

E.coli infection causes neonatal septicaemia, neonatal diarrhoea, postweaning diarrhoea, oedema disease, cystitis and mastitis in pigs and can colonise existing lesions elsewhere in the body. Some strains form part of the normal faecal flora, whilst others are pathogenic.

Infections occur at different ages:

Septicaemia

"Colisepticaemia" is commonest in the newborn piglet 0-4 days of age and may be associated with diarrhoea.

Enteritis (Enteric colibacillosis) is associated with diarrhoea at three main periods in the pig's life:

1. Neonatal diarrhoea (0-4 days of age)
2. Neonatal - weaning diarrhoea. Between the neonatal period and weaning i.e. 4 days - 3-4 weeks.
3. Post-weaning diarrhoea or post-weaning enteritis associated with weaning.

Oedema disease usually occurs in pigs which have recently been weaned (see Bowel Oedema).

Mastitis and cystitis occur in adult sows.

E.coli disease in the young pig

Incidence

The organism occurs in every pig. Associated disease occurs when specific pathogenic strains enter a susceptible population or when management factors lead to an increase in challenge or a decrease in specific immunity. E.coli is identified as the cause of over 50% of all reported cases of pig enteritis in the UK and in many other countries.

Aetiology

E.coli is a normal inhabitant of the gut and is restricted to the lower small intestine and large intestine in mature healthy animals. The organism is a short Gram-negative rod or coccobacillus with flagellae, fimbriae or pili and sometimes a capsule. It grows aerobically and anaerobically on a wide variety of media to produce 3-5 mm colonies within 24 hours. Some are haemolytic on sheep blood agar and most isolates ferment lactose. Its identity is confirmed by biochemical tests and these can be used to separate the species into biotypes. Further classification is by serotyping based on 'O' or cell wall antigens, 'K' or capsular antigens 'H' or flagellar antigens and 'F' or fimbrial antigens. Monoclonal antibodies and DNA probes produced against pathogenic determinants allow pathotypes to be identified. Organisms may be further classified within strains by antibiotic resistance patterns (antibiograms) or plasmid profiles for epidemiological purposes. Analysis by other systems such as multilocus enzyme electrophoresis may not agree with serotypes.

E.coli can survive drying for months, is killed by heating to 66°C for 30 minutes and by most disinfectants. It is sensitive to a wide range of antimicrobials but resistance to most of them has been recorded.

Characters of pathogenic E.coli strains

Strains of E.coli with particular combinations of O and K antigens are associated with particular syndromes. Neonatal septicaemia strains are often non-haemolytic on sheep blood and include those such as 08 K87, K88 and 078 K80. They may be serum resistant due to the production of columinic acid and rarely adhere to intestinal epithelium.

E.coli strains involved in enteric disease possess a number of pathogenic features.

a) Fimbriae

Fimbriae or pili are filamentous structures 2.1-7.0 nm in diameter which allow the organisms to adhere to the brush borders of intestinal epithelial cells. Fimbriae associated with enteric disease include F4(K88) in the ab, ac or ad forms, (MW 27.5 kDa), F5 (K99), F6 (987P), F41 F107 (15.1 kDa). Others such as 2134P are being defined. Pili such as F165 (MW 18.5 kDa) are present on septicaemic strains and F107 on Bowel Oedema strains. Genes for most fimbriae have been sequenced and the proteins are being defined. The genes may be located on transmissible plasmids (F4, F5 and F6) or the chromosome (F41). An E.coli strain may possess genes for more than one fimbrial type but some of these such as F6 and F41 may only be expressed in appropriate conditions.

b) Toxins

Toxins produced by enterotoxigenic E.coli and are: LTp or heat labile toxin, MW 91.5 kDa which is antigenic and occurs in two parts, LTa and LTb; STa and STb, heat stable toxins which are non-antigenic (STap, MW 1.8-2.0 kDa) or poorly antigenic (STbp, MW 5.0 kDa) and VTIIv/SLTIIv or Verotoxin/Shiga-like toxin MW 70 kDa, and antigenic. The genes for these toxins are located on plasmids. Other toxins have been described such as a cytotoxin (Cytotoxic Necrotising Factor) and the haemolysin (Hly).

c) Outer Membrane Proteins

A 94 kDa outer membrane protein has been associated with the eae gene and with attachment to ileal brush borders and their effacement. The presence of many of these pathogenic determinants on plasmids means that they can occur in more than one strain.

A typical diarrhoea-producing strain is Abbotstown, 0149 K91, F4 (K88) ac which produces LT and STa, others are 09 K103 (987P), 0147 K89, F4 (K88). F5 (K99) and F6 (987P) strains do not produce LT but produce STa (STb). Recent studies with DNA probes have demonstrated that various combinations of determinants such as F4 (K88) STb LT, F4 (K88), F6 (987P) STb, LT, STa, F5 (K99) F41 STa (STb) and F4 (K88)-ve LT+ve can occur. The verocytotoxin may also occur in some isolates. It is present in all bowel oedema strains which include 0139 K82(B), 0138 K81(B), 0141 F107 (K85(B)) F4 (K88) ac and 041 K85(B).

Pathogenesis

The way in which E.coli causes disease has been the subject of considerable study. Bowel Oedema will be treated separately but the factors affecting a) the production of lesions by E.coli and b) the factors which allow the organism to reach numbers high enough to cause disease are both outlined below.

a) Pathogenic strains of *E.coli* produce their effect in the young pig by:-

i) direct invasion of the upper respiratory tract or anterior small intestine in the non-immune piglet to cause septicaemia. Strains involved in this way include 08, K87, F4 (K88) and 078, K80. Both capsule and F165 have been shown to be necessary for septicaemia in 0115K F165. Many strains are serum-resistant. Other enterobacteria may contaminate the umbilicus and cause septicaemia.

ii) attaching to the brush borders of the cells of the mucosal epithelium by their adhesive antigens or to the overlying mucus. The brush border and mucus receptors for several fimbrial types have been characterised and the genetics of some of them have been studied. Phenotypes A, B, C, D and E have been identified for F4 (K88) fimbriae. Phenotype A is associated with 210 and 240 kDa proteins which binds all three K88 variants ab, ac and ad; Phenotype B with the same proteins and binds K88 ab and K88 ac; Phenotype C binds K88 ac and K88 ad; Phenotype D binds K88 ad and Phenotype E none of the three forms. The expression of these receptors is under genetic control. Homozygotes with the genotype SS and heterozygotes Ss are susceptible to attachment and to F4 (K88) ac ab-mediated *E.coli* diarrhoea. Homozygotes with the genotype ss are resistant. A similar system Dd exists for F4 (K88) ad. Attachment sites for F4 (K88) antigen are more common in the anterior small intestine and also in younger pigs. F4 specific glycoprotein receptors of 90 kDa, 61 kDa and 28 kDa in mucus appear to increase with age. Attachment by F5 (K99) and F6 (987P) bearing *E.coli* strains occurs lower down the small intestine, particularly to sialic acid residues in the ileum. Receptors for both determinants have been defined and the expression of the receptors has been shown to be under genetic control.

iii) producing enterotoxin. Enterotoxigenic *E.coli* (ETEC) closely adherent to the brush border produce enterotoxins which affect cell membrane receptors which contain a ganglioside compound. LT stimulates the production of 3'5' cyclic AMP by adenyl cyclase and this acts on the ion-transport systems within the membrane to cause active secretion of chloride ions into the lumen. These are followed passively by water and sodium ions. The effect of LT toxin is sustained and it also affects tissues outside the gut. STa enterotoxin affects the cyclic guanosine monophosphate (GMP) transport system with a similar net result, but produces a more immediate reaction than LT toxin. STb appears to cause alterations in the apical epithelium of villi and to impair active alanine absorption. It is sensitive to trypsin. Some of the secreted fluid is reabsorbed lower down the intestine but the large intestinal capacity to absorb it is overcome and diarrhoea results. Metabolic acidosis and dehydration occur leading to circulatory collapse and death. Some strains of enterotoxigenic *E.coli* (ETEC) possess the gene for SLTIIv/VT but this toxin makes no contribution to enteritis.

iv) multiplication in the small and particularly the large intestine where they invade and destroy the epithelial cells of the mucosa to cause enteritis and subsequent diarrhoea. Systemic spread may occur. Cytotoxins are produced by some of these *E.coli* strains. (Colonisation and Necrotising Factor, CNF). Others attach to the brush border and efface microvilli becoming attached by pedestals. (Attaching and Effacing *E.coli* AEEC). These strains may also destroy epithelial cells. Haemorrhagic lesions may result from enterohaemorrhagic *E.coli* (EHEC)/

b) *E.coli* populations cause disease and reach high numbers in the pig intestine when the defence mechanisms (gastric acidity, other bacterial populations and antibody protection) are deficient in some way or when stress or infection with other infectious agents reduces their protective effect.

i) Genetic factors. The resistance of certain strains of pig to F4 (K88) infection because of the phenotype of their brush borders has been noted above. This type of resistance also occurs with F5 and F6 adhesions and similar systems apply for mucus receptors.

ii) Gastric acidity does not reach high levels until 3 or 4 days after birth. This may allow higher than normal numbers of *E.coli* to enter the small intestine.

iii) Gut flora changes. The intestine of the new born pig is bacteriologically sterile and the first organisms to colonise it multiply rapidly to reach high numbers. Some of these bacteria, e.g. lactobacilli and streptococci, are considered harmless but some strains of *E.coli* can produce disease at this stage. After colonisation, a balance forms between the members of the normal flora. Colonisation with *E.faecium* and pig strains of lactobacilli has been shown to reduce mortality from *E.coli* diarrhoea but not to prevent colonisation or to prevent the occurrence of diarrhoea.

iv) Non-specific colostral protection. It is becoming clear that fat globules in milk, whey proteins other than immunoglobulins and substances such as lactoferrin act together with maternal leucocytes in the milk to reduce the effect of *E.coli* disease in a non-specific manner.

v) Specific immune protection. The piglet can absorb colostral antibodies until 36 hours after birth, but until it does so, it is susceptible to septicaemia caused by environmental *E.coli*. The passive immunity obtained in this way protects against systemic invasion by *E.coli* strains experienced by the sow and lasts for 6-10 weeks. Passive immunity in the form of IgA, IgG and IgM antibodies directed against *E.coli* encountered by the sow is present in the milk and the IgA antibodies are adsorbed to the mucosa of the piglet's intestine. Here they prevent the adhesion or penetration of pathogenic *E.coli* and neutralise LT toxin thus preventing diarrhoea. In addition to anti-adhesive and antitoxic activity, the multiplication rate of *E.coli* in the lumen is reduced and phagocytosis by neutrophils is increased. Dams with the genotype ss do not form antibody to F4 (K88) and any progeny with the genotype Ss are unprotected against F4 (K88)-bearing pathogens. From 1-2 weeks of age, the piglet intestine is capable of producing antibodies to *E.coli* and from 2 weeks of age IgM and IgA antibodies are produced in gradually increasing quantities until, by 6 weeks of age, the full IgA response to intestinal antigens is operating. This response is protective against *E.coli* strains present in the normal intestine and feed but pathogenic strains of *E.coli* not previously experienced by the sow or the piglet may still colonise the gut and cause disease. However, the acute diarrhoea and septicaemia seen in the neonatal piglet is less common in older pigs because of increasing antibody protection. Diarrhoea may occur in piglets of 3-4 weeks of age at a time when passively-acquired IgG antibody levels in the serum are falling. IgA antibodies in the milk are still present, but their efficiency may be reduced by the presence of solid food in the diet. At this time, the piglet's own immune competence in terms of IgG and IgA antibody production is not yet sufficient to reduce the severity of *E.coli* infections.

vi) Infection with other agents. Infections with rotavirus, epidemic diarrhoea virus, coccidia, cryptosporidia and bacterial agents other than *E.coli* may also be important predisposing factors and cause syndromes which may be confused with *E.coli* infections or occur with *E.coli* in the field.

vii) Intestinal motility and secretions. The normal flow of food and secretions may exert a "flushing" effect of bacterial populations in the lumen. If interrupted, e.g. by stress or weaning, E.coli numbers may build up sufficiently in the small intestine to cause disease. Frequent small feeds reduce the severity of diarrhoea when compared with 1 or 2 daily feeds.

viii) Environmental and management factors. Changes such as chilling have now been shown to affect the duration of diarrhoea by an indirect effect through cortisol levels on immunity. Starvation, water, deprivation, other forms of stress and change in diet disturb the normal balance and allow pathogenic E.coli strains to multiply in the small intestine and cause disease. Dirty accommodation increases the number of infecting bacteria and makes clinical disease more likely.

From this point onwards the syndromes caused by *E.coli* will be considered separately.

Neonatal *E.coli* Septicaemia

Clinical signs

One or more newborn piglets in a litter may become ill within 12 hours of birth and die within 48 hours. Affected piglets stand apart from the rest of the litter with drooping tails, sink into recumbency and die after a period of unconsciousness, sometimes accompanied by convulsions and paddling movements. The body temperature may be high in the earlier stages of the disease but becomes subnormal before loss of consciousness occurs. Once body temperature has fallen below 35°C euthanasia should be considered.

Pathological findings

The post-mortem findings are not very specific. Piglets may be in good bodily condition, sometimes with cyanosis of the extremities. The carcase muscles may appear congested, the spleen may be enlarged and the stomach is usually filled with curd. When animals have not died immediately, there may be fibronopurulent polyserositis, polyarthritis and meningitis. Pneumonia may be present. Occasionally the intestine may be distended with pale contents indicating the presence of concurrent neonatal diarrhoea.

E.coli can be isolated from liver, spleen and heart blood in cases of septicaemia. The isolates may be identifiable as a pathogenic serotype.

Epidemiology

Neonatal septicaemia results from the infection of non-immune piglets - those which have not ingested colostrum or those which ingest colostrum lacking specific antibody. The organism is present in dirty farrowing accommodation or in the intestinal flora of the sow, having established itself too recently to give rise to immunity. Continuous farrowing, inadequate cleaning and poor environmental temperature control all increase the likelihood of infection. The introduction of a new strain to a farm may precipitate a 3-month long outbreak. Similarly the disease may occur in the progeny of recently-purchased gilts or sows. 0115 F165 *E.coli* may be responsible.

Diagnosis

Piglets with neonatal septicaemia can be distinguished by their good condition from those dying of starvation. Deaths occur only during the first 12-48 hours from this cause. The isolation of *E.coli* from freshly-dead carcases may confirm. Other causes of neonatal death should be considered. Strains associated with septicaemia such as 08K87, K88, 0781K80 and 0115 K-F165 may be isolated in pure culture from heart blood, liver and spleen as well as from gut.

Treatment

Affected piglets may be given parenteral or oral antimicrobial. The prognosis for affected piglets is poor. The remainder of the litter should be treated, also depressed piglets of similar age in adjacent litters. Suitable agents for injection include ampicillin, amoxycillin, streptomycin, gentamycin (where registered), apramycin, spectinomycin, neomycin, oxytetracycline and chlortetracycline, chloramphenicol, cephalosporins, fluoroquinolones such as enrofloxacin (where registered), baquiloprim and trimethoprim: sulphonamide. Long acting formulations of ampicillin, amoxycillin and oxytetracycline may be used to continue therapy.

Oral dosers may be used for 3-5 days, to treat the apparently unaffected litter with products which are active systemically. These include amoxycillin, ampicillin, trimethoprim sulphonamide. Supportive treatment using electrolyte replacers, correct heating etc., should be given.

Control

Ensure that colostrum has been taken and that temperature is adequate. No specific vaccines are yet available. If supplementary feeding of piglets is necessary, colostral substitutes may be of value.

Neonatal Diarrhoea

Clinical signs

Piglets affected by neonatal enteric colibacillosis show varying degrees of watery diarrhoea before death or recovery. Affected piglets may still suck but often stand with drooping tails and appear shrunken, lose the bloom from their skin and have erect coat hairs. Loss of flesh is apparent, particularly over the hips and backbone. The diarrhoeic faeces may be extremely difficult to see on casual inspection as it is often pale, creamy yellow in colour. Dried crusts of diarrhoeic faeces may be seen on the thighs or perineum and there may also be scalding about the anus. Affected pigs may enter a coma and die or recover without subsequent loss of condition after 3-6 days. Diarrhoeic faeces may be present in creeps and on the bars of slatted floors. Blood-stained diarrhoea may occur in some outbreaks.

Outbreaks of neonatal diarrhoea and septicaemia occur in farrowing houses where successive litters, particularly those of gilts or newly purchased sows, may be affected. In some cases the morbidity may reach 70% of all piglets born. Mortality from the septicaemic form approaches 100% of the affected piglets and 70% of piglets affected with diarrhoea in the first few days of life may die. Mortality rates then decrease rapidly until less than 10% mortality occurs in affected pigs over 2 weeks of age. Piglets which are extremely dehydrated and which do not respond to treatment should be killed.

Pathology

The carcase is dehydrated and the liver dark in colour. The stomach usually contains milk curd and may have infarctions of the wall, the small intestine is dilated, flaccid and mildly congested. In freshly-killed or very recently dead animals, the villi may be intact and finger-like in some enterotoxic diarrhoeas and in others some degree of villous atrophy may have occurred. The jejunum is the principal area affected by F4 (K88)+ve strains and the lower jejunum and ileum by F5 (K99)+ve and F6 (987P)+ve strains.

Blood may be present in the large intestinal contents where CNF-producing strains are involved. Both enterocolitis and interstitial pneumonia have been recorded in experimental infections. Microvillous effacement and pedestal formation my be visible in histological sections of the colons of freshly-killed piglets with AEEC.

Strictly enterotoxigenic *E.coli* strains are isolated only from the gut.

Epidemiology

Infection may originate from the sow, from residual contamination in poorly-cleaned pens or by lateral spread from adjacent affected litters. Failure to ingest colostrum and chilling predispose to the condition as does genetic susceptibility to F4 (K88), F5 (K99) or F6 (937P)-bearing organisms. The widespread use of vaccination of sows has reduced the prevalence of F4 (K88) in neonatal diarrhoea. It may also be more common in gilt litters.

Diagnosis

Watery diarrhoea in neonatal piglets may be confused with that caused by T.G.E., epidemic diarrhoea, rotavirus, *Clostridium perfringens* type A or type C, or *Campylobacter coli*. The piglets do not vomit (T.G.E. and epidemic diarrhoea), other pigs on the farm are rarely affected (T.G.E. and epidemic diarrhoea) and there is little gastritis and little villous atrophy (T.G.E., epidemic diarrhoea rotavirus and other viruses). In most cases there is no blood (*C.perfringens* type C, type A), no necrosis of the small intestinal mucosa (Clostridia) and no mucoid small intestinal or colonic contents (*C.coli*). Coccidial and cryptosporidial infections do not occur until the end of this period.

Where blood is present in the intestine, the condition may be distinguished from *C.perfringens* type C disease by the age of onset (earlier) and the pattern of mortality (100% of the affected litter in the clostridial disease), Confirmation depends upon bacteriology.

Laboratory confirmation of neonatal *E.coli* diarrhoeas can be obtained from faecal samples submitted as swabs or as whole faeces. The isolation of a pathogenic serotype in profuse or pure culture may suggest *E.coli* diarrhoea but, unless examinations for virus, other bacteria and protozoa are carried out, the identification of *E.coli* as the cause is only presumptive. It is better to send a carcase or a live piglet to the laboratory as T.G.E. and epidemic diarrhoea can then be ruled out and the characteristic post-mortem findings may be seen. Specific antibody or monoclonal antibody to pilus antigens has been used to identify pathogenic serotypes in frozen sections which may also be used for T.G.E. and epidemic diarrhoea diagnosis. The isolation of apparently pure cultures of pathogenic serotypes from the small intestine provides strong confirmatory evidence for the diagnosis of *E.coli* disease. ELISA tests for pilus antigens [F4 (K88), F5 (K99), F6 (987P) and F41] may be used on faeces, intestinal contents or swabs. Isolated colonies may be examined using reverse passive latex agglutination tests for pilus antigens F4, F5, F6 and F41 (Fimbrex, Central Veterinary Laboratory) and for LT and ST enterotoxins. F5 and F6 pilus antigens may only be expressed when cultures are grown on Minca medium.

DNA probes have been used to determine the pathogenic determinants of isolates and they are frequently serotyped using polyclonal sera to common pathogens e.g., Abbottstown. Polymerase chain reaction primers have now been described for most pathogenic determinants of *E.coli* but their use in diagnosis is not yet routine.

Treatment

Neonatal diarrhoea and other scours due to *E.coli* in sucking pigs may be treated parenterally using the agents listed for septicaemia oral therapy for 3-

5 days is preferable with those and the following agents: neomycin preparations and furazolidone, spectinomycin apramycin, sulfametopyrazine and enrofloxacin. Electrolyte replacement with Lectade GSL (S.K. Beecham) or other electrolyte preparations should be available or be given if piglets cannot drink. Maintaining adequate environmental temperature is helpful.

Failure of treatment may be due to antimicrobial resistance. Antimicrobial sensitivity should be determined. If organisms are sensitive and there is response to therapy, reconsider the diagnosis.

Control

Farrowing accommodation should be clean, dry and should be disinfected and, if possible, fumigated between farrowings. All-in-all-out husbandry (batch farrowing) should be practised. The sow may be scrubbed on entry to reduce contamination and creep heating should be arranged so as to ensure an even temperature of 35°C, 95°F for the first week of life. Soft sterilised sawdust bedding will improve comfort. All piglets should take colostrum. If this is not available, colostrum substitutes may be of value. Supplementary feeding should be carried out using proprietary sow milk replacer for best results. Water should be available and electrolyte solutions may be provided if neonatal diarrhoea occurs commonly. Oral medication given as soon as colostrum has been taken may prevent outbreaks in unprotected litters.

The prime method of prevention is by vaccination of the sow prior to farrowing to provide passive immunity in the colostrum.

Killed _E.coli_ vaccines given parenterally may induce serum antibody which is passed on to the piglets in the colostrum. Vaccines may be of the mixed pathogenic serotype variety (Porcovac, Hoechst) or contain strains carrying pathogenic determinants and enterotoxin antigens or the purified pathogenic determinants themselves. Examples available in the UK include Gletvax 6 Mallinkrodt, _C.perfringens_ type C, F4 (K88) ab, ac, F5 (K99) and F6 (987P), Suvaxyn _E.coli_ P4 Solvay Duphar veterinary adjuvanted pili F4 (K88, K99, 987P F41), Porcovac Plus Hoechst (mixed killed cells supplemented by K88 ab, K88 ac, K99, 987P and LT fragment B with alum adjuvant)] and Nobivac Porcol 5, Intervet (LT toxoid, K88 ab, K88 ac, K99 and 987P in an oil adjuvant). A primary course requires two doses 4 to 6 weeks apart with boosters every six months. Vaccination within two weeks of farrowing is not advised for most sow vaccines.

Killed oral vaccines containing 7 enteropathogenic serotypes (Intagen F. Hoffman La Roche) have been combined with vaccination of the sow prior to farrowing with a killed _E.coli_ vaccine to produce a similar effect. F4 (K88) plasmid may be eliminated from _E.coli_ in the gut of vaccinated pigs directly or by selection in the population. Autogenous vaccines from the farm of origin may be prepared and given dead or live (Kohler type) in some countries (but not in Britain). The live vaccine must be given some time prior to farrowing to avoid mortality and loss of productivity in the litter. Immunity from such vaccines may only last for a single lactation.

Recent experimental studies suggest that the inclusion of F41 antigens improves protection. STb has been shown to be poorly immunogenic.

Passive immunisation using hyperimmune sera to _E.coli_ may still be available in some countries and provide some degree of protection. The most common form of passive immunity is provided by colostrum substitutes which are given to neonatal piglets by stomach tube at birth. These may contain porcine or bovine antibodies to _E.coli_ (not necessarily to pathogenic determinants) and may be of value in the control of neonatal diarrhoea problems.

The efficacy of all biological methods of control varies and although mortality is reduced and loss of productivity is prevented, protection may not be complete. The failure of ss genotype dams to recognise K88 antigen in vaccines may be partly responsible, also the involvement of serotypes of *E.coli* not included in the vaccines and the uneven intake of colostrum and protective milk in sucking piglets which can reduce protection. Failure of a vaccination programme should involve re-examination of the diagnosis, the methods of administering the vaccine, environmental factors such as temperature and hygiene and the intake of colostrum in neonates. Finally, confirmation of the compatibility of vaccines and the serotypes/pathotypes present on the farm should be assessed, as changes in fimbrial types have occurred in *E.coli* populations following vaccination programmes.

Probiotics are commonly given to piglets soon after birth but whatever their claimed efficacy in the prevention of neonatal diarrhoea, they do not protect non-immune piglets against experimental challenge.

E.coli diarrhoea between the neonatal period and weaning (3 week scour, milk scour).

Clinical signs

A greyish or whitish diarrhoea may occur in unweaned piglets between 10 and 28 days of age. Affected animals become emaciated and hairy and may remain permanently stunted. Diarrhoea of this type may also occur, sometimes with fever, in piglets of any age fed on milk replacer diets or where creep feed of unsuitable quality is given. This is traditionally attributed to *E.coli* and the organisms may be present but many other agents have been incriminated.

Whole litters are rarely affected, but the larger animals in almost every litter may be affected on some farms. Mortality is usually less than 20%. Haemorrhagic gastroenteritis may occur from 8 days onwards. Affected piglets die suddenly or after the passage of a brownish diarrhoea.

The faeces of recovering animals becomes progressively firmer but usually remains white. The most common indication for humane slaughter is chronic stunting.

Pathology

Similar to that of neonatal diarrhoea. In most cases pathogenic *E.coli* is isolated from lesions of coccidiosis, rotavirus infection or coronavirus infection, as a secondary invader.

Epidemiology

Primary *E.coli* outbreaks are most likely in this age group in the litters of gilts or when a new serotype is introduced to a herd. In most cases the disease which occurs in successive litters is initiated by coccidia or rotavirus and infection persists from neonatal diarrhoea.

Diagnosis

The demonstration of features of *E.coli* enteritis described under neonatal diarrhoea and the isolation of pathogenic *E.coli* in pure and profuse culture suggest primary *E.coli* diarrhoea.

The above features may distinguish *E.coli* enteritis from other conditions, but in this age period (from 4 days-weaning), mixed infections are not uncommon. Sudden death, with or without brownish diarrhoea and congested intestines may indicate haemorrhagic enteritis. As coccidiosis, cryptosporidium and *C.perfringens* type C secondary infection can all occur in this age group, the appropriate bacteriological and histological findings should be present before diagnosis is confirmed.

Treatment

As neonatal diarrhoea, ensuring that electrolyte is present in the pen. Recently antimicrobials have been included in sterilised peat but no controlled studies of uptake have been carried out.

Control

Sow vaccination may have a residual effect on *E.coli* in pigs of this age and medicated first creep given fresh in small quantities daily may reduce the occurrence of disease. Water medication and electrolyte may also reduce the involvement of *E.coli* in diarrhoea at this age.

Postweaning Enteritis Post weaning diarrhoea)

Clinical signs

Postweaning diarrhoea occurs within 10 days of weaning, often within 4-5 days of the change of diet. Affected pigs pass greyish, brownish, or watery diarrhoeic faeces with no traces of blood. Haemorrhagic diarrhoea is extremely uncommon. Mucus is rarely present. The diarrhoea is usually transient and resolves within 3-5 days but it may persist, and deaths from dehydration or septicaemia may occur in adverse husbandry conditions. In some cases fever (up to 40.6°C, 105°F) may occur over a period of 4 or 5 days and affected animals may be anorexic and depressed. Chronic post-weaning enteritis may cause permanent stunting in recovered pigs. Faeces may be difficult to see in flat decks or in veranda houses. The feeders in flat decks and the corners of the dunging areas in veranda houses should be examined for signs of diarrhoea in full-slatted accommodation. Where inspection is difficult, affected animals may be identified by their dehydrated appearance, and perineal staining.

20-50% of all weaned pigs may be affected, but mortality from the uncomplicated disease is less than 10% of those affected unless complications occur. Even when diarrhoea is only transient, marked reduction in the rate of daily liveweight gain may occur in the remainder of an affected group.

Chronically stunted or severely dehydrated animals which are unable to rise should be killed.

Pathology

The carcase is usually dehydrated, the eyes sunken and there may be some faint cyanosis of the extremities. The serous surfaces are sticky, the liver is congested and the stomach full of feed in most cases. The gastric mucosa may be congested (a non-specific change) and the small intestine is dilated and congested with watery, buff-coloured contents which can be seen through the wall. The mucosal epithelium is congested and the villi are intact. The colon and rectum contain fluid faeces or are empty.

Histological examination may be useless due to autolysis, but in freshly-killed piglets, the villi appear intact, are often congested and may sometimes be covered with adherent bacteria. Varying degrees of cell shedding may be seen. In haemorrhagic enteritis associated with attaching and effacing *E.coli*, characteristic palisades of attached organisms may be seen on the brush border with effacement of the microvilli and cup and pedestal formation of the lumenal surface. This type of lesion may be seen in the duodenum. Haemorrhage and ulceration may occur in the large intestine in this rare form of the disease.

Pure growths of ß-haemolytic F4 (K88)-positive *E.coli* can usually be isolated from the anterior small intestine or F5 (K99)-positive or F6 (987P) E.coli from the posterior small intestine in enteric colibacillosis but not from other organs outside the gut. Isolates may subsequently be identified as known pathogenic serotypes or pathotypes. It is not uncommon for more than one pathotype to be present in affected animals after recovery but only pure cultures are usually present during acute disease.

Epidemiology

The mixing of immune carrier and non-immune piglets at weaning, the loss of maternal immune protection, the change of environment and contact with poorly cleaned pens or drainage from pens containing other affected pigs contribute to the development of the disease. The purchase of pigs, their mixing and introduction to new diets and cold dirty pens or houses with an existing problem may be contributory factors in outbreaks.

On a national scale, a particular *E.coli* serotype may be associated with outbreaks of clinical disease and may then be succeeded by other serotypes. However, certain serotypes have been isolated consistently from enteric colibacillosis over long periods of time. Examples include 0149 K91 F4 (K88) ac (Abbottstown) which still accounts for many outbreaks in the UK.

Diagnosis

The clinical findings of a grey-brown watery diarrhoea 3-5 days after weaning are suggestive. T.G.E. and epidemic diarrhoea rarely affect the post-weaning age group alone and are rarely associated with fever or mortality. In salmonellosis, high fever, necrotic material in the faeces, discoloured skin and a septicaemic carcase may be seen. The post-mortem appearance in *E.coli* post-weaning enteritis is characteristic. The isolation of pure cultures of pathogenic *E.coli* confirm the diagnosis. Spirochaetal diarrhoea has an incubation period of 6-7 days or more, and the slightly mucoid appearance to the faeces and the restriction of lesions to the large intestine distinguishes it from *E.coli*. Spirochaetes are present in large numbers in the faeces. In rotavirus diarrhoeas the agent may be identified and where *C.perfringens* type A or other clostridia are involved large numbers of sporulating *C.perfringens* type A are present and enterotoxin or specific cytotoxins are identifiable by vero cell assay or the Reverse Passive Latex Agglutination test. Cryptosporidial infection is usually chronic and does not affect pigs so acutely.

Treatment

Severely affected pigs may be treated parenterally using the products listed for neonatal septicaemia but therapy is normally given in feed or water. Water medication is preferable using antimicrobials such as ampicillin, amoxycillin, apramycin, neomycin, tetracyclines, trimethoprim:sulphonamide combinations, spectinomycin, furazolidone, gentamycin and cephalothin (where registered). Treatment should be continued for 3-5 days and should be started as soon as clinical signs are noted.

In feed medication at therapeutic levels can also be given either after the outbreak has begun or over the period of risk and should be continued for at least 10 days and preferably for 3-5 weeks. Agents for in-feed medication include chlortetracycline, oxytetracycline, apramycin, neomycin, sulphonamide, trimethoprim: sulphonamide and enrofloxacin. Recently furazolidone has been banned from infeed use in the UK.

Treatment should be accompanied by correction of environmental temperature, and by disinfection of the pen towards the end of the treatment period and may be supplemented by fluid replacement with Lectade GSL, (S.K. Beecham) or antibiotic containing proprietary electrolyte-replacing solutions. If there is no response to treatment which has previously been effective, re-examine diagnosis and check antimicrobial sensitivity of *E.coli* as antimicrobial resistance can develop readily in this organism.

Non-antimicrobial treatment. Experimental studies have been carried out with enterotoxin antagonists and these show some promise but are not yet available.

Bacteriophage treatment. Experimental and field studies suggest that phage suspensions specific for enteropathogenic *E.coli* strains can be used in treatment.

Control

Recently-weaned pigs should be maintained at an even temperature for the first week. If kept dry and warm in clean surroundings, postweaning enteritis is less likely to occur. Dusty surroundings and chilling exacerbate morbidity. Affected piglets should be treated promptly and other litters of susceptible age watched. Avoid change of feed at weaning and reduce quantity slightly. Ensure feed is clean and fresh. The use of totally digestible diets may also reduce diarrhoea at weaning. Some suggestions have been made that the use of large amounts of creep feed fed before weaning may reduce any immunological component of enteric disease at weaning. There is little evidence for this view. Lactic acid in the diet may reduce gastric pH and reduce the multiplication of *E.coli*. Probiotics containing porcine lactobacilli, toyocerin and *E.faecium* may reduce the severity of disease but do not prevent it in controlled experiments.

Medication at treatment level may be given over the period of risk. Water medication is preferable as it does not require a change of ration.

Some "growth promoters" (or permitters) with an effect on *E.coli* may be incorporated in the feed (creep or weaner ration) over the period of risk and may help prevent the development of the disease. Examples include carbadox and olaquindox (Bayonox, Bayer where registered) Treatment may also be given over this period.

Vaccination of the sow may have some residual effect if weaning is at 3-4 weeks of age but protection of the piglet at weaning requires vaccination of the piglet. Vaccines used for sows may be used to vaccinate piglets in the first week of life. Oil adjuvanted vaccines should be avoided unless there is a specific claim for protection. Endotoxin levels in vaccines containing whole cells may be unsuitable for piglets. Live, unattenuated vaccines should not be used. Experimental studies suggest that protection is not complete.

Intagen (F. Hoffman La Roche) can be incorporated in pre-starter creep and weaner rations to protect the weaned animal against *E.coli* component of post-weaning diarrhoea. It is safe and relies upon the stimulation of enteric IgM and IgA antibody to pathogenic strains of *E.coli*.

References

Attridge, S., Hackett, J., Morona, R., Whyte, P. (1988). Vaccine 6, 387-389. Towards a live oral vaccine against enterotoxigenic *E.coli* of swine.
Brinton, C.C., Fusco, P., Wood, S. and Jayappa, H. (1983). Vet.Med. S.A.C. 78, 962-966. A complete vaccine for neonatal swine colibacillosis and the prevalence of *E.coli* pili on swine isolates.
Broes, A., Fairbrother, J.M., La Riviere, S., Jacques, M. and Johnson, W.M. (1988). Infection & Immunity 56, 241-246. Virulence properties of enterotoxigenic *E.coli* 08 KX105 strains isolated from diarrhoeic piglets.
Conway, P.L., Welin, A., Cohen, P.S. (1990). Infection & Immunity 58, 3178-3182. Presence of K88 specific receptors in porcine ileal mucus is age specific.
Cupere, F. de., Deprez, P., Demeulenaere, D., Muyle, E. (1992). J.Vet Med., Series B 39, 277-284. Evaluation of the effect of 3 probiotics on experimental *E.coli* enterotoxaemia in weaned piglets.
Dean, E.A. (1990). Infection & Immunity 58, 4030-4035. Comparison of receptors for 987P pili of enterotoxigenic *E.coli* in the small intestines of neonatal and older pigs.
Dean, E.A., Whipp, S.C. and Moon, H.S. (1989). Infection & Immunity 57, 82-87. Age specific colonisation of the porcine intestinal epithelium by 987P piliated enterotoxigenic *E.coli*.
Dubreuil, J.D., Fairbrother, J.M., Lalier, R., La Riviere, S. (1991). Infection & Immunity 59, 198-203. Production and purification of heat stable enterotoxins from a porcine *E.coli* strain.
Erickson, A.K., Willgohs, J.A., McFarland, S.Y., Benfield, D.A. and Francis, D.H. (1992). Infection & Immunity 60, 983-988. Identification of brush border glycoproteins that bind the K88 ac adhesion of *E.coli* and correlation of these glycoproteins with adhesive phenotype.
Fairbrother, J.M., Broes, A., Jacques, M., La Riviere, S., Am.J.Vet.Res. (1989). 50, 1029-1036. Pathogenicity of *E.coli* 0115 K "V165" strains isolated from pigs with diarrhoea.
Faubert, C., Drolet, R. (1992). Canadian Vet..J. 33, 251-256. Haemorrhagic gastroenteritis caused by *E.coli* in piglets. Clinical, pathological and microbiological findings.
Helie, P., Morin, M., Jacques, M., Fairbrother, J.M. (1991). Infection & Immunity 59, 814-821. Experimental infection of newborn pigs with an attaching and effacing *E.coli* O45K "E65" strain.

131

Hornes, E., Wateson, Y., Olsvik, O. (1991). J.Clin.Micro. 29, 2375-2379. Detection of E.coli heat stable enterotoxin genes in pig stool, specimens by an immobilised colourimetric nested PCR.
Kelly, D., O'Brien, J.J., McCracken, K.J. (1990). Res.Vet.Sci. 49, 223-228. Effect of creep feeding on the incidence, duration and severity of post-weaning diarrhoea.
Kortbeek Jacobs, J.M.C., Kooten, P.J.S. van, Donk, J.A. Vander Dyk, J.E., van, Rutten, V.P. (1984). Vet.Microbiol. 9, 287-299. The effect of oral immunisation on the population of lymphocytes migrating to the mammary glands of the sow.
Kuyogushima, M., Ginsburg, V., Kiwan, H.C. (1989). Arch.Biochem. 270, 391-397. E.coli K99 binds to N-glycolyl sialoparagloboside and N glycolyl GM3 found in piglet small intestine.
Metcalf, J.W., Krogfelt, K.A., Krivan, H.C., Cohen, P.S., Laux, D.C. (1991). Infection & Immunity 59, 91-96. Characterisation and identification of a small intestine mucus receptor for the K88 ab fimbrial adhesin.
Mills, K.W., Teitze, K.L., Phillips, R.M. (1983). Am.J.Vet.Res. 2188-2189. Use of an ELISA for detection of K88 pili in fecal specimens from swine.
Morris, J.A., Sojka, W.J. and Wells, G.A.H. (1982). Vet.Rec. 111, 165-166. K99 and 987P adhesins on E.coli enteropathogenic for piglets.
Nagy, L.K., Painter, K.R. and Mackenzie, T. (1985). Vet.Rec. 116, 123-125. Vaccination with K88, K99 and 987P. Evaluation of procholeragenoid against experimental colibacillosis in piglets of vaccinated dams.
Rose, R., Moon, H.W. (1985). Infection and Immunity 48, 818-823. Elicitation of enteroluminal neutrophils by enterotoxigenic and non-enterotoxigenic strains of E.coli in swine.
Smith, H. and Huggins, M.B. (1983). J.Gen.Microbiol. 129, 2659-2675. The effectiveness of phages in treating experimental E.coli diarrhoea in calves, piglets and lambs.
Woodward, M.J., Kearsley, R., Wray, C., Roeder, P.L. (1990). Veterinary Microbiology 22, 277-290. DNA probes for the toxin genes in E.coli isolated from diarrhoeal disease in cattle and pigs.
Wray, C., Piercy, D.W.T., Carroll, P.J., Cooley, W.A. (1993). Res.vet.Sci. 54, 290-298. Experimental infection of neonatal pigs with CNF toxin-producing strains of E.coli.

Oedema disease

Definition

Oedema disease or bowel oedema is seen in pigs especially after weaning. It is characterised by the occurrence of sudden death and the development of oedema and nervous signs in variable numbers of pigs in a pen. It is caused by enteric infection with certain serotypes of E.coli which produce a toxin with effects on the arterial walls.

Incidence

Occurs worldwide and on individual farms it may be important, but not common in Britain at present.

Aetiology

The syndrome is caused by infection with *E.coli* strains capable of expressing VTII (SLT IIv) or enterotoxaemic *E.coli* (ETEEC). They usually belong to serotypes 0139: K12: H1, 0138 K81 NW, 0141 K85 ab H4 and 0141 K85 a, c H_4, but VT may be present in other strains along with enterotoxins. 86% *E.coli* isolates from cases of oedema disease have been shown to express F107 fimbriae (major subunit protein MW 15.1 kDa) although this is clearly not the only adhesin.

Pathogenesis

The *E.coli* strains responsible for Oedema Disease multiply throughout the small intestine and adhere to the brush borders of the epithelial cells. Adhesion appears to be governed by a genetic mechanism and pigs phenotypically resistant to Oedema Disease have been found to possess epithelial cells resistant to adhesion by F107+ve *E.coli* and *vice versa*.

E.coli levels reached 4×10^9 per ml in the mid jejunum and the organism clusters on and adheres to the villous epithelium. *E.coli* levels are greatest 2 days post-infection and prior to the appearance of clinical signs of oedema disease. Toxin is produced and absorbed and causes hypertension following which angiopathy develops in the submucosal arterioles.

Lesions in the blood vessels begin 2 days post-infection with swelling and vacuolation of endothelial cells followed by sub-endothelial deposition of fibrin, perivascular oedema, microthrombus formation, necrosis of the tunica media and endothelial proliferation. There may also be damage to the submucosal nervous plexuses. These changes in the arterial walls appear to be responsible for the oedema seen in the tissues in this disease and for the nervous signs and central nervous system lesions. The toxin appears to damage cells by inhibition of protein synthesis and both lesions and the syndrome can be reproduced by giving as little as 3ng of pure toxin/kg intravenously although 6ng/kg is required to kill pigs.

Enterotoxin production by VT producing strains of *E.coli* may result in concurrent diarrhoea and catarrhal enteritis has been recorded in some outbreaks of oedema. Recovery from infection may be accompanied by the development of antibody to both F107 fimbriae and to a lesser extent to VT.

Clinical signs

The disease usually occurs within 10 days of weaning and affects one or more of the better piglets in the group. Outbreaks often commence with one or more pigs being found dead and others may have varying degrees of nervous disturbance may be present. Affected pigs appear dull, may appear blind and may show head pressing. General incoordination and loss of balance occur later and may be noted at feeding time. Affected animals lag behind others and are less able to reach the trough. Lateral recumbency with paddling movements leading to coma and death normally follow within 4-36 hours of the onset of clinical signs. Affected pigs may have oedema of the eyelids, nose and ears and early cases may have a peculiar, squeaky voice. Body temperature may reach 40°C, 104°F, early in the disease but rectal temperature is often normal at the onset of clinical signs. Neither constipation nor diarrhoea is a constant feature, but a short period of diarrhoea may precede the onset of oedema disease proper. Affected pigs may recover completely apart from a check in growth or remain with a head tilt, gait disturbance or paralysis. Paralysed animals should be killed humanely, as should those where gait disturbances are sufficiently severe for physical damage to develop.

Pathological findings

Dead animals are usually in good condition with full stomachs. Cyanosis is rarely present and oedema of the eyelids and face may be visible in recently dead animals. The most constant finding is oedema of the wall of the greater curvature of the stomach, where it occurs between the mucosa and the muscle layers. Jelly-like areas of oedema may also be present in the mesocolon, in the larynx and in the kidney capsule. Clear fluid may be present in the body cavities. Ischaemia of the kidney cortex and congestion of the medulla may be noted and all the carcase lymph nodes may be oedematous. Oedema disappears rapidly once the carcase is opened and may disappear after death. It may be absent if enteritis is also present. Histological findings usually confirm the presence of oedema in the stomach wall and in the brain where the perivascular spaces may be very pronounced. In chronic cases encephalomalacia is seen. The underlying lesion is hyaline degeneration and fibrinoid necrosis in arteries and arterioles. Proliferative arteriopathy develops as the lesions age and may be seen in pigs which have not died until several days after the onset of the disease. Histological lesions may be present in sub-clinically affected animals.

Epidemiology

The disease may affect 10-30% of recently weaned pigs with up to 100% mortality in the affected animals, and is normally restricted to pigs in this age group. The use of treatment may postpone its onset. The disease does not appear to spread from herd to herd and it was rare in Britain but is now increasing in incidence, particularly in early weaned pigs and in those which receive rations with no feed additives. Recent outbreaks have caused 30% mortality for some weeks and may be associated with changes in the susceptibility of breeding stock.

Diagnosis

The clinical signs and the post-mortem findings in recently dead animals are distinctive. When cases of sudden death occur alone, the condition must be distinguished from other causes of such deaths such as mulberry heart disease, Hertztod and anthrax. The absence of high fever and the presence of oedema enable the nervous signs to be differentiated from those of Teschen-Talfan disease, streptococcal meningitis, salt and organic arsenical poisoning. The high, squeaky voice is of use here. Oedema of the colonic mesentery may be seen in early cases of spirochaetal diarrhoea and swine dysentery, but the involvement of the colon in those diseases is diagnostic.

The isolation of serotypes of *E.coli* such as 0139 K81, 0139 K12 and 0141 K58 from the small intestine may be confirmatory and the demonstration of verotoxins in culture supernates also confirms. DNA probes for verotoxin have been used to identify potentially pathogenic strains.

Treatment

Affected pigs rarely recover, but some courses of treatment are frequently adopted and may be of value to the group they are:

a) <u>antibiotic therapy</u> - usually injection or water treatment with a tetracycline streptomycin, enrofloxacin ampicillin and other antimicrobials effective against *E.coli*, on the basis that reduction of *E.coli* numbers in the gut may prevent further cases. (For antimicrobials see Postweaning Enteritis above).

b) <u>reduction of blood pressure in clinically affected animals.</u> The value of this has not been fully established and in such animals nursing may be of more value. Melperone 4-6mg/kg may be of value

c) <u>reduction of feed intake.</u> Restriction of feed intake or the inclusion of bran or other roughage in the diet may reduce the *E.coli* load in the remainder of the group.

<u>Control</u>

Control is based on the prevention of the build up of pathogenic *E.coli* populations in the gut. Pigs on an affected farm should be weaned by removal of the sow and placed on a low level diet. It has been suggested that increasing creep levels before weaning may be of value and increasing roughage levels afterwards may reduce the incidence. Unfortunately, the use of sufficient roughage to inhibit *E.coli* colonisation depresses growth and leaves treated pigs susceptible as colonisation never reaches levels required to induce immunity. Weaning with scrupulous attention to hygiene and environment has been coupled with frequent small feeds of digestible rations after weaning in some UK herds. The amounts of feed are gradually increased.

Treatment levels of antimicrobials effective against colibacillosis may be included in the drinking water or feed (see Postweaning enteritis above) during the period of risk. The use of growth promoters such as olaquindox and carbadox also appears to reduce the incidence. Recent studies have shown that antibody to both F107 fimbriae and VTIIv may be protective. The inactivated toxin is antigenic but is difficult to detoxify and alteration of the molecule has been found to reduce its toxigenicity but retain antigenicity. No vaccine is yet available commercially.

It is not yet possible to select resistant pigs on a commercial scale.

<u>References</u>

Awad Masalmeh, M., Schuh, M., Kofer, J. and Quaryi, E. (1989). Deutscher Tierartzliche Wochenschrift 96, 397-432. Uberprufung der Schutzwirkung eines Toxoid P impfstoffes gegen die Oedemakrankheit des Absetzferkels im Infektionsmodell.
Bertschinger, H.U. and Pohlenz, J. (1983). Vet.Path. 20, 99-110. Bacterial colonisation and morphology of the intestine in porcine *E.coli* enterotoxaemia (Oedema Disease).
Bertschinger, H.U. and 7 authors (1990). Vet.Microbiol. 25, 267-281. Adhesive fimbriae produced *in vivo* by E.coli 0139 K12(B) H1 associated with enterotoxaemia in pigs.
Bertschinger H.U., Stamm, M., Vogell, P. (1993). Vet.Micro. 35, 79-89. Inherited resistance to Oedema Disease.
Imberechts, H., Greve, H de., Lintermans, P. (1992). Vet.Microbiol. 31, 221-233. The pathogenesis of edema disease in pigs.

Imberechts, H. and 11 other authors (1992). Inf. & Immun. 60, 1963-1971. Characterisation of F107 fimbriae of E.coli 107/86 which causes oedema disease in pigs and nucleotide sequence of the F107 major fimbrial subunit gene.

MacLeod, D.L., Gyles, C.L. (1991). Vet.Microbiol. 29, 309-318. Immunisation of pigs with a variant Shiga-like toxin II variant toxoid.

MacLeod, D.L., Gyles, C.L., Wilcock, B.P. (1991). Vet.Path. 28, 66-73. Reproduction of Edema Disease of swine with purified Shiga-like toxin II variant.

Methiyapun, S., Pohlenz, J.F.L., Bertschinger, H.U. (1984). Vet.Path. 21, 516-520. Ultrastructure of the intestinal mucosa in pigs experimentally inoculated with an edema disease-producing strain of E.coli (0139: K12 H1).

Stamm, M. and Bertschinger, H.U. (1992). Proc. IPVS. 12, 242. Identification of pigs genetically resistant to oedema disease by testing adhesion of E.coli expressing F107 to intestinal epithelial cells.

Salmonellosis

Definition

Salmonellosis caused by *Salmonella choleraesuis* occurs as outbreaks of septicaemia, acute enteritis or chronic enteritis and wasting in weaned pigs of 10-16 weeks of age. Morbidity and mortality may be high in affected groups. Infection with other salmonellae may be inapparent, cause mild enteritis or more severe disease resembling that caused by *S.choleraesuis*.

Incidence

The incidence of salmonellosis varies from country to country. In Denmark where national monitoring is carried out 11.8% herds were infected in 1993. In the UK where isolation is reported about 140-150 isolations are reported annually. These figures are typical of EU countries. Infections in EU countries are rarely due to *S.choleraesuis* in contrast to the situation in the mid-West of the US where most outbreaks are due to *S.choleraesuis*. Only one isolation of *S.choleraesuis* has been reported in the UK recently (1993).

Aetiology

Salmonellosis is caused by Gram-negative bacteria of the genus Salmonella. These grow readily on MacConkey and other bile agars and do not ferment lactose (*S.arizona* may do so). They are classified into named serotypes by the antigenic factors present on their O or somatic antigens and the antigens on their H or flagellar antigens. Final differentiation within 'species' is carried out by phage typing, plasmid profiling and resistance pattern. Recent changes to the nomenclature of this group mean that the only species of pathogenic salmonella is *S.choleraesuis* and all others are serotypes. In this book the serotypes will be referred to by their conventional names. *S.typhimurium*, *S.derby*, *S.saintpaul*, *S.infantis*, *S.heidelberg*, *S.typhisuis* and *S.cholereasuis* may all ocur in pigs.

Pathogenesis

S.choleraesuis is primarily a pig pathogen, capable of infecting pig herds for long periods. Clinically-normal carrier animals appear to carry the organism in the gut mucosa or mesenteric lymph nodes. Invasion of the mucosa and subsequent systemic spread often occurs after stresses such as weaning or transportation.

Infection normally follows ingestion of the organism which then multiplies in the small intestine to reach high numbers (*S.typhimurium*). Organisms may adhere to the epithelium (*S.typhimurium*) and enter enterocytes to pass through them or multiply within them to cause cell death. The genetic control of this process of adhesion and invasion is currently being studied, but may be associated with the possession of a 50 kbp plasmid (*S.choleraesuis*). *S.choleraesuis, S.infantis* and invasive strains of other serotypes may also be taken up by the epithelium of Peyer's patches and reach the mesenteric lymph nodes 24 hours after infection and become distributed systemically.

S.choleraesuis and some other serotypes are carried by macrophages in which they may multiply. Organisms may be released in organs such as the liver to form micro-colonies surrounded by necrosis and macrophages. Those which remain within macrophages cause endothelial damage and microthrombus formation throughout the body. The effects of this are most severe where end arteries occur. Systemic effects of the disease are also related to the sites of multiplication. Enteric lesions are associated with loss of the enterocytes and the resulting catarrhal enteritis. The effects of systemic infection on submucosal blood vessels contributes to enteritis in invasive strains (*S.choleraesuis*) and enterotoxin production has been reported in *S.typhimurium* infection. The inflammatory gastrointestinal lesions may become necrotic. Infection is followed by the development of systemic antibodies from day 7 post-infection, peaking at 28 days post-infection and declining but still demonstrable 80 days post-infection. Cellular immunity also develops and animals are immune to challenge but often remain carriers.

Clinical signs

Pigs of all ages can be affected although outbreaks are commonest in pigs aged between weaning and 3 or 4 months. The septicaemic form is commonest among younger pigs. Animals may be found dead (mortality almost 100% in this form) or be depressed, dull with weakness and even nervous signs. Affected animals often bury themselves in straw and show mauve-red cyanosis of the ears, limbs and the centre of the back. Affected pigs have a temperature of 40.6-41.7°C, 105-107°F and die within 24-48 hours. The acute enteric form also occurs in younger pigs and may follow septicaemia in animals which do not die. Affected animals pass a thin watery, yellowish diarrhoea and may be dull and fevered (40.6-41.7°C, 105-107°F. Pneumonic signs, weakness and nervous signs such as paralysis and tremor may occur. In severely affected cases, skin discolouration is present. Recovered pigs may slough affected ears or tails. In the chronic enteric form affected pigs appear severely emaciated and may have intermittent fever. There is persistent diarrhoea.

Infection with serotypes other than *S.choleraesuis* rarely result in death except in sucking pigs. Diarrhoea is the most prominent clinical sign although fever may occur. The diarrhoea is initially brownish (or creamy in sucking piglets) and rarely contains blood. It may contain necrotic material and sometimes has a characteristic smell.

Chronically affected animals may become stunted and some may develop the rectal stricture syndrome in which the rectum may be occluded. Euthanasia should be carried out on septicaemic animals which are moribund, those with acute respiratory distress, on chronic wasted pigs and on those with complete rectal stricture.

Pathological findings

Septicaemic form. The carcases may be in good condition and may show discolouration of the skin and ears. Few gross lesions may be seen, but multiple haemorrhages, enlarged haemorrhagic lymph nodes and enlarged spleens often occur. Widespread focal necrosis and hyaline capillary thrombosis is seen histologically.

Acute enteric form. Skin discolouration may be present. The gut appears inflamed and the contents may be watery with some necrotic material. There may be infarction or ulceration of the gastric mucosa and the mucosa of both small and large intestines may be inflamed and necrotic in later cases. The mesenteric lymph nodes may be enlarged and haemorrhagic. The lungs may be pneumonic and hepatised, the liver is usually pale and there may be petecchiae on the kidneys.

Chronic enteric form. The gut is thickened and the mucosa is usually necrotic. Button ulcers are occasionally seen at the ileocaecolic junction and the mesenteric lymph nodes are usually haemorrhagic. "Typhoid nodules", the result of necrotic foci, may be seen in the liver.

Diarrhoeic form due to salmonellae other than *S.choleraesuis.* Varying degrees of inflammation of the small intestinal mucosa, enlargement, ulceration of the Peyer's patches and lymphadenitis may be present but the changes are not specific. Necrosis of the Peyer's patches and later of the mucosa of both small and large intestine may follow. Rectal strictures associated with mega-colon may be identified. Salmonellae may be isolated from the parenchymatous organs in septicaemic disease and from the mesenteric lymph nodes, gall bladder and intestinal mucosa in the enteric form.

Epidemiology

S.choleraesuis infection may be enzootic on some farms and then appears only in weaned pigs 12-16 weeks of age. Infection is usually introduced to a herd by the purchase of carrier pigs or animals infected by contact at markets. Recent studies suggest that tonsillar carriage or survival in the environment may be uncommon on infected farms. The reason for the marked difference in incidence and prevalence of this condition between EU countries and mid-Western states of the US is unknown.
Outbreaks of salmonellosis due to other Salmonella serotypes may result from contamination of feed by rodents or birds or from contaminated animal protein. The widespread use of pelleted or heat-treated feeds in the UK has reduced this source of infection.
Infection may be introduced with weaners, store pigs or breeding stock or in infected faeces contaminating transport or clothing. Spread within farms occurs by the faecal oral route along lines of drainage contact, within pens and by faecal contamination of food and water. Diarrhoeic faeces contains 10^9 organisms/gram and the infective dose may be as low as 10^3 organisms.

Salmonellae may be recovered from carrier pigs where they persist on the tonsils and are shed in the faeces from the gall bladder and intestinal mucosa for up to 22 weeks post-infection. Piglets may be infected from carrier sows. Non-immune sows introduced to an infected herd develop disease. Salmonellae are present in slurry, flies, rodents and in dust within pig housing but the relative importance of these sources in initiating new infections will depend upon the husbandry system.

Salmonellae in faeces and in septicaemic bacteraemic and carrier pigs contaminate meat at slaughter and may give rise to human disease. Experimental studies have shown that *S.typhimurium* can be recovered from 93.5% tonsils, 71% caecums, 55% mandibular lymph nodes and 45% ileocaecocolic lymph nodes at slaughter 20-28 weeks after infection. Comparable figures have been obtained from natural outbreaks. *S.infantis* may persist in many carcase organs. Man may also be infected from contact with live pigs or contaminated effluents.

Diagnosis

The peracute form may be suspected where there is a history of infection on a farm but must be differentiated from erysipelas (skin lesions) and from classical and African swine fever. Post-mortem laboratory examination may rule out these other conditions but they should always be considered. The isolation of salmonellae from all parts of the carcase, especially spleen, lung, intestine and mesenteric lymph node, may suggest salmonellosis but does not rule out the swine fevers.

The presence of necrotic material in the faeces of diarrhoeic animals may suggest salmonellosis or swine dysentery Fever is not a feature of the latter and the faeces usually contains mucus as well as fresh blood. the isolation of the organism from faecal samples or swabs in profuse culture confirms the diagnosis. Indirect culture confirms the presence of infection but may merely indicate carriage. At post-mortem examination the presence of small intestinal inflammation, enlarged mesenteric lymph nodes, necrosis of Peyer's patches and typhlocolitis or rectal stricture may suggest salmonellosis.

Isolation of *S.choleraesuis* or other salmonellae is significant in the absence of other pathogens. Enrichment media used for isolation could contain brilliant green and not selenite which inhibits *S.choleraesuis*. Spleen, liver, lung, mesenteric lymph nodes and small intestine from affected pigs should be submitted for bacteriological diagnosis. The isolation of a few colonies of a *Salmonella spp.* from faeces, slurry or lymph nodes, especially following enrichment may not indicate significant infection of the animal or involvement of the organism in any disease syndrome. It may indicate concern for public health and any isolations of salmonellae from pigs must be reported under the Zoonosis Order 1975. The isolation of large numbers of organisms on direct culture may well be significant.

The presence of past infection may be confirmed by the presence of serum antibody. Agglutination tests and ELISA tests may be carried out on serum and on meat juices.

Treatment

Affected animals may be treated individually by the daily injection of a suitable antibacterial agent. Tetracyclines, streptomycin, apramycin, neomycin, ampicillin, amoxycillin, spectinomycin, trimethoprim:sulphonamide, enrofloxacin, danofloxacin and chloramphenicol (not UK) are all effective. After initial individual treatment, the affected group should be given a course of treatment by water medication with one of the following drugs : the tetracyclines; streptomycin; neomycin; apramycin ampicillin; amoxycillin, nitrofurazone; furazolidone; trimethoprim:sulphonamide, enterofloxacin, danofloxacin or chloramphenicol (not UK), for 3-5 days or until 2 days after the cessation of clinical signs. Carrier animals may remain after the cessation of treatment. In feed medication may also be given but all inappetent animals must be treated individually.

Failure to respond to antimicrobial treatment may suggest that the organism responsible is resistant to the antimicrobial used and isolation and antimicrobial sensitivity testing should be carried out.

Control

Isolation, the use of salmonella-free stock, the use of clean feed and water, rodent control and netting against birds may all help prevent the introduction of salmonellosis to a farm.

Control on infected farms may be difficult Strategic medication in feed or water may be given when disease is expected using the agents listed above at therapeutic levels. The use of carbadox or olaquindox in feed may suppress the disease. All-in-all-out housing, coupled with isolation of batches by disinfectant barriers and thorough cleaning and disinfection between batches may reduce the spread. Rodent, bird and fly control may also help. The use of organic acids and probiotics has been suggested but prevention may not be effective on every farm.

Vaccination is possible. A number of live attenuated *S.choleraesuis* and *S.typhimurium* vaccines have been described. Such vaccines given at least 14 days prior to exposure (introduction to an infected farm or house, or housing) may protect against clinical disease. Effective live vaccines may not be available in all countries but Aro-negative vaccines are being developed. Killed vaccines are also protective. In limited studies Bovivac (Hoechst) a killed *S.typhimurium* and *S.dublin* vaccine appears to be protective against *S.typhimurium* infection.

Eradication of the organism is difficult but has been achieved by complete depopulation or, in a limited number of instances, by treatment of a whole herd, coupled with disinfection.

Decisions on control and treatment may be aided by carrying out bacteriological examination of the herd and the farm to determine the distribution of infection.

Clinically-affected animals should not be sent for slaughter.

References.

Kramer, T.T., Roof, M.B., Matheson, R. (1992). Am.J.Vet.Res. 53, 444-448. Safety and efficacy of an attenuated strain of *S.choleraesuis* for the vaccination of swine.
Laval, A., Morvan, H., Desperez, G., Corbion, B. (1991). Rec.Vet.Med. 167, 835-848. La salmonellose du porc.
Nielsen, B., Baggesen, D., Bager, F., and Lind, P. (1994). Proc.Int.Pig.Vet.Soc. 13, 218. Serological diagnosis of salmonella infections in swine by ELISA..

Maguire, H.C.F., Codd,A.A., Mackay, V.E., Rowe, B. and Mitchell, E. (1993). Epidemiology and Infection 110, 239-246. A large outbreak of human salmonellosis traced to a local pig farm.

Reed, W.M., Olander, H.J., Thacker, H.L. (1985). Am.J.Vet.Res. 46, 2300-2310. Studies on the pathogenesis of *Salmonella heidelberg* infection in weanling pigs.

Reed, W.M., Olander, H.J., Thacker, H.L. (1986). Am.J.Vet.Res. 47, 75-83. Studies on the pathogenesis of *S.typhimurium* and *S.choleraesuis.* var kunzendorf infection in weanling pigs.

Wood, R.L., Pospischil, A., Rose, R. (1989). Am.J.Vet.Res. 50, 1015-1021. Distribution of persistent Salmonella typhimurium infection in the internal organs of swine.

Wood, R.L., Rose, R., Coe, N.E., Ferris, K.E. (1991). Am.J.Vet.Res. 52, 813-819. Experimental establishment of persistent infection in swine with a zoonotic strain of *S.newport.*

Wray, C., McLaren, I.M., Beedell, Y.E. (1993). Vet.Micro. 35, 313-319. Bacterial resistance monitoring of salmonellae isolated from animals. National experience of surveillance schemes in the UK.

Swine Dysentery

Definition

Swine dysentery is an infectious mucohaemorrhagic colitis of pigs characterised clinically by wasting and the passage of diarrhoeic faeces containing varying amounts of mucus, blood and necrotic material. A proportion of untreated affected pigs may die.

Incidence

Occurs worldwide. There are few recent figures but in 1982 40% of herds in the US were considered to be infected. 1984 figures for the UK suggested that 27% of sows were in infected herds and the disease is still the second most commonly diagnosed enteric disease of pigs in the UK. The increasing number of herds founded using swine dysentery-free breeding stock, the use of such pigs exclusively in feeding enterprises and separate site weaning and rearing operations have reduced the incidence in Europe and the US to below these historic levels.

Whole sectors of an industry such as breeding companies and their multiplying herds may be free from the disease.

Aetiology

A large anaerobic spirochaete, *Serpulina (Treponema) hyodysenteriae* initiates swine dysentery and can be isolated from field cases of the disease. *S.hyodysenteriae* is 6-I0 μ in length, flexible and active when viewed by phase contrast microscopy and stains readily with aniline dyes. The cell contains a protoplasmic cylinder 350 nm in diameter with pointed ends and 8-16 fibrils inserting at each end all surrounded by an envelope. The organism can be grown on horseblood agar in atmospheres containing 5% CO_2 and 95% H_2 and forms colonies 1 mm in diameter surrounded by ß-haemolysis after 48 hours' incubation. ß-haemolysis results from the secretion of a powerful haemolysin stimulated by the presence of ribonucleic acid.

S.hyodysenteriae is indole-positive and alpa- galactosidase-negative and may be distinguished from other spirochaetes using specific antisera (specific antigens include a 36 kdA protein, 10 kDa envelope protein and a 46 Da envelope periplasmic flagellar protein). Multiloccus enzyme electrophoresis has also been used to confirm identity. The organism is distinct from other spirochaetes on 16 SrRNA analysis, DNA:DNA hybridisation, using whole cell DNA probes and by restriction enzyme analysis (REA). The species can be sub-divided into serogroups A-I based on lipopolysaccharide antigens and these can be further sub-divided into serotypes. It is sensitive to drying and acid pH <6.0 and is readily destroyed by heat but can survive in organic matter for days or weeks.

Pathogenesis

Infection with *S.hyodysenteriae* is by the oral route. The organism is protected from stomach acid by mucus in dysenteric faeces and reaches the large intestine. There, invasion of the mucus and crypts of the mucosa occurs within 2 hours of exposure but attachment to brush borders does not appear to be a feature of the early disease. The bacteria multiply in the crypts, invade goblet cells and epithelial cells and damage or disrupt them. Invasion through epithelial cell junctions has also been described. Epithelial cells may be damaged by the haemolysin (tly) and tly-negative mutants are of lowered pathogenicity. A cytotoxin and lipopolysaccharide may also be involved in the damage to the cells.

An inflammatory response develops associated with mast cell degranulation. The outcome of this inflammatory change is to cause failure by the colonic epithelium to re-absorb chloride and sodium ions. The resulting fluid and ion loss leads to diarrhoea containing blood and mucus and to death by dehydration or ion imbalance. A phagocytic response occurs within 2-3 days of the onset of clinical disease and serum antibody can be demonstrated within 7-10 days of the onset of clinical signs and persists for up to 19 weeks. Serum antibody may be related to protective immunity and IgG, IgA and IgM antibody in the lumen of the large intestine may reduce the rate of mucosal colonisation. IgA immunity to envelope antigens has been demonstrated in sow's milk and appears to protect sucking piglets. Healing lesions may persist as local foci of inflammation for 40-50 days after clinical recovery and the intestinal mucosa may remain infected although grossly normal.

Studies of *S.hyodysenteriae* infections in gnotobiotic pigs indicate that the organism can cause the disease alone. In lesions in conventional pigs are colonised by a number are colonised by bacteria such as *Campylobacter coli*, *Bacteroides vulgatus*, *Acetivibrio ethanolgignens* and *Fusobacterium necrophorum* which may aid in the development of the lesion. Only *S.hyodysenteriae* will initiate the disease.

Clinical signs

The first signs of the disease include twitching of the tail, abdominal discomfort, hollowing of the flanks, slight reddening of the skin and slight inappetence. A transient fever of 40-40.6°C, 104-105°F may occur, but usually disappears at the onset of the diarrhoea which persists throughout the course of the disease. Diarrhoea may be the clinical sign first noted. Blood, mucus and, later, pieces of necrotic material appear in the faeces which are yellowish in colour at first and later become brownish-red, liquid in consistency and foul-smelling. When recovery begins after 7-14 days, motions containing large quantities of mucus are produced.

Affected pigs show a marked and rapid loss of bodily condition and appear thin with sunken eyes, hollow flanks and prominent ribs and backbones. The coat may be rough, the tail limp and the perineum stained with faeces. Affected pigs show a variable reduction in appetite but all continue to drink. The feed conversion rate and daily liveweight gain may be permanently depressed. Permanently stunted pigs may pass khaki liquid faeces. The depression in bodily condition may cause depression of reproductive performance in outbreaks of disease in sows.

Pigs of all ages are affected although the peak incidence is in weaned pigs of 6-12 weeks of age. The disease can be particularly severe in sows at farrowing or mid-lactation. Production depression on an affected farm may result in an extension of the rearing time from birth - 100 kg of up to 30 days and a 15% increase in farm costs. The presence of passive or incomplete active immunity, treatment of inadequate duration or level and the use of some growth promoters may all reduce the severity of the clinical signs.

Animals with chronic disease, low rectal temperatures (<38°C) and chronic khaki diarrhoea should be killed on humane grounds.

Post mortem findings

Pigs which have died from swine dysentery are usually in poor bodily condition, and the carcase may appear pale and faintly cyanotic.

The large intestine is the only organ consistently affected. It is usually flaccid and may appear dark or congested with a shiny surface due to oedema of the serosa. The mesenteric lymph nodes are frequently pale and swollen but are rarely congested. The contents are fluid, foul smelling and contain varying proportions of mucus, undigested food and necrotic material and are brownish-red in colour. The appearance of the mucosa varies with the age of the lesion. In early cases it is swollen and congested, later becoming covered with blood-streaked mucus and patches of fibrinous diphtheritic material. There is an extensive layer of necrotic material in older lesions and this may become dislodged in patches to expose the bleeding mucosa.

In some cases the liver may appear swollen and friable and the gastric mucosa may appear inflamed. The stomach contents may be fluid or contain fibrous material. Microscopic lesion are confined to the large intestinal mucosa which is inflamed. The mucosal epithelium is displaced and the underlying capillaries are exposed or covered with a layer of cellular debris, fibrin, bacteria and red blood cells. Spirochaetes can be demonstrated in the crypts of the colonic mucosa in the earliest lesions in silver-stained, fluorescent antibody or enzyme-linked antibody treated sections. Large spirochaetes can be demonstrated in wet smears of the lesions and S.hyodysenteriae can be isolated from them in profuse culture.

Epidemiology

Swine dysentery is transmitted to healthy, susceptible pigs by the ingestion of the faeces of affected or carrier animals. The incubation period of the disease in the field varies between 7 and 60 days but is usually 4-14 days in experimentally infected animals. Carriers may remain infected and may be able to transmit the disease for at least 90 days after clinical recovery. Farms on which an outbreak of the disease has occurred remain infected unless depopulation and disinfection or a whole herd treatment have been carried out. Pigs of all ages are affected although the peak incidence is in weaned pigs of 6-12 weeks of age. The disease can be particularly severe in sows at farrowing or mid lactation. The disease is usually introduced to farms by the purchase of infected pigs spreads slowly from pen to pen by means of drainage channels or movement of infected pigs, pig-to-pig contact or on infected boots and implements.

Morbidity may reach 75% of all pigs on the farm and mortality varies between 5 and 25%. Some immunity results from infection with swine dysentery and recovered pigs rarely suffer relapses upon re-infection. Antibodies to the causal spirochaete have been identified in the sera, colonic secretions and colostrum of recovered animals and may be detected on a herd basis by agglutination and ELISA tests.

S.hyodysenteriae can persist in moist faeces at 5°C for up to 40 days and in faeces diluted 1:10 with tapwater for up to 60 days. It can persist in slurry for at least 3 days and in soil for up to 41 days at -20°C, 18 days at 14°C, 2 days at 22°C and less than 5 hours at 37°C. Transmission to susceptible pigs from infected soil is difficult. Drying or disinfectants such as formalin, phenols and hypochlorites eliminate the organism from contaminated pens within hours. Recent studies show that oxidising disinfectants such as Virkon S and Farm Fluid S (Antec) act within minutes.

Mice, rats, flies and dogs have been shown to carry the organism experimentally, and dogs, rats, mice and flies have been identified as carriers in the field. S.hyodysenteriae isolated from mice on infected farms have been shown to be pathogenic for pigs and the organism can be maintained in mouse populations.

<u>Diagnosis</u>

Swine dysentery is usually diagnosed on the basis of the history of the outbreak, the clinical signs shown by affected pigs and the post-mortem findings. The examination of Gram-stained air-dried or wet smears of faeces for the spirochaete may be useful in confirmation. Isolation of the organism may be attempted using spectinomycin blood agar containing 400ug spectinomycin/ml or selective media containing additional antibiotics, but care should be taken in assessing the results as weakly-haemolytic spirochaetes may also be isolated. A direct fluorescent antibody test using acetone-fixed faeces smears has been widely used in the UK. The fluorescent antiserum is prepared in rabbits and absorbed with non-pathogenic spirochaetes in order to enhance specificity. Spirochaetal isolates may be confirmed as S.hyodysenteriae by growth inhibition tests using specific antisera or by slide agglutination tests using similar sera. Enzyme analysis using the API ZYM system is useful as S.hyodysenteriae isolates lack alpha-galactosidase. They are indole-positive. Multilocus enzyme electrophoresis is able to distinguish between S.hyodysenteriae and other spirochaetes and increasing use is made of monoclonal antibodies to specific proteins in fluorescent antibody, agglutination and ELISA tests for S.hyodysenteriae isolates. DNA probes and polymerase chain reaction primers using DNA sequences from 16 S tRNA have been described. Specific tests are rarely commercially available and a combination of characters may have to be used.

Isolates may be serotyped. Serological tests such as microtitre agglutination tests and ELISA tests can be used on a herd basis to identify infected herds. Current studies suggest that neither is completely accurate and neither can identify individual infected animals. The main problem is that these tests may detect antibody to common antigens present in non-*S.hyodysenteriae* spirochaetes and statistical interpretation may be required. Herd infection can also be detected using an ELISA for faecal antigen which can detect 10^2 organisms/ml of faeces or slurry in spite of drug treatment or prolonged storage which makes isolation impossible. Herd monitoring can be carried out using rectal faeces swabs or samples from recently weaned pigs, for culture or immunofluorescence, serum ELISA, faecal ELISA and by culturing 10 sites in the colonic mucosa of slaughter pigs. The polymerase chain reaction may be useful and primers capable of identifying 10 ng of DNA in faeces have been described.

The presence of fresh blood and mucus in the diarrhoea differentiate this condition from most other enteric conditions. Salmonellosis is often associated with fever, post-weaning *E.coli*, *S*almonella, and spirochaetal colitis and diarrhoeas rarely contain thick mucus or frank blood. T.G.E. and epidemic diarrhoea occur in explosive outbreaks rather than spreading slowly from pen to pen. Faecal blood in gastric ulceration and proliferative haemorrhagic enteropathy is altered and blackish. At post-mortem examination the restriction of lesions to the large intestine rules out all but spirochaetal diarrhoea which is a milder disease or *Trichuris suis* infection.

Swine dysentery may occur with other diseases and then be atypical. In this situation and following incomplete drug treatment, laboratory examination is required for confirmation of Experimental animal infection or detailed study of the organisms may be necessary for this.

Treatment

Treatment is best administered in the drinking water, but individual treatment of severely-affected animals by injection should be given. This is particularly necessary if feed medication is to be used. The treatments given below may not all be available in any one country for regulatory reasons.

Tiamulin is extremely effective when given by injection at 10 mg/kg, in the drinking water at 60 ppm for 5 days (Tiamutin, Leo, Sandoz/Biochemie) to give 8.8 mg/kg body weight, and in the feed at 120 ppm for 14-21 days. Resistant to tiamulin is rare in the field and only low levels 2.0 µg/ml have been identified *in vitro*. It should not be given in conjunction with monensin, salinomycin or norasin.

Lincomycin may be used as a feed additive (110 g/ton, 21 days), by injection at 10 mg/kg in the drinking water at 34 ppm and in combination with spectinomycin (Lincospectin soluble, Upjohn) in the drinking water. This last product is not registered for use in pigs in the UK. Resistance to lincomycin occurs.

Nitroimidazole drugs are also extremely effective. Dimetridazole (Emtryl Rhone Merieux) should be given at 260 ppm in the drinking water for 5-7 days and in the feed at 500 ppm for 7-14 days. Ronidazole may be given for 3-5 days in the drinking water at 60 ppm and at 120 ppm in the feed. Strains resistant to dimetridazole have been identified. Ronidazole is not available in the UK and dimetridazole is no longer available in some countries.

Macrolides may be given by intramuscular injection (tylosin Tylan, at 15 mg/kg) in the drinking water (tylosin at 200 ppm for 7-10 days) or in the feed (tylosin at 100 ppm for 21 days). Resistance to tylosin is widespread amongst

S.hyodysenteriae isolates in Britain and elsewhere but where organisms are sensitive it is effective.

Organic arsenicals such as sodium arsanilate in the drinking water (175 ppm, 6 days), arsanilic acid (500g/tonne, 21 days), sodium amino arsonate and monosodium 3-nitro 4-phenyl arsonate have also been used.

All animals in drainage contact should be treated at the same time and disinfection of pens or a move to clean pens after treatment will give best results.

Control

a) Medication

The disease may be prevented using medication at therapeutic levels just after weaning and mixing. Groups of treated pigs should enter cleaned, dried and disinfected accommodation and may be maintained in isolation until slaughter. Treatment into all-in-all-out systems is very effective and can maintain a rearing or finishing herd free from the disease even when infected breeding stock are present.

Continuous low level medication can be used for a period using carbadox in feed at 50 ppm (to 35 kg only, not UK) or at any time during the rearing and finishing period using tiamulin at 30-40g/tonne, lincomycin at 44g/tonne, dimetridazole at 200g/tonne and ronidazole at 60g/tonne. Interruption of feed intake resulting from intercurrent disease or management changes may result in the appearance of clinical or sub-clinical disease which should be treated promptly. Failure to respond to treatment may be due to the development of resistance or to the presence of other enteric pathogens such as salmonella.

b) Management

General hygiene reduced the spread of the disease within a unit. The use of all-in-all-out husbandry, coupled with proper cleaning, disinfection and drying helps reduce the spread. Spread from house to house can be reduced by disinfecting pathways and by using disinfectant foot dips and separate implements. Slatted floors, solid partitions between pens, control of flies and rodents and lowering of slurry levels all reduce the spread of the disease.

The use of multiple site rearing may reduce the incidence of disease and, coupled with treatment at movement (Medicated Early Weaning see Enzootic Pneumonia), "Isowean" or introduction to a clean drainage unit/house may reduce the number of disease outbreaks dramatically.

Prompt treatment of clinical disease also reduces spread. The use of a 77% rice, 21% animal protein diet has recently been shown to prevent the onset of infection but has not been tested generally.

c) Vaccination

No vaccines are currently (1994) registered for use in the UK. Killed whole cell vaccines made from one or more serotypes and enriched with envelope proteins have been used in the field. They appear to reduce the prevalence of disease, to improve performance and reduce the number of treatments required. They do not appear to prevent disease completely or to prevent infection. Experimental vaccines composed of digests of *S.hyodysenteriae*, subunits such as envelopes and flagellal proteins, live naturally-attenuated and transposon mutants of the tly gene have all bee shown to produce protection.

d)   Eradication

Eradication has been carried out in a number of ways:

Depopulation and restocking

The scale or slaughter of the stock is followed by cleaning manure disposal, disinfection, an empty period to allow drying (best in summer) and, rodent and fly control. The clean unit is then restocked with swine dysentery-free pigs (usually originally hysterectomy derived) from a breeding company and maintained in isolation except for the purchase of disease-free breeding stock.   Such herds remain disease-free indefinitely.
Depopulation may take place as a single event or pigs may be moved to other holdings to reduce the unprofitable time. Similarly clean breeding stock may be maintained on a clean unit to occupy the cleaned and disinfected unit immediately it is safe to restock.
Treatment of the whole herd accompanied by disinfection and rodent control. A number of agents (tylosin, dimetridazole, ronidazole, lincocin and tiamulin have been shown to eliminate *S.hyodysenteriae*. Treatment of the whole herd at the recommended rate (extended to double the usual period for safety), followed by cleaning, disinfection and the isolation of all farrowing sows and their litters until both have undergone full periods of treatment has eliminated the disease. Partial depopulation helps the cleaning process and allows for the increase in growth rate which follows successful eradication. Breeding stock should be bought from clean herds.

e)   Partial eradication accompanied by control

Where hygiene and management are good, the breeding stock may be treated and the organism eliminated. Treated pigs are isolated from the contaminated ruminant of the herd by a disinfectant barrier along drainage lines which are moved forward ahead of the clean piglets being born. Sufficient space for cleaning must be cleared, partial depopulation of the feeding herd and clinical disease should be suppressed by prompt treatment or continuous medication.
Such schemes are often cost effective, the cost being recouped within 6 months and may reduce finishing periods by 7-21 days. Isolation and treatment of all incoming animals should be practised.
Isolation of the herd and the purchase of clean breeding stock is essential for continued success.

f)   Medicated Early Weaning and 'Isowean'

The use of medicated early weaning (see Enzootic Pneumonia) and the movements of pigs at intervals in the 'Isowean' system may allow the maintenance of swine dysentery-free finishing enterprises. These may be used as sources for swine dysentery-free breeding stock although hysterectomy-derived stock is safer.

g)   Monitoring for freedom from swine dysentery

A number of programmes have been devised to monitor the success of eradication campaigns and the continued freedom from infection of breeding companies. Herds to be monitored should not use treatments which can suppress swine dysentery or growth promoters such as carbadox and olaquindox and salucomycin which can affect its appearance. Farm staff should monitor freedom from clinical signs of swine dysentery and report for investigation any outbreaks of other diarrhoeas. A quarterly veterinary inspection which includes inspection of slatted pens and rectal faecal examination confirms this procedures. A regular programme of monitoring any dead pigs post-mortem helps pick up early or mild intestinal lesions.

This programme can be augmented by serology (where available) using blood samples from slaughtered pigs or those aged more than 10-12 weeks. Inspection of colons at slaughter may be carried out. culture of colonic lesions from slaughtered pigs or those which have died may be carried out on a regular basis. Diarrhoeic faeces or rectal samples taken at quarterly inspections can be examined for *S.hyodysenteriae*. Animals with post-weaning diarrhoea, those recently mixed and young gilts at service are most likely to yield evidence of infection in a sub-clinically-infected herd. Monitoring may be by faecal ELISA, PCR, or culture but the laboratory carrying out the examination must be capable of distinguishing between *S.hyodysenteriae* and other spirochaetes.

References

Alexander, T.J.L., Taylor, D.J.   (1969). Vet. Rec. 85, 59-63. The clinical signs, diagnosis and control of swine dysentery.
Alexander, T.J.L., Thornton, K., Boon, G., Lysons, R.J. and Gush, A.F. (1980). Vet.Rec. 106, 114-119.   Medicated early weaning to obtain pigs free from pathogens endemic in the herd of origin.
Argenzio, R.A., Whipp, S.C. and Glock, R.D. (1980). J.Infectious Dis. 142, 676-684. Pathophysiology of swine dysentery: Colonic transport and permeability studies.
Combs, B.G., Atyeo, R.F., Hampson, D.J. (1994). Proc. IPVS 13, 148. Use of polymerase chain reaction for the identification of *Serpulina hyodysenteriae*.
Egan, I.T., Harris, D.L. and Joens, L.A.(1983). Am.J.Vet.Res. 44, 1323-1328. Comparison of the microtitration agglutination test and the ELISA for the detection of herds affected with swine dysentery.
Fernie, D.S., Ripley, P.H. and Walker, P.D. (1983). Res. in Vet.Sci. 35, 217-221. Swine dysentery: Protection against experimental challenge following single dose parenteral immunisation with inactivated *T.hyodysenteriae*.
Glock, R.D. (1984). Modern Vet.Practice 65, 611-614.
Glock, R.D. and Harris, D.L. (1972).   Vet.Med. Small Anim.Clin. 67, 65-68. Swine dysentery II.   Characterisation of lesions in pigs inoculated with *Treponema hyodysenteriae* in pure and mixed culture.
Hampson, D.J., Mhoma, J.R.L., Combs, B., Buddle, J.R. (1984). Epidemiology and Infection 102, 75-84. Proposed revision to the serological typing system for *T.hyodysenteriae*

Harris, D.L., Glock, R.D., Christensen, C.R. and Kinyon, J.M. (1972). Vet.Med. S.A.C. 61-68. Swine dysentery I. Inoculation of pigs with *Treponema hyodysenteriae* (new species) and reproduction of the disease.

Huurne, A.A.H.M.ter, Hyatt, D.R., Joens, L. and de Rea, J.M. (1994). Proc. IPVS 13, 150. Development of a swine dysentery vaccine based on a *Serpulina hyodysenteriae* tlyA-deletion mutant.

Jensen, N.S., Casey, T.A., Stanton, T.B. (1990). J.Clin.Microbiol. 28, 2717-2721. Detection and identification of *T.hyodysenteriae* by using oligodeoxynucleotide probes complementary to 16S rRNA.

Joens, L.A. and Marquez, R.B. (1986). Infection and Immunity 54, 893-896. Molecular characterisation of proteins from porcine spirochaetes.

Lemcke, R.M. and Burrows, M.R. (1981). J. Hygiene 86, 173-182. A comparative study of spirochaetes from the porcine alimentary tract.

Lymbery, A.J., Hampson, D.J., Hopkins, R.M., Combs, B., Minoma, J.R.L. (1990). Vet.Microbiology. 22, 89-99. Multilocus enzyme electrophoresis for identification and typing of *T.hyodysenteriae* and related spirochaetes.

Lysons, R.J., Kent, M.A., Bland, A., Sellwood, R., Robinson, W.F., First, A. 1991). J.Med.Micro. 34, 97-102. A cytolytic haemolysin from *T.hyodysenteriae*: a probable virulence determinant in swine dysentery.

Lysons, R.J. and Lemcke, R.M. (1983). Vet.Rec. 112, 203. Swine dysentery: to isolate or to fluoresce!

Rees, A.S., Lysons, R.J., Stokes, C.R., Bourne, F.J. (1989). Res.Vet.Sci. 47, 263-269. Antibody production in the pig colon during infection with *T.hyodysenteriae*.

Schmall, L.M., Argenzio, R.A. and Whipp, S.C. (1983). Am.J.Vet.Res. 44, 1309-1316. Pathophysiologic features of swine dysentery: cyclonucleotide independent production of diarrhoea.

Siba, P.M., Pethick, D.W. and Hapson, D.J. (1994). Proc.Int.Pig Vet.Soc. 13, 149. Dietary Control of Swine Dysentery.

Taylor, D.J., Alexander, T.J.L. (1971). Brit.Vet.J. 127, 58-61. The production of dysentery in swine by feeding cultures containing a spirochaete.

Taylor, D.J., Lysons, R.J., Bew, J., Stevenson, R. and Lemcke, R.M. (1985). Vet.Rec. 116, 48-49. Survival of *Treponema hyodysenteriae* in samples of dysenteric pig faeces sent by post and stored at room temperature.

Windsor, R.S. and Simmons, J.R. (1981) . Vet.Rec . 109, 482-484. Investigation into the spread of swine dysentery in 25 herds in East Anglia and assessment of its economic significance in 5 herds.

Wood, E.N. and Lysons, R.J. (1988). Vet.Rec. 122, 277-279. The financial benefits from the eradication of swine dysentery.

Spirochaetal Diarrhoea

Definition

A syndrome in which infection with spirochaetes other than *S.hyodysenteriae* results in diarrhoea, sporadic dysentery and depression of weight gain in young weaned pigs.

Incidence

Increasingly recognised and apparently widespread. Seen in France, Sweden, Poland, Germany, Britain, Australia, U.S. and Canada. Clinical disease seen in minimal disease pigs, following withdrawal of antibiotics and where non-immune pigs are mixed with carriers. It is particularly common where no growth promoters are used.

Aetiology

A number of strains or species of weakly ß-haemolytic spirochaetes have been isolated from the faeces or colonic mucosa of pigs. Extensive studies by electron microscopy, antigenic analysis, biochemical profiles, restriction endonuclease analysis, multilocus enzyme electrophoresis and sequence analysis of 16S rRNA. At present there is no coherent scheme for their classification but they appear to fall into at least two groups, the completely non-pathogenic spirochaetes and those which have caused some disease.

Serpulina innocens is a name that has been given to some of these harmless weakly haemolytic fermentative spirochaetes but this group contains more than one species on ultrastructural grounds alone. Other spirochaetes isolated from pigs with diarrhoea and from rodents have been shown to cause diarrhoea in experimental pigs. All of these are distinct from S.*hyodysenteriae* on ultrastructural, biochemical or antigenic grounds.

One type of these organisms, 6-l0µ in length, 0.25µ in diameter and with 5-7 fibrils in the axial filament has been shown to be pathogenic for pigs. Others, designated 'S.*hyodysenteriae* biotype 2' or 'intermediate type' have been designated as such because of biochemical differences from S.*hyodysenteriae* and their ability to cause spirochaetal diarrhoea.

Pathogenesis

Pathogenicity has not been studied exhaustively but colonisation of the colonic mucosa and consequent failure of colonic absorption appear to be more important than epithelial invasion in this condition. Organisms appear to produce colonic failure by colonising the lumenal border of large intestinal epithelial cells very densely. Spirochaetal cells are arranged end on and may be invaginated into the cell membrane displacing the brush border. Large micro colonies of the organisms develop in the crypts. Spirochaetal colonisation is associated with mild inflammation and is followed by plasma cell accumulation in the lamina propria.

Recovery and resistance appear to occur as for swine dysentery. In addition to primary infections, the organism colonise lesions of the colon in cases of proliferative haemorrhagic enteropathy, *Trichuris suis* infection, swine dysentery and other enteric diseases.

Clinical signs

Clinical signs are seen most commonly in young, weaned animals, but may occur in non-immune animals of any age. The incubation period varies from 5-20 animals have a slight fever (40°C, 105°F) appear "tucked up" and may be off their feed. Recovery occurs within 7-10 days and mortality is rare. A marked reduction in the rate of daily liveweight gain may occur and recovered animals may appear hairy. In some units older animals may also be affected and chronic diarrhoea may occur.

Pathology

The large intestinal serosa may be oedematous and the colon contents fluid. The mucosa is thickened with excess clear mucus or local bleeding points and some diphtheritic material. In recovering animals, islands of necrotic material may be seen on the mucosa. The mucosa is oedematous with dilated crypts which may be filled with silver-stained organisms. Spirochaetes other than *S.hyodysenteriae* can be isolated from the mucosa. The particular small spirochaete described above may be isolated or demonstrated in a false brush border on the cells of the mucosal epithelium or, in complicated infections invading pre-existing lesions caused by other pathogens.

Epidemiology

Appears to spread in the same way as swine dysentery. The studies of mouse and rat spirochaetes and their ability to infect pigs suggest that infections in newly-established hysterectomy-derived nucleus herds may be of rodent origin.

Diagnosis

Spirochaetal diarrhoea should be suspected when a chronic, non-fatal diarrhoea with little or no blood and some clear mucus occurs in recently weaned pigs in S.P.F. herds or following withdrawal of a growth promoter. Confirmation is difficult, but the post-mortem findings, the isolation of weakly haemolytic spirochaetes negative to the biochemical antigenic and nucleic acid criteria for *S.hyodysenteriae*. It may be possible to identify them as *S.innocens* in which case they may not be a primary cause of the colitis or it may be possible to identify them as intermediate type Serpulinas, as belonging to the pathogenic group of small spirochaetes designated "*Anrguillina coli*" or as one of the other pathogenic spirochaetes recently described. The techniques available include enzyme analysis (API Zym), growth inhibition, multilocus enzyme electrophoresis, immunofluorescence and immunoperoxidase using specific monoclonal antibody and the polymerase chain reaction capable of detecting 10^4 cells. An important reason for confirming the identity of the spirochaete is when spirochaetosis is identified in herds where swine dysentery is thought to have been eradicated or to be absent.

Treatment and control

Similar to that used for swine dysentery. Tylosin and other macrolides are often effective and olaquindox is more effective against spirochaetal diarrhoea than against swine dysentery. All animals in drainage contact should be treated and treatment should be followed by cleaning and disinfection. Rodent control is particularly important during management for this disease. It is not yet clear whether the organism or the disease can be eliminated from an individual animal or herd other than by medicated early weaning.

There is no vaccine.

References

Binek, M. and Szynkiewicz, Z.M. (1984). Comparative Immunology, Microbiology and Infectious Diseases 7, 141-148. Physiological properties and classification of strains of Treponema spp. isolated from pigs in Poland.
Felstrom, C., Uhlem, M., Pettersen, B., Gunnarrson, A., Johansson, K.E. (1994) Proc.IPVS. 13, 146. Classification of intestinal porcine spirochaetes by sequence analysis of 16Sr RNA and biochemical methods.
Jacques, M., Girard, C., Higgins, R., Goyette, G. (1989). J.Clin.Micro. 27, 1139-1141. Extensive colonisation of the porcine colonic epithelium by a spirochaete similar to T.innocens.
Lee, B.J. and Hampson, D.J. (1994). Proc.IPVS. 13, 198. A monoclonal antibody reacting with the cell envelope of spirochaetes from intestinal spirochaetosis.
Lee, J.I., Hampson, D.J., Lymbery, A.J., Harders, S.T. (1993). Vet.Micro. 34, 273-285. The porcine intestinal spirochaetes: identification of new genetic groups.
Lymbery. A.J., Hampson, D.J., Hopkins, M., Combs, B. and Mohoma, J.R.L. (1990). Vet.Micro. 22, 89-99. Multilocus enzyme electrophoresis for identification and typing of T.hyodysenteriae and related spirochaetes.
Mohan Romanathan, Duhamel, G.E., Mathieson, M.R., Messier, S. (1993). Vet.Micro. 37, 53-64. Identification and partial characterisation of a group of weakly ß-haemolytic intestinal spirochaetes of swine distinct from S.hyodysenteriae.
Park, N.Y., Chung, C.Y., McLaren, A.J., Atyeo, R.F. and Hampson, D.J. (1994). Proc.IPVS. 13, 192. Polymerase chain reaction for identification of spirochaetes associated with intestinal spirochaetosis.
Taylor, D.J., Simmons , J.R. and Laird, H.M. (1980). Vet. Rec. 106, 324-332. Production of diarrhoea and dysentery in pigs by feeding pure cultures of a spirochaete differing from Treponema hyodysenteriae.

Campylobacter enteritis

Definition

Campylobacters cause a mucoid creamy diarrhoea which may contain blood in piglets 3 days - 3 weeks of age. They may also cause enteritis in non-immune weaned pigs, and contribute to inflammatory conditions of the ileum and large intestine. Mucus in the faeces in other enteric conditions may indicate their presence.

Incidence

The organisms are ubiquitous worldwide but clinical signs are rarely ascribed to the infection. 100% pigs may be infected with C.coli but not all may be infected with the other species.

Aetiology and Pathogenesis

C.coli is a microaerophilic curved Gram-negative rod forming sprawling watery colonies of blood agar after 48 hours. It is catalase-positive, grows at $43^{\circ}C$ but not at $25^{\circ}C$ and does not produce H_2S on T.S.I. medium and is hippurate negative. Following infection, multiplication occurs in the small intestine, particularly the ileum where the organism is closely associated with the mucosa. A brief bacteraemic phase may occur but the organism does not appear to penetrate the epithelium in any numbers. Recent studies suggest that the organism may produce a cytotoxin which could cause the inflammatory changes seen. Colonisation of the large intestine occurs. Clinical signs begin after an incubation period of 1-3 days after infection.

Other campylobacters are also present in the porcine intestine. *C.hyointestinalis*, *C.jejuni*, *C.mucosalis* and *C.laridis* have all been identified and may reach high numbers and be associated with enteritis, particularly in weaned pigs.

Clinical signs

Affected piglets may have a mild fever (to 40.6°C, 105°F) which may be maintained for 2-3 days. A watery or creamy diarrhoea containing mucus with occasional streaks of blood is present. These clinical signs may continue for some days. In weaned pigs *C.coli* infection may be associated with chronic mucoid diarrhoea in which no blood is seen. In both forms of the disease loss of condition occurs but mortality is rare.

Infection may not cause clinical signs in immune pigs but experimental infection of hysterectomy-derived, colostrum-deprived or gnotobiotic pigs with *C.coli*, *C.jejuni*, *C.hyointestinalis* or *C.sputorum* may produce diarrhoea after 1-4 days.

Pathological findings

In neonatal pigs gross changes are slight and are confined to the small intestine which is slightly inflamed with thickening of the ileum, especially of the terminal portion. The mesenteric lymph nodes are prominent. The ileal mucosa is mildly inflamed and mucoid contents may be present at this site or in the caecum. The mucosa of the large intestine is usually mildly inflamed or normal. Stunting of the ileal villi may be seen. Histological changes are slight, the most prominent being massive enlargement of the lymphoid tissue in the terminal ileum. Crypt abscesses may be present. The ileal thickening results from the lymphoid hyperplasia and not from any proliferation of the mucosal epithelium. In weaned pigs, thickening of the small intestine, particularly of the terminal portion, may be prominent. Large intestinal changes resembling chronic mild swine dysentery may be seen. *C.coli* may be isolated on selective medium from the small intestine in large numbers, and curved Gram-negative rods seen in smears made from the mucosal surface.

Epidemiology

Pigs in most farms are infected with *C.coli*. Infection takes place by the faecal/oral route in piglets from maternal faeces, contaminated water or horizontal transmission. Maternal immunity normally prevents clinical disease but does not prevent colonisation. Infected animals remain carriers for long periods and pass 10^3-10^4 organisms/g faeces for months. Carriage is in the gall bladder, ileal mucosa and large intestinal mucosa.

Introduction of a campylobacter species to which immunity is absent can result in outbreaks of diarrhoea. *C.jejuni*, *C.laridis* from other species or from water may cause disease.

Contamination of pigmeat with campylobacters may lead to human infection. *C.coli* infection is relatively rarely identified in man in the UK.

Diagnosis

C.coli infections should be suspected when a mucoid diarrhoea containing blood stained mucus occurs in piglets with little mortality and some loss of condition. To confirm, the organism must be present in profuse culture in the ileum and other causes of diarrhoea, such as rotavirus, epidemic diarrhoea, *Clostridium perfringens*, *E.coli*, coccidia and cryptosporidia should be eliminated to reach a diagnosis of primary *C.coli* infection. Histological lesions of proliferative intestinal adenopathy (P.I.A.) should be absent. Colonic lesions should be distinguished from P.I.A., spirochaetal diarrhoea and swine dysentery.

Isolation has recently been supplemented by DNA probes and PCR for *C.jejuni*, *C.sputorum* and *C.hyointestinalis*.

Treatment

Oral treatment with neomycin, other amino-glycosides, tetracyclines, microlides and enrofloxacin may all eliminate or markedly reduce Campylobacter infection.

Control

Control has rarely, if ever, been attempted in the pig. Low level antimicrobial treatment would be the most appropriate method, coupled with hygiene and chlorination of water supplies.

References

Mafu, A.A., Higgins, R., Nadeau, M., Cousseau, G. (1989). J.Food Production 52, 642-645. The incidence of salmonella, campylobacter and *Yersinia enterocolitica* in swine carcases and slaughterhouse environment.
Olubunmi, P.A. and Taylor, D.J. (1982). Vet.Rec. 111, 197-202. Production of enteritis in pigs by the oral inoculation of *Campylobacter coli*.
Taylor D.J. and Olubunmi, P.A. (1981). Vet.Rec. 109, 112-115. A re-examination of the role of *C.fetus* subsp. *coli* in enteric disease of the pig.
Vitovci, J., Kondela, B., Sterba, J., Tomancova, I., Matyas, Z., Vladiz, P. (1989). Zbl.fur Bakt. 271, 91-103. The gnotobiotic piglet as a model for the pathogenesis of *C.jejuni* infection.

Helicobacter pylori

This organism has been isolated from the pig stomach and has been shown to infect gnotobiotic pigs in experiments. Its significance in the pig is unknown although it is likely to be involved in gastritis. Porcine isolates may give rise to human infections.

References

Eaton, K.A., Morgan, D.R., Krakowka, S. (1989). Inf. and Immun. 57, 1119-125. Campylobacter pylori virulence factors in gnotobiotic pigs.

Arcobacter cryoaerophila

This campylobacter-like organism, which grows at 25°C has been isolated from the vagina, uterus and aborted foetuses in cases of infertility and abortion. It has also been isolated from enteritis.

Proliferative Enteropathy

Definition

An infectious bacterial condition in which proliferative changes occur in the epithelium of the small and large intestinal mucosa. The condition underlies necrotic enteritis, regional ileitis and proliferative haemorrhagic enteropathy. Affected pigs appear pale, may be stunted and may die suddenly with clotted blood in the lumen of the small intestine.

Incidence

The disease has been described in Canada, USA., Taiwan, Japan, Australia and Europe, including Britain, where it is particularly noticeable in herds which were originally hysterectomy-derived.

Aetiology

Proliferative enteropathy is caused by one obligate intracellular bacterium currently known as Ileal Symbiont (IS) *intracellulare*. The organism resembles *Desulfovibrio desulfuricans* using 16S rDNA (91% homology) but may eventually be named *Ileobacter* (1994). It is a Gram-negative curved rod I.5 μm in length with tapered ends which multiplies by septation within cells. At present it is cultured in a rat enterocyte cell line 1EC-18 in the cells of which it forms micro colonies after 7-14 days. The organism can be sub-cultured in this cell line and can survive outside the cells but not multiply. Pure cultures of the organism harvested from these cell cultures have been given to conventional and gnotobiotic pigs and reproduce the lesions of the disease within 21 days. Monoclonal antibodies and DNA probes confirm that this organism is present in the lesion and the association between organism and lesion has been confirmed statistically with an odds ratio of ≥ 14 and an estimated attributable fraction of $\geq 92\%$.

Pathogenesis

Infection is oral and the organism enters epithelial cells of the crypts of the small intestine. The bacteria lie adjacent to the apices of the epithelial cells and enter by endocytic vacuole formation. The vacuoles may fuse with lysosomes but the organisms survive and enter the cytoplasm in which they become more electron lucent and divide by septation. They are located near mitochondria and rough endoplasmic reticulum. Numbers increase until micro colonies of >50 organisms are present within a cell. Infected cells survive parasitisation with only minor changes to mitochondrial structure but eventually rupture apparently by apoptosis to extrude the organisms. Those shed to the exterior are electron dense and may enter other cells or pass out in the faeces.

These developments in the intestinal epithelial cells are responsible for the microscopic and gross changes seen in the pig gut. The earliest changes occur as hyperplasia of the glandular epithelium of the small intestine. Goblet cells disappear, the epithelial cells become elongated with many mitoses and the crypts elongate and branch. They may be filled with polymorphs. Capillaries dilate and then rupture at the apex of the villi. Blood loss into the lumen occurs leading to anaemia. These changes can take place in germ-free gnotobiotic pigs but colonisation with *Bacteroides vulgatus* and pathogenic *E.coli* increase their severity.

These changes in the mucosal epithelium may regress it, may become necrotic (necrotic enteritis, sometimes caused by salmonellosis or nicotinic acid deficiency) or may continue to proliferate to give rise to a benign adenomatosis. Mucosal proliferation and erosion may result in changes in the terminal ileum, the muscular coats of which become hyperplastic to give regional ileitis or hosepipe gut. The presence of infection and lesions in the large intestine may lead to failure of colonic absorption.

The development of serum antibody occurs from 60 days after exposure to the agent. During this period the organisms may be demonstrated in the apical cytoplasm of affected cells. Haemorrhage in proliferative haemorrhagic enteropathy occurs at the same time as destruction of the organisms and other mucosal changes and may be immunomediated.

Clinical signs

The clinical disease is most commonly seen in recently-weaned pigs and lasts for about 6 weeks. It has an incubation period of 3-6 weeks and can occur in animals of any age from 3-4 weeks to adults. The first signs are failure to gain weight or loss of weight and capricious appetite. Affected pigs appear pale, may vomit, are anaemic (P.C.V. as low as 20%) and may have blackened faeces due to melaena. After 4-6 weeks they may recover completely. Some pigs may suddenly die. These usually appear pale with a low body temperature (37.8°C,100°F,) within 1-2 hours of death and may be of any age from 6-10 weeks upwards. Breeding stock may die when the disease first enters a herd (particularly with proliferative haemorrhagic enteropathy, see below). Some animals remain stunted. Morbidity may reach 12% and mortality 6% in such cases. Affected pigs may appear thin, pale and pass loose granular faeces which spread on concrete like portions of wet cement in cases where other infections are present (see intestinal spirochaetosis and campylobacter enteritis).

The presence of the disease in breeding herds may lead to a decrease in production of up to 8%, partially due to abortion which follows 6 days after clinical signs develop in pregnant sows. There are two indications for humane slaughter: when animals are suffering from severe blood loss, hypothermia, and are unable to rise, and severely stunted pigs with chronic disease.

Pathological findings

Pigs which die from the disease are pale with a thickened small intestine which may appear dark or pale, swollen, reticulated and flaccid from the serosal surface. The lesions of proliferative enteropathy occur in the ileum and upper third of the spiral colon. The wall of the gut may be thickened and flaccid. The surface of the mucosa may be thrown into folds reminiscent of those seen in Johne's disease of cattle and the tips of these rugae may show bleeding points. Plaques of thickened mucosa resembling that of the affected small intestine may be seen in the large intestine and polyps may also be present.

In necrotic enteritis the lining of the intestine may be covered in yellow or greyish masses of friable necrotic material closely adherent to the surface.

In regional ileitis ("hosepipe gut") the wall of the lower small intestine is smooth and rigid, particularly in the terminal region of the ileum. Upon section, the muscle layers are thickened and the lining is ulcerated or covered in granulation tissue.

In proliferative haemorrhagic enteropathy the lesions are largely restricted to the small intestine. The lower third is distended and filled with clotted blood mixed with food. Bleeding points can only be seen using a dissecting microscope and are very localised. the mucosa is often highly folded. The contents of the large intestine are blackish and tarry. The carcase is pale and the blood watery.

In histological sections, the affected mucosa is thicker than normal and contains branched crypts packed with dividing cells. There is a marked absence of goblet cells. Affected tissue may lie next to normal tissue, particularly at the edge of a polyp. In silver-stained sections the apical cytoplasm of the cells lining the crypts may be seen to contain large numbers of bacteria which may be identified as IS.intracellularis with specific fluorescent antibody or using DNA probes.

Other bacteria such as campylobacters may be present in lesions in both small and large intestine. Their presence may affect the pathological findings.

Epidemiology

The recent identification of the organism will allow the details of the epidemiology to be determined. The organism has been identified in faeces by the polymerase chain reaction and by dot blot hybridisation. It is clear that infected animals shed the organism in the faeces but details of its ability to survive in the environment are not yet available. It is possible that it may survive in rodents and other small mammals as pure cultures have been used in experimental infections in hamsters and similar organisms have been identified in these species.

One means of transmission of disease from herd to herd is in carrier pigs, but the role of vectors is not clear. The development of disease within an affected farm is affected by immunity and clinical signs rarely occur in piglets and recovered animals remain immune. Disease is most obvious when non-immune animals are introduced to an infected herd, when the disease is introduced to a non-immune herd and when courses of treatment delay infection until near slaughter.

Diagnosis

Based on the clinical signs of failure to thrive and the occurrence of pale pigs with altered blood in the faeces in proliferative haemorrhagic enteropathy. This occult blood may be detected using biochemical methods. the point at which the disease develops may be determined clinically by sequential weighing. The presence of the infection can be confirmed by PCR using 16S rDNA probes on faeces or dot-blot hybridisation of bacterial DNA extracts.

The disease may be identified by post-mortem examination of pigs which die on farm or at the slaughter house. The gross lesions of ileal thickening, mucosal lesions and blood in the lumen are suggestive and can be confirmed as P.E. by histopathology and by the demonstration of organisms in the apical cytoplasm of the epithelial cells of affected gut in smears of intestine stained by

Koster's method (red bacilli), use of specific antibody in immunofluorescence or immunoperoxidase or by the use of DNA probes or PCR.

Treatment

Feeding affected pigs or those at risk on a ration containing antibiotics such as tetracyclines, sulphonamides or tylosin may be of value. Treatment with injectable long-acting tetracycline appears to cure clinically affected pigs. In some cases, the use of these drugs merely postpones the onset of the disease. A regime in which tetracycline treatment in feed at 300-400 ppm for two weeks (or 4 days in water) is followed by no treatment and then by another course of treatment has been suggested on the basis that organisms are eliminated and re-infection in the majority of pigs is prevented by immunity following the initial exposure. Chlortetracycline, penicillin and sulphamethazine combinations (Cyfac, ASP250 Cyanamid) may be useful. Recently *in vitro* tests have suggested that tiamulin is effective against the organism. When spirochaetosis, salmonellosis or other bacterial disease is present, the treatment should be modified accordingly.

Control

The introduction of genetic material into nucleus herds free from the disease should be hysterectomy, AI or embryo transfer. Within a herd the disease may be suppressed by continuous low level medication using one of the products named above or by carrying out a treatment regime intended to stimulate natural immunity. Any form of treatment may leave a variable proportion of the animals non-immune and susceptible to disease.

References

Gebhart, C.J., Barns, S.M., McOrist, S., Lin, G.F. and Lawson, G.H.K. (1993). Int.J.Systematic Bact. 43, 533-538. Ileal symbiont intracellularis, an obligate intracellular bacterium of porcine intestines showing a relationship to *Desulfovibrio* species.
Jasni, S., McOrist, S., Lawson, G.H.K. (1994). Res.vet.Sci. 56, 186-192. Experimentally-induced proliferative enteritis in hamsters : an ultrastructural study.
Jones, G.F., Davies, P.R., Rose, R., Ward, G.E., Murtaugh, M.P. (1993). Am.J.Vet.Res. 54, 1980-1985. Comparison of techniques for diagnosis of proliferative enteritis of swine.
Love, R.J., Love, D.N. (1977). Vet.Rec. 100, 473. Control of proliferative haemorrhagic enteropathy in pigs.
McOrist, S., Boid, R., Lawson, G.H.K. (1989). Inf. and Imm. 57, 957-962. Antigenic analysis of Campylobacter species and an intracellular Campylobacter-like organism associated with porcine proliferative enteropathies.
McOrist, S., Boid, R., Lawson, G.H.K., McConnell, I. (1987). Vet.Rec. 121, 421-422. Monoclonal antibodies to intracellular Campylobacter-like organisms of porcine proliferative enteropathies.
McOrist, S., Gebhart, C.J. and Lawson, G.H.K. (1994). Proc.I.P.V.S. 13, 155. The aetiology of porcine proliferative enteropathy (ileitis).
McOrist, S., Lawson, G.H.K. (1989). Res.vet.Sci. 46, 27-33. Reproduction of proliferative enteritis in gnotobiotic pigs.

McOrist, S., Lawson, G.H.K., Roy, D.J., Boid, R. (1990). FEMS Microbiology Letters 69, 189-193. DNA analysis of intracellular campylobacter-like organisms associated with porcine proliferative enteropathies.

Rowland, A.C. and Lawson, G. (1974). Res.vet.Sci. 17, 323-330. Intestinal adenomatosis in the pig : Immunofluorescence and electron microscopic studies.

Rowland, A.C. and Lawson, G.H.K. (1975). Vet.Rec. 97, 178-180. Porcine intestinal adenomatosis : A possible relationship with necrotic enteritis, regional ileitis and proliferative haemorrhagic enteropathy.

Yersinias in enteritis and human health

Definition

Yersinias (principally *Y.enterocolitica*) are capable of causing enteritis and typhlocolitis in weaned pigs and contaminating carcases to cause human food poisoning.

Incidence

Worldwide, tonsillar carriage of *Y.enterocolitica* appears to vary but is often 60% of pigs at slaughter.

Aetiology

Clinical disease in pigs is principally associated with *Y.enterocolitica* and *Y.pseudotuberculosis* and human food poisoning with *Y.enterocolitica* of biotypes 2, 09, biotype 4, 03 and biotype 1, 08. Yersinia are Gram-negative coccobacilli which form 1-2 mm colonies on blood agar after 48 hours at 37°C but which also grow at temperatures as low as 4°C. They are divided into biotypes and serotypes (usually the O group).

Pathogenesis

Oral infection with Yersinia species can lead to infection of the tonsils and multiplication in the ileum and large intestine. *Y.enterococlitica* is capable of expressing virulence determinants such as a 220 kDa outer membrane protein and an enterotoxin. *Y.pseudotuberculosis* is more commonly associated with septicaemic spread and the development of micro abscesses in liver, spleen, mesenteric lymph nodes and gut as well as the enteric lesions. Infection may localise on the tonsil and the anal ring.

Clinical signs

Y.enterocolitica is associated with mild fever (40°C, 104°F), diarrhoea which may be watery and dark in colour and with blood-stained mucus on solid faeces. It has also been recovered from lesions in cases of rectal stricture. Diarrhoea may last only 4-5 days. *Y.pseudotuberculosis* is associated with dullness, inappetence, oedema and blood-stained diarrhoea and has been isolated from rectal stricture. Poor feed conversion has been reported.

In man *Y.enterocolitica* is associated with enteritis and appendicitis. Pigs normally recover spontaneously and rarely require humane slaughter.

Pathology

No gross or microscopic findings are associated with tonsillar carriage. *Y.enterocolitical* may give rise to a catarrhal enteroiolitis in which micro colonies of the organism may be seen surrounded by neutrophils. Similar findings with button ulcers of the colon, micro-abscesses in gut wall, mesenteric lymph nodes, liver and more obvious inflammatory lesions are found in *Y.pseudotuberculosis* infection.

The organisms may be isolated from tonsil, systemic lesions and gastrointestinal tract in affected pigs.

Epidemiology

Both species may be carried by pigs for long periods of times on tonsils and *Y.enterocolitica* may be detectable in faeces for up to 30 weeks after recovery from clinical disease. The organism may survive in the environment and is capable of infecting other species such as rodents, flies and man. It has been identified in water.

In slaughter houses infection from tonsils, tongues and gut contents may contaminate carcases directly or indirectly by way of equipment. Workers may be exposed. O3 from pigs appears to be identical with that isolated from human enteritis as Restriction Endonuclease Analysis types were identical in one study.

Diagnosis

The clinical signs are not particularly suggestive of this infection and diagnosis is usually suspected following post-mortem examination or bacteriology. Isolation from faeces may require enrichment in phosphate buffered saline at 4°C. Both organisms may be isolated directly from parenchymatosis organs and may be demonstrated in tissue by DNA probes. Antibody may be present in serum and may interfere with testing for *B.suis*.

Treatment

Y.enterocolitica enteritis may respond to treatment with tetracyclines, synthetic penicillins, furazolidone and enrofloxacin in water or feed medication.

Control

Low levels of the above antimicrobials may suppress infection in pigs at risk but control of rodents, hygiene and prompt treatment of outbreaks reduces the incidence. The control of rodents and flies is important.

Vaccination using autogenous vaccines has been described.

Transmission to man may be controlled by hygiene amongst abattoir workers and by care during evisceration, removal of tongues and tonsils and by cleaning of machinery, flooring and prevention of splashing.

References

Andersen, J.K. (1988). Int.J.Food Micro. 7, 193-202. Contamination of freshly slaughtered pig carcases with human pathogenic *Y.enterocolitica*.
Barcellos D.E.S.N. de and Castro, A.F.P. de, (1981). Br.Vet.J. 137, 95-96. Isolation of *Y.pseudotuberculosis* from diarrhoeas in pigs.

160

Erwerth, W. and Natterman, H. (1987). Monatshefte fur Veterinarmedezin 42, 319-324. Histopathologische Untersuchungen bei der experimentellen oralen *Y.enterocolitica* Infektion des jungschweines.

Fukushima, H. Wakamura, R., Ito, Y. and Saito, K. (1984). Vet.Micro. 9, 375-389. Ecological studies of *Y.enterocolitica*. II Experimental infection with *Y.enterocolitica* in pigs.

Harper, P.A.W., Homitzky, M.A.Z., Rayward, D.G. (1990). Aust.vet.J. 67, 418-419. Enterocolitis in pigs associated with *Y.pseudotuberculosis* infection.

Neef, N.A., Lysons, R.J. (1994). Vet.Rec. 135, 58-63. Pathogenicity of a strain of *Y.pseudotuberculosis* isolated from a pig with porcine colitis syndrome.

Nesbakken, T. (1988). Int.J.Micro. 6, 287-293. Enumeration of *Y.enterocolitica* O:3 from porcine oral cavity and its occurrence on cut surfaces of pig carcases and the environment in a slaughterhouse.

MYCOPLASMA INFECTIONS

A number of species of Mycoplasmas and some related organisms have been isolated from pigs, but only three species have been repeatedly associated with clinical syndromes in the field. They are: *M.hyopneumoniae* the causal agent of enzootic pneumonia, *M.hyorhinis* which causes polyserositis and arthritis in younger pigs, and *M.hyosynoviae* which causes arthritis in pigs of over 35 kg. liveweight.

Other mycoplasmas isolated from pigs include the following species: *M.flocculare* (from the respiratory tract), oral cavity; *M.hyoarthrinosa* (from joint lesions); *M.hyogenitalium* (from the uterus of a sow), *M.sualvi* and *M.hyopharyngis* from intestinal and vaginal samples. Other mycoplasmas may be isolated occasionally and include *M.salivarium*, *M.gallisepticum*, *M.iners*, *M.bovigenitalium*, *M.buccale*, *M.mycoides* and *M.arginini*. Acholeplasmas do not require sterols for growth and *A.laidlawii*, *A.granularum*, *A.axanthum*, *A.oculi* and others have been isolated from the upper respiratory tract, joints and conjunctivitis but have primarily been isolated (*A.laidlawii*) from faeces.

Ureaplasmas have been isolated from the genital tracts of sows and from boar semen.

Anaerobic mycoplasmas unique to the pig have been demonstrated in large intestinal contents and the large intestinal mucosa.

Enzootic Pneumonia

Definition

Enzootic pneumonia is a contagious pulmonary disease of the pig caused by *Mycoplasma hyopneumoniae* and characterised clinically by coughing, unthriftiness and very low mortality.

Incidence

The disease is found throughout the world and is an important cause of economic loss. Herds free from enzootic pneumonia have been established and maintained in many countries. Infected herds are more common than those with clinical signs or lesions at slaughter as management, treatment and, recently, vaccination have all affected the incidence.

Aetiology

Experimental infection with pure cultures of *M.hyopneumoniae* causes enzootic pneumonia. *M.hyopneumoniae* is 200-500 nm in size, and may be seen in Giemsa-stained smears as a delicate pleomorphic organism in the form of cocci, rings, signet rings, bipolar and triangular shapes. The cell surface bears fimbriae which are more numerous in vivo that *in vitro*. The organism can be grown only on complex media containing porcine serum but little if any penicillin (it is inhibitory) in aerobic and microaerophilic conditions (5-10% carbon dioxide) and can form colonies after 2-10 days on solid media. It requires cholesterol for growth and ferments glucose but not arginine or urea. Growth inhibition studies on solid media suggested antigenic differences between strains and isolates of *M.hyopneumoniae* and the existence of different strains has been confirmed by restriction endonuclease analysis and polyacrilamide gel electrophoresis. *M.hyopneumoniae* is antigenically related to *M.flocculare* and *M.hyorhinis* in the same subcluster of *M.fermentans*. A number of antigens are specific to *M.hyopneumoniae*. They include a 36 kDa lactate dehydrogenase protein, 40, 43, 64, 74 and 97 kDa antigens which can be used to distinguish *M.hyopneumoniae* from *M.flocculare* and *M.hyorhinis* which may occur in the lesions of enzootic pneumonia. *M.hyopneumoniae* is inactivated within 48 hours of drying on cloth or hair but may persist for up to 17 days in rain water at 2-7°C. It is sensitive *in vitro* to penicillin G (important for isolation) and to tiamulin, tylosin, lincomycin, other macrolides such as spiramycin. fluorinated quinolones such as enrofloxacin, ciprofloxacin and danofloxacin and to a lesser extent to tetracyclines.

Pathogenesis

Infection with *M.hyopneumoniae* takes place by the inhalation of infected aerosols produced by infected pigs or by direct contact, and the mycoplasma becomes established in the respiratory tract where it localises on the ciliated cells of the tracheal, bronchial and bronchiolar epithelium. Attachment appears to depend upon fimbriae produced by the mycoplasmas which bind them to the microvilli and to each other. It persists in these sites for a period of weeks or months and initiates the sequence of pathological changes described below. These changes appear to be due to the presence of the organism on the surface of the epithelium where it often lies between the cilia and the apical cytoplasm of the cells. Cilia on infected cells are clumped by mycoplasma and are then shed. The apical cytoplasm of the denuded cells then bulges and the cells degenerate. A cytotoxic effect associated with the cell membrane has been demonstrated. The cytotoxin appears to be a heat-sensitive antigenic protein inactivated at 100°C for 15 minutes. Penetration of the organism into the tissues does not usually occur. Recent studies in gnotobiotic and SPF pigs show that systemic spread is possible following intravenous inoculation and may result in arthritis.

Infection of the ciliated epithelium of the respiratory tract appears to prevent normal clearance of secretory products from the tract. The lesions have been considered to result from the pooling of such material in the lobes of the lung. The earliest lesions appear 3 days after experimental infection as small dark red areas in anterior lung lobes. These areas enlarge after seven days and coalesce by 13 days post infection to give consolidation of the anterior lobes of the lung. The mediastinal and bronchial lymph nodes become greatly enlarged.

Three weeks after infection, the consolidated areas lose their reddish colour and become greyish pink, gradually fading to grey by the 8th week post infection and disappearing by 80-100 days after infection. At their maximum extent they occupy a mean of 5.7% of consolidated lung volume (28 days p.i.) in uncomplicated infection. Histological changes first appear 3 days after infection with inflammation associated with congestion of the capillaries of the alveolar septa, and the accumulation of neutrophil polymorphs in the airways and lamina propria of bronchioles. Five days post infection lymphocytes and macrophages appear, and by the 7th day, lymphoid accumulation about the bronchi and bronchioles becomes marked and the alveoli contain many large mononuclear cells, polymorphs, lymphocytes and plasma cells. There is hyperplasia of the bronchiolar epithelium, and proliferation of type 2 pneumocytes. Later changes include proliferation of the lymphoid tissue to cause occlusion of some bronchioles. Hypertrophy of the bronchial glands occurs and mucus and a mononuclear cell exudate are found in the airways. This results in the only measurable effects on respiratory function - a decrease in the respiratory:expiratory resistance ratio from 1.08 (normal) to 0.6, reduced oxygen consumption and hyper-ventilation. Affected animals eventually recover and the lesions regress, so that older sows (after 2-4 litters) may be free from infection in experimental studies.

IgA antibody develops in the tracheal mucosa and may be demonstrated in secretions from 30 days p.i. followed by IgG. Alveolar washes contain IgG from 45 days p.i. and levels peak at 80 days p.i. Serum antibody develops 8-46 days p.i., and may peak at 70-80 days p.i., persisting for at least a year. Antibody is passed by immune sows to their piglets in the colostrum and may be demonstrated in piglet serum for at least four weeks after birth. It protects against infection.

Secondary infection with *M.hyorhinis* and *Pasteurella multocida* is common and in the case of *P.multocida* may affect the extent of the lesions and the severity and duration of clinical signs. Other organisms such as *Haemophilus parasuis* and *Actinobacillus pleuropneumoniae* may also invade the lesions.

Clinical signs

Two distinct clinical syndromes occur in enzootic pneumonia, a rare, acute form associated with the reintroduction of the disease into a S.P.F. herd, and the common, chronic type found in herds where the disease is enzootic. In many S.P.F. herds, however, reinfection with *M.hyopneumoniae* has resulted in clinical signs and has had no effect on daily liveweight gain or feed efficiency.

Acute Form

Pigs of all ages may be affected and may show anorexia, pyrexia of 40.6-41.7°C, 105-107°F and respiratory distress accompanied by coughing. Some adults and up to 50% of piglets may die, often before coughing is apparent. Boars may not work and there may be delayed weaning to service intervals and other reproductive disturbances.

Chronic Form

In most cases few clinical signs of infection are apparent. Young pigs of 3-10 weeks of age become infected and within 10-16 days develop clinical signs. These begin with transient diarrhoea and a dry cough, although sneezing may be observed in sucking pigs. A low fever may occur. Later the clinical signs consist of a barking cough, particularly in finishing pigs. Coughing is most obvious when the animals are disturbed first thing in the morning. Coughing spreads gradually to most members of the group (over a period of 3-14 weeks) and lasts for about 50 days. Signs of respiratory embarrassment are rare unless secondary infection occurs. Secondary infection can lead to outbreaks of pneumonia and coughing which is particularly severe in 2-4 month old pigs.

An important clinical sign is the gradual development of uneven size amongst animals of the same weaning weight because of unequal infection in a litter. This leads to delay in marketing a batch and to husbandry problems. Uncomplicated infection depresses growth rate by as much as 15.9% from 5 to 85 kg with worsening of feed conversion ratios by as much as 13.8%. Effects are often less dramatic than this with an average reduction in feed efficiency of 0.2. Adverse environmental factors such as dusty atmospheres, chilling or high humidity may exacerbate these effects on growth. The production effects appear to be proportional to the volume of lung affected and both are more severe when other infections are present.

Animals with severe respiratory distress sufficient to cause prostration, failure to suck (if piglets), and subnormal rectal temperatures and congestion of the extremities should be killed humanely.

Pathological findings

Evidence of enzootic pneumonia is usually found incidentally at slaughter or after death from other causes, e.g. complicated pneumonia. Lesions are found bilaterally in the apical, cardiac and intermediate lobes and in the anterior parts of the diaphragmatic lobes and are fawn/pink or plum-coloured and clearly demarcated from the normal lung tissue. The bronchial and mediastinal lymph nodes are enlarged. Lung lesion scores can be constructed to give quantitative results from lung maps.

Histological examination normally shows marked peribronchial and peribronchiolar lympho-reticular hyperplasia. There is proliferation of cells on the alveolar walls and many type 2 pneumocytes and macrophages occur in the lumen of the alveoli. Plasma cells also occur in the alveolar lumen. In older lesions, alveolar collapse may occur.

Mycoplasmas are present in Giemsa-stained impression smears made from the lesions but they are difficult to identify as *M.hyopneumoniae* by their morphology. Isolation of the organism is not feasible in many cases, as *M.hyorhinis* often grows more profusely and masks *M.hyopneumoniae* colonies. If isolation attempts are made, presumptive *M.hyopneumoniae* colonies may be identified by a fluorescent antibody method or the growth inhibition test. The methods described by Friis (1975) or Friis *et al.* (1991) are most widely used for isolation. *M.hyopneumoniae* may also be identified in lung tissue using immunofluorescence on smears or on frozen sections. Organisms can be seen as a yellow-green granular layer on the surface of the bronchial and bronchiolar epithelium. Immunoperoxidase techniques can demonstrate organisms in fixed sections.

Epidemiology

Enzootic pneumonia is normally transmitted to susceptible pigs by direct contact with infected animals or by their inclusion in the same air-space. Young pigs normally become infected from carrier sows soon after birth or when introduced into an airspace containing infected animals. Maternal immunity may protect piglets from infection and the infection of a group may be uneven, taking several weeks under some circumstances. The organism becomes progressively less easy to isolate from 85 days post-infection and many gilts of 8 months of age may be free from infection and by the second or third parity infection is rare.

The widespread use of serological testing has confirmed that spread of infection within a unit depends upon the husbandry system and that clinical signs and slaughterhouse monitoring of lungs do not reflect the onset or prevalence of infection very well. Differences in the onset of infection of 3-4 weeks may occur in different houses on the same unit. Infection is transmitted most rapidly within common airspaces in continuous stocking systems with open pen divisions, and least frequently in all-in-all-out systems and outdoor systems. It may die out in small (<25 sow) herds. Aerosol spread between buildings can occur but occurs less frequently when buildings are 10 m apart.

Spread between buildings on clothing and implements is also possible, but the organism does not appear to persist in human respiratory passages or to occur in reservoir hosts such as rats and mice.

Infection is usually introduced to uninfected farms by the purchase of carrier pigs but aerosol transmission between units may occur up to 3.2 km (2 miles). Sources of aerosol infection include infected farms (especially units with more than 500 animals) and infected pigs being transported past the farm. Transmission of infection between farms by man, other animals or fomites appears to be rare.

Diagnosis

Enzootic pneumonia is normally diagnosed on the basis of findings in a herd rather than in an individual animal. The most useful criteria are:

1.   The presence of a chronic pneumonia in the herd, particularly in fattening pigs, resulting in uneven growth rate and poor feed conversion efficiency but with no mortality.

2.   Clinical signs in the 2-4 month old age range - a dry non-productive cough without fever or respiratory distress.

3.   Post-mortem findings of a sharply demarcated, "cuffing" type of pneumonia in the anterior lung lobes. The histological findings are not specific, but help to confirm the diagnosis.

4.   Confirmation by laboratory tests is essential for diagnosis, especially in monitoring schemes. Infection can be confirmed by:

     Culture from freshly collected lung tissue with and without lesions from apical and cardiac lobes. Access to a competent laboratory is required and the methods of Friis *etal.* (1991) may be most appropriate.

Immunofluorescence uses the same material as culture and specific monoclonal or absorbed polyclonal antisera.

Polymerase chain reaction (PCR) using swabs from all three stem bronchi of both lungs and primers from the 16S rRNA gene.
Antigen ELISA using specific monoclonal antibody can be used on the same swab samples.

All three of these methods are equivalent to culture at 14 and 28 days post-infection but their sensitivity declines to 60-90% by day 57 p.i. and 11-40% by day 85 p.i.
DNA probes have been described but may only be 60% as efficient as immunofluorescence.

Immunoperoxidase may be used on fixed sections.

Antibody may be detected in serum using a number of tests. Most repeatable and specific results have been obtained with ELISAs using the 36 kDa engineered lactate dehydrogenase enzyme as antigen. Monoclonal blocking ELISA.s and Tween 20 ELISAs are also available.

All of these three serological tests (and others using fractions extracted from M.hyopneumoniae) are specific for that organism and do not cross-react with M.flocculare, M.hyorhinis or M.hyosynoviae in use. Antibody levels are first detectable at 10 days post-infection and remain detectable for at least 80 days post infection.
The Complement Fixation test (CFT) may still be used but is less specific and sensitive than the commercially-available ELISAs.
Other agents commonly complicate enzootic pneumonia. M.hyorhinis and P.multocida are common invaders, the latter frequently being present in the more severe and prolonged cases of enzootic pneumonia with the most extensive lesions. PRRS may also be present. Enzootic pneumonia can be differentiated from Haemophilus infection, pleuropneumonia and swine influenza by the lack of fever except, possibly, in non-immune herds, and from parasitic infection such as Ascaris and Metastrongylus infections by the post-mortem findings. The lesions of enzootic pneumonia are distinctive but may need to be differentiated from those caused by Chlamydia.

Treatment

Infection with mycoplasmas is difficult to eliminate entirely, but the clinical manifestations of enzootic pneumonia can be reduced by treatment with a number of drugs. Water medication with tetracyclines will prevent infection with mycoplasmas and treatment with tylosin or spiramycin may also reduce infection. Tiamulin, (Tiamutin, Dynamutilin) 10-15 mg/kg has been shown to reduce and eliminate lesions from infected pigs when given in the water, and in the feed, but may not eliminate the mycoplasma. Treatment may have to be continued for 5-10 days. Best results have been obtained by tiamulin treatment using injectable drug at 15 mg/kg for three successive days. It may also be used with chlortetracycline. Lincomycin and spectinomycin:lincomycin combinations may also be of value. Fluorinated quinolones such as ciprofloxacin and danofloxacin are active against M.hyopneumoniae. The only one of these products currently (1995) registered in UK is enrofloxacin (Baytril

Bayer) which is available in parenteral and oral forms for use at 2.5 mg/kg. The lung lesions of enzootic pneumonia take some time to regress after treatment and are not completely eliminated by treatment although significant production improvement can be expected.

Control

a) Husbandry methods to mitigate the effect

1. All-in, all-out policy for buildings or units. Each house should be emptied at the same time, fumigated and re-filled.
There are clear advantages in this practice and productivity is higher and general disease levels are lower. The effects are particularly marked if all-in, all-out husbandry is applied to whole sites. When combined with treatment of a batch upon entry, this practice may reduce economic effects considerably.

'Isowean' (PIC)
This name is given to a system in which piglets are weaned at three weeks, moved to a clean site and reared for four weeks. They are then moved to clean grower sites and the rearing site cleaned ready for a new batch. After 4-6 weeks in grower sites, pigs move to clean finisher sites. This application of the all-in, all-out principle may be accompanied by treatment at entry and has reduced disease losses dramatically.

2. Low stocking densities for housed pigs. Each pig is allowed individual accommodation and forced ventilation is used. Expensive, but when applied to groups with good ventilation, enzootic pneumonia may be reduced   Studies have shown that ammonia does not predispose to *M.hyopneumoniae* infection but exacerbates complicated lesions.

3. Pigs in extensive systems rarely develop enzootic pneumonia, but finishing pigs by this method is uneconomic. Infection may persist in animals reared outdoors.

b) Vaccination

A number of vaccines have been produced and evaluated. Most have been parenteral and consist of killed organisms or extracts of them, combined with aluminium hydroxide. Aerosol vaccination, oral vaccination, intraperitoneal vaccination with oil-adjuvanted killed organisms, and the use of live lapinised vaccines have all been described. The vaccines which are now commercially available (not UK 1995) Suvaxyn M-hyo (Duphar) and Respisure/Stellamune (SKB) have been tested in a number of countries. In controlled trials they reduce the number and extent of lesions by 50% and improve daily liveweight gain, feed conversion and days to slaughter to a variable extent. Responses are most satisfactory when pigs are vaccinated at 3 and 5 weeks as opposed to 1 and 3 weeks.

c) Treatment

1. Continuous medication

Low levels of medication may be given continuously e.g., tiamulin at 40 ppm in feed to suppress the development of clinical signs and lesions.

2. Pulse medication

Treatment may be given at therapeutic levels to all pigs in a building or in the finishing portion of the herd. Treatment usually lasts for two days in each week, allowing for withdrawal periods for units sending pigs for slaughter weekly.

3. Strategic medication

Treatment may be given at therapeutic level to all pigs entering an airspace. This is particularly effective when coupled with all-in, all-out husbandry.

Any of the products listed above could be used but combinations such as tiamulin and chlortetracycline may be more effective on some units where enzootic pneumonia is complicated.

d) Serum profiling

The availability of ELISAs for serum antibody testing has allowed antibody profiles to be constructed for herds and individual houses within a herd. These allow the time of infection (10 days prior to initial antibody detection) to be identified and allow vaccination (where available) or treatment measures to be applied precisely.

e) Eradication

Enzootic pneumonia may be eradicated in four main ways:

1. Hysterectomy and isolation

Piglets removed by hysterectomy and reared apart from the dam in isolation are free from enzootic pneumonia and many other infective conditions. Complete repopulation of herds by this means is rarely a practicable proposition on the average farm, but has been used to provide enzootic pneumonia (and other disease) free stock for repopulation. The nucleus herds of large hybrid organisations are mostly enzootic pneumonia-free, are maintained in strict isolation and are given new blood lines only by hysterectomy. Isolation should include at least 3.2 km separation from the nearest infected unit under U.K. conditions for it to be effective for long periods. Isolated units should be sited away from main roads and visiting personnel and transport should be closely controlled.

In the U.K. many herds of this type are monitored for infection by means of quarterly or six-monthly clinical inspections, the recording of incidents of respiratory disease and the examination of lungs from pigs at slaughter with further investigation of any circumstance which suggests enzootic pneumonia or infection with *M.hyopneumoniae*. A regular programme of serological monitoring is now possible. Monitoring of finishing pigs should be supplemented by sampling of sows and their colostrum. In some circumstances new blood may be introduced by A.I. or embryo transfer which pose little risk of infection.

Breakdown rates of 4-10% p.a. have been recorded in such schemes in the U.K., Switzerland, Denmark and the U.S.A.

2. Slaughter and re-stocking

    Enzootic pneumonia-free stock is available in Britain and other countries, on a commercial basis. Farms should be cleared of all pigs, cleaned, disinfected and fumigated, left free from pigs for four weeks and then repopulated with disease-free animals. The sources of these animals are usually the nucleus or multiplying herds of commercial hybrid organisations, many of which are free from the disease.

3. Treatment and isolation as means of eradication

    Medicated early weaning: Tiamulin has recently been used in two ways for the eradication of enzootic pneumonia from pig herds. In the Medicated Early Weaning technique, farrowing sows are treated with tiamulin and their litters snatched or weaned at 5 days and reared artificially. For the first 10 days of life, oral therapy with tiamulin at 10 mg/kg is given. Mortality can be high, but the organism is apparently eliminated in most cases.

    The piglets produced can be reared in isolation and tested for the development of antibody before introduction to a clean herd.

    Whole herd treatment after partial depopulation. Breeding stock can be treated with tiamulin in the feed (at 200 ppm) or in drinking water to give 10 mg/kg daily for 10 days following removal of weaned, growing or finishing pigs. Provided no untreated pigs are present on the farm, pigs may remain free from enzootic pneumonia for years. The absence of infection can be confirmed by serological and clinical monitoring of the new finishing herd.

4. Segregation and isolation

    This method is laborious. The progeny of older sows (more than 2 parities) are often free from infection and can be reared in isolation. They may be protected from disease by colostral immunity and remain carriers. Exhaustive serological testing and slaughter monitoring of these pigs may be required to confirm that an enzootic pneumonia-free herd has been produced.

    Piglets reared and later finished on successive all-in, all-out isolated sites (Isowean) may also be free from infection, but careful monitoring is needed before they could be introduced to nucleus or multiplying herds.

References

Alexander, T.J.L., Thornton, K., Boon, G., Lysons, R.J. and Gush, A.F. (1980). Vet.Rec. 106, 114-119. Medicated early weaning to obtain pigs free from pathogens endemic in the herd of origin.

Barford, K., Sorensen, V., Feld, N.C. (1994). Proc.IPVS 13, 189. Evaluation of a monoclonal blocking ELISA detecting antibodies on a single pig level.

Bereiter, M., Young, T.F., Foo, H.S. and Ross, R.F. (1990). Vet.Microbiol. 25, 177-192. Evaluation of the ELISA and comparison to the complement fixation test and radial immunodiffusion enzyme assay for detection of antibodies against *M.hyopneumoniae* in swine serum.

Blanchard, B., Vena M.M., Cavalier, A., Lannic, J. le., Gouranton, J., Kobisch, M. (1992). Vet.Micro. 30, 329-341. Electron microscopical observations of the respiratory tract of SPF piglets inoculated with *M.hyopneumoniae*

Clark, I.F., Scheidt, A.B., Mayrose, V.B., Armstrong, C.H. and Knox, K. (1990). Proc.IPVS 11, 91. Prevention of the development of enzootic pneumonia within an infected swine herd.

Doster A.R. and Lin, B.C. (1988). Am.J.vet.Res. 49, 1719-1721. Indirect immunoperoxidase used to identify *M.hyopneumoniae* in porcine lung.

Feenstra, A.A., Sorensen, V., Friis, N.F., Jensen, N.E. and Bille Hansen, V. (1994). Proc.IPVS 13, 187. Experimental *M.hyopneumoniae* infection in pigs.

Friis N.F. (1975). Nord.Vet.Med. 27, 337-339. Some recommendations concerning primary isolation of *M.suipneumoniae* and *M.flocculare*.

Friis, N.F., Ahrens P. and Larsen, H. (1991). Acta.Vet.Scand. 32, 425-429. *M.hyosynoviae* isolation from the upper respiratory tract and tonsils of pigs.

Geary, S.J. and Walczak, E.M. (1983). Infection and Immunity, 41, 132-136. Isolation of a cytopathic factor from *M.hyopneumoniae*.

Goodwin, R.F.W. (1985). Vet.Rec. 116, 690-694. Apparent reinfections of enzootic pneumonia-free pig herd : search for possible causes.

Goodwin, R.F.W. and Whittlestone, P. (1967). Vet Rec. 81, 643. The detection of enzootic pneumonia in pig herds 1. Eight years' general experience with a pilot control scheme.

Haldimann, A., Nicolet, J., Frey, J. (1993). J.Gen.Microbiol. 139, 317-323. DNA sequence determination and biochemical analysis of the immunogenic protein P36, the lactate dehydrogenase (LDH) of *M.hyopneumoniae*

Hannan, P.C.T., O'Hanlon, P.J., Rogers, N.H. (1989). Res.Vet.Sci. 46, 202-211. *In vitro* evaluation of various quinolone antibacterial agents against veterinary mycoplasmas and porcine respiratory pathogens.

Simon, F., Semjen, G., Dubos Kovacs, M., Laczay, P. and Cserep, I. (1990). Proc.IPVS. 11, 96. Efficacy of enrofloxacin against enzootic pneumonia of swine.

Sorensen, V., Barfod, K., Ahrens, P., Feenstra, A.A., Pedersen, M.W., Feld, N.C. and Jensen, N.E. (1994). Proc.IPVS. 13, 188. Comparison of four different methods for demonstration of *M.hyopneumoniae* in lungs of experimentally inoculated pigs.

Sorensen, V., Barfod, K., Feenstra, A.A. and Feld, N.C. (1994). Proc.IPVS 13, 190. The humoral immune response to *M.hyopneumoniae* infection in pigs in reltion to clinical signs and pathological lesions.

Sorensen, V., Barfod, K., Feld, N.C. (1992). Vet.Rec. 130, 488-490. Evaluation of a monoclonal blocking ELISA and I.H.A. for antibodies to *M.hyopneumoniae* in SPF pigs.

Sorensen, V., Barfod, K., Feld, N.C., Vraa-Andersen, L. (1993). Revue Scientifique et Technique - Office International des Epizooties 12, 593-604. Application of ELISA for the surveillance of *M.hyopneumoniae* infection in pigs.

Stark, K.D.C., Keller, H., Eggenburger, E. (1992). Vet.Rec. 131, 532-535. Risk factors for the reinfection of pig breeding herds with enzootic pneumonia.

Strasser, M., Frey, J., Besteti, G., Kobisch, M., Nicolet, J. (1991). Inf. and Imm. 59, 1217-1222. Cloning and expression of a species-specific early immunogenic 36 kDa protein of *M.hyopneumoniae* and *E.coli*.

Vraa-Andersen, L., Christensen, G., Kuiper, R. (1994). Proc.IPVS. 13, 192. Vaccine efficacy with Suvaxyn *M.hyo* in Denmark.

Infection with Mycoplasma hyorhinis

Definition

M.hyorhinis causes polyserositis and arthritis in pigs of 3-10 weeks of age and some strains have been shown to cause pneumonia and to occur in otitis media.

Incidence

The clinical syndrome is rarely identified but is probably widespread in Britain as *M.hyorhinis* is a common inhabitant of the nasal cavity of pigs and can be isolated from up to 60% of pigs. It is commonly present in the lesions of enzootic pneumonia (40-60%) It is usually absent from hysterectomy-derived herds maintained in isolation.

Aetiology

M.hyorhinis forms colonies on the same media used for *M.hyopneumoniae* within 1-2 days. However, *M.hyorhinis* cannot always be grown on conventional mycoplasma media and may need to be cultured on media containing cells such as BHK-21 or lysates of them or on mink S and L cells in which a characteristic cytopathic effect is produced. M.hyorhinis produces phosphatase and reduces tetrazolium unlike either of the other two common porcine mycoplasmas. Slight antigenic differences between isolates have been identified.

Some of these have been shown to be due to a variable surface lipoprotein Vlp, three forms of which exist, able to produce 10^4 antigenic variations. The genes for these proteins have been cloned.

Pathogenesis

M.hyorhinis enters the body, by the respiratory tract often from lesions of enzootic pneumonia, causes a septicaemia and settles out on serous surfaces and in the joints where it causes inflammation. Complement-fixing and metabolic inhibition antibodies are produced.

Clinical signs

An incubation period of 3-10 days is followed by subclinical infection or a slight fever, less than 40.6°C, 105°F, which is present for 4-5 days. Affected pigs are often 3-10 weeks of age and show a reduction in appetite and a marked reduction in growth rate, a hairy coat. Many stretch or breathe in an unusual fashion when disturbed. Arthritis and swelling of the joints may occur, and many pigs remain affected for up to 6 months. Recovery begins 4 weeks after infection. Up to 25% of the pigs may be affected in an outbreak.

Infection commonly complicates enzootic pneumonia without any apparent exacerbation of the condition and pasteurellosis where it may exacerbate clinical signs. It has been isolated repeatedly from otitis media.

Affected animals rarely require humane destruction but it might be indicated following fibrous pericarditis or prolonged lameness unresponsive to antimicrobial treatment.

Pathological findings

At post-mortem examination, affected pigs are seen to be thin, with fibrinous pericarditis, pleurisy and peritonitis. In later cases, adhesions may be present between the organs in the affected cavity. Joint lesions occur, particularly in the tarsus, stifle, carpus and shoulder. Affected joints contain large amounts of serofibrinous or serosanguineous synovia, and villous hypertrophy of the synovial membranes and erosion of the articular cartilages is often present. The villous hypertrophy is associated with accumulations of plasma cells and lymphocytes.

Inflammatory changes in the respiratory tract include a subacute catarrhal bronchopneumonia which resolves spontaneously and eustachian tube inflammation. Organisms adhere to the cilia.

Antibody develops following infection.

Epidemiology

Infection spreads between pigs by aerosol or direct contact and between farms principally by infected carrier pigs.

Diagnosis

Distinguished from Glasser's disease, streptococcal meningitis and arthritis and *A.pleuropneumoniae* infection by the absence of fever and low mortality, and from M.hyosynoviae by the age affected. Post-mortem findings, bacteriology and immunofluorescence on frozen sections of respiratory tract will confirm.

Control and treatment

The use of hyperimmune gamma globulin has been described for both treatment and prevention of *M.hyorhinis* infection but it is rarely available and not in UK. Antimicrobials suitable for use in enzootic pneumonia may be of value and eradication using the methods used for enzootic pneumonia may also be effective.

Reference

Friis, N.F., Feenstra, A.A. (1994). Acta Vet Scand 35, 93-98. *M.hyorhinis* in the aeriology of serositis amongst piglets.

Kazama, S., Yagihashi, T., Morita, T., Awakura, T., Shimada, A., Umemura, T. (1994). Res.Vet.Sci. 56, 108-110. Isolation of *M.hyorhinis* and *M.arginini* from the ears of pigs with otitis media.

Levy, J.A., Sumner, P.E. and Hooser, L.E. (1982). J.General Microbiology 128, 2817-2820. Rapid tissue culture method for detection of *M.hyorhinis*.

M.hyosynoviae Infection

Definition

M.hyosynoviae causes an arthritis in pigs weighing between 35 kg and 115 kg and is a frequent cause of lameness in recently purchased breeding stock.

Incidence

It was reported to be responsible for 23% of cases of arthritis in fattening pigs over 35 kg liveweight in Iowa. It has been identified in Britain by clinical signs, and confirmed by serology and isolation and is now common in pigs from some suppliers.

Aetiology

M.hyosynoviae differs from the other two major pig mycoplasmas by fermenting arginine but not glucose or urea. It is best isolated in anaerobic conditions when it can outgrow M.hyorhinis. It may survive drying for up to 4 weeks but is more sensitive in vitro to tiamulin than other mycoplasmas.

Pathogenesis

It is commonly found on the tonsils of healthy carrier sows and occurs in the pharyngeal region in 7-8 week old pigs. Infection is by the oronasal route and has taken place in many herds by 10-12 weeks of age. Septicaemia develops 2-4 days after intranasal inoculation and the organism settles out in the joints to a variable extent to produce the characteristic clinical and pathological findings. It may also occur in the lungs.

Clinical signs

Few clinical signs are apparent. No fever is noted, and the only apparent effect is alteration in the gait of the affected pigs. Acute lameness may also occur in one or more limbs. Affected animals usually weigh more than 35 kg. Bursitis may develop but external signs may not be apparent. Affected pigs limp, shift weight from one leg to another or may be unable to rise. In Britain, non-immune gilts or boars introduced into infected herds are chiefly affected with sudden lameness 7-21 days after introduction.

Humane slaughter may be indicated when chronically-affected animals are unable to rise. These acute signs may last for 3-10 days and then decrease.

Pathological findings

The synovial fluid from affected joints is yellowish-brown in colour and may contain flakes of fibrin but the articular surface usually remains normal. Swelling and hyperaemia is seen in the synovial membrane of affected large limb joints. Polyserositis is absent. M.hyosynoviae can be isolated from affected joints, lymph nodes and mucous membrane secretions during the acute stage of the disease and from tonsils and pharynx in carriers.

Diagnosis

Acute lameness in older fattening pigs or recently introduced breeding stock with no fever or evidence of polyserositis. Isolation and identification of the organism confirms. Selective media (Friis 1991) may be required to suppress *M.hyorhinis*. ELISA demonstration of circulating antibody may also be used. Erysipelas and osteochondrosis should be eliminated before reaching a diagnosis.

Treatment

Treatment of animals with early clinical signs with tiamulin at 15 mg/kg by injection on 2-3 successive days has been found useful. Isolation of the organism from the joints of such treated animals is difficult. Those at risk such as animals in contact should also be treated. Tylosin or lincomycin may also be used for a similar period.

References

Blowey, R.W. (1993). Pig Vet.J. 30, 72-76. *M.hyosynoviae* arthritis.
Burch, D.G.S. and Goodwin, R.F.W. (1984). Vet.Rec. 115, 594-595. Use of tiamulin on a herd of pigs seriously affected with *M.hyosynoviae* arthritis.
Friis, N.F., Ahrens P., Larsen, H. (1991). Acta Vet.Scand. 32, 425-429. *M.hyosynoviae* isolation from the upper respiratory tract and tonsils of pigs.
Madeiro, C.A. (1984). Vet.Rec. 115, 446. *M.hyosynoviae* treatment in pigs.

M.arthritidis infection

M.arthritidis, a rodent mycoplasma, has been isolated from joints in an outbreak of conjunctivitis, severe polyarthritis and infertility in a boar stud.

Reference

Binder, A., Aumuller, R., Likitsecharote, B., Kirchhoff, H. (1990). J.Vet.Med. Series B. 611-614. Isolation of *M.arthritidis* from the joint fluid of boars.

Bordetella bronchiseptica infections

Definition

B.bronchiseptica colonises the ciliated epithelium of the upper respiratory tract early in life to cause rhinitis characterised by sneezing, mild turbinate atrophy and some reduction in the rate of daily liveweight gain. *B.bronchiseptica* also colonises the lower respiratory tract to cause a persistent purulent bronchitis and a pneumonia which may persist in the absence of nasal changes to cause depression of the daily rate of liveweight gain.

Incidence

Infection with *B.bronchiseptica* was present in 91% of pig herds in one survey in southern England and the infection is present in all pig rearing countries, often at a similar prevalence. One study from Italy found it in 75/76 farms

Aetiology

B.bronchiseptica is a small (0.5 x 0.8-I.0 µm) Gram-negative aerobic bacillus and is motile. It produces ß-haemolytic 1-2 mm grey colonies on some nutrient blood agars but on richer media is non-haemolytic. On MacConkey agar it produces non-lactose fermenting colonies and usually takes 48 hours to become fully visible. The organism is urease positive, and utilises citrate and glucose.

B.bronchiseptica exists in 4 colony phases, I to Vir-. Phase 1 colonies contain fully virulent organisms. The pathogenic determinants produced include fimbriae, the mannose-resistant haemagglutinin, (filamentous hamagglutinin, FHA) and the 68 kDa outer membrane protein pertactin all involved in adhesion. A number of toxic factors are also produced; the haemolysin is an adenyl cyclase; a cytotoxin has been described, an osteocytic toxin and the Dermonecrotoxin (DNT) of 14 kDa has been cloned. Phase II, III organisms may not express all these characters and may be isolated from pigs. All variants, including Vir- may be derived from Phase I organisms *in vitro.* but reversion to Phase I can only take place *in vivo.* There are antigenic differences between isolates but they have not been fully defined.

The organism survives drying and in water for 3 weeks, is sensitive to disinfectants and to antibiotics such as trimethoprim, sulphonamide ampicillin and fluorinated quinolones such as enrofloxacin.

Pathogenesis

Phase I *B.bronchiseptica* infect pigs by aerosol or contact and colonise the ciliated epithelium of the nasal cavity.

It is not clear whether infection of the lower respiratory tract occurs directly or as a result of inhalation or postnasal drip from the infected nasal cavity. The organism attaches to the cilia, microvilli and epithelial cell surfaces by means of surface structures which appear as a fuzzy or stringy structure visible in electron-micrographs and proliferates to reach high numbers ($4x10^{10}$). When levels exceed $3x10^5$, the cilia are lost in the region of greatest bacterial growth and a neutrophil reaction occurs. Toxic substances which include adenyl cyclase and DNT diffuse into the tissue and cause changes in osteoblasts of the bones of the nasal cavity within 7 days of infection. Osteoid fibres are reduced and turbinate atrophy has occurred within 14-21 days. In other parts of the body, bony changes and changes in cartilages have been seen but it is not clear whether these are directly attributable to the toxin or to indirect effects of altered nutrition and chronic inflammation. Turbinate atrophy usually resolves in uncomplicated infections by the time of slaughter and within 70 days in experimental infections in gnotobiotic pigs.

In the lower respiratory tract, a bronchopneumonia may develop early in the disease process. It affects the cranial and middle lobes of the lung in particular but may occur as discrete patches in other lobes. The pneumonic areas may contain the bacteria but these are usually restricted to the bronchi where they cause a mucopurulent exudate. The organisms persist in the trachea, bronchi and bronchioles for at least 2-3 months after infection. Lung lesions often resolve by collapse and scarring.

Immunity to infection may develop and is passed on to the offspring as passive immunity. Neither type of immunity appears to eliminate infection and passive immunity can be overwhelmed by heavy challenge. Immunity does appear however to reduce the bony changes and restrict lower respiratory tract infection to the bronchioles, bronchi and trachea. Infection with other bacteria such as *P.multocida, Mycoplasma hyorhinis, Haemophilus parasuis* can occur in the nose and *Haemophilus parasuis* and mycoplasmas commonly occur in the bronchitis or bronchopneumonia.

Clinical signs

Outbreaks of sneezing occur in baby pigs from 1 week of age and this may be paroxysmal with snorting and sometimes epistaxis. Tear staining is often seen and mucopurulent exudate may be seen on the nostrils, hanging from them or on the pen floor. Occasionally signs of twisting of the snout may develop in uncomplicated infections but this and other persistent changes of atrophic rhinitis such as brachygnathia superior (shortening of the upper jaw) and complete turbinate atrophy are more common in Progressive Atrophic Rhinitis. There may be coughing in the pneumonic form which may begin within 3-4 days of infection and be accompanied by mild fever (to 40°C, 104°F), anorexia and loss of condition and increased respiratory rates. Mortality can occur at this stage in uncomplicated infections and may reach 30%.

Uncomplicated infections with *B.bronchiseptica* have been shown to cause reductions in the rate of daily liveweight gain of 16-19% when compared with minimal disease controls and from 26-30% in conventional pigs. In complicated infections these figures could be exceeded in non-immune pigs but in immune pigs may be reduced as would be the severity of the clinical signs. In the progeny of immune sows they may be restricted to sneezing amongst piglets.

Humane destruction may be indicated in young pigs with severe pneumonia and loss of condition or in wasted sucking piglets. It need not be considered unless treatment has proved ineffective.

Pathology

The pathology of uncomplicated *B.bronchiseptica* infection is that of a catarrhal rhinitis accompanied by some failure of the conchal bones and ethmoturbinates to develop and/or some distortion of the nasal septum. The nasal mucosa may be covered in exudate, inflamed and in the later stages may be metaplastic. In all cases, a purulent bronchitis can be demonstrated and in cases of bronchopneumonia, areas of consolidation and reddening may be seen in the cranial and middle lung lobes or as red, pneumonic areas elsewhere. These lesions frequently heal by collapse and fibrosis and leave fissures in the lung. The bronchitis can be demonstrated in the absence of gross lung lesions.

Histological changes include a catarrhal rhinitis with loss of the epithelium and heavy infiltration with inflammatory cells. In chronic cases metaplasia and loss of the goblet cells occurs. Fibrous tissue occurs in the submucosal tissues and there is a decrease in the numbers of osteoblasts. In the lower respiratory tract a catarrhal exudate is present in the bronchi and in pneumonic lesions there is congestion, intra-alveolar haemorrhage and accumulation of neutrophils. The healing lesion contains macrophages and fibroblasts. Bacteria may be seen adhering to surviving ciliated epithelium.

B.bronchiseptica can be isolated from the nasal cavity, trachea, bronchi and bronchial lymph nodes in early cases, but only from the ethmoturbinate and sometimes from the bronchi in chronic cases or carriers. Other organisms, e.g. *P.multocida* may also be isolated.

Epidemiology

B.bronchiseptica infection is usually introduced to a herd by the purchase of infected carrier pigs from an infected herd. These pigs may be clinically normal. On rare occasions the organism may be introduced on clothing or hair on which the organism may be in dust or dried nasal secretions. A number of animal species such as dogs, rodents and man can carry the organism in their respiratory tracts. These organisms can cause disease in pigs but are less likely to colonise the nose in the numbers required for disease than porcine strains. Restriction endonuclease studies confirm that pig *B.bronchiseptica* strains differ from those of other species.

Spread within a farm is by aerosol and by direct and indirect contact. It is enhanced by poor ventilation, by the presence of large numbers of pigs within an airspace and by the weight of infection. In immune herds airborne organisms are most common from 14 days of age in farrowing accommodation and throughout the rearing period.

Evidence from nasal inoculation studies in gnotobiotic pigs suggests that 3×10^5 organisms may be required to cause infection to become established. The development of pneumonia, atrophy of the turbinate changes and distortion of the nasal septum depend upon a number of factors. The most important of these is probably the state of immunity of the pig when infected. Maternal immunity is passed to the piglet and protects against gross changes but not against the establishment of infection. The piglets of non-immune mothers or those with a poor immune status (usually gilts) may develop severe disease. In herds which are rapidly expanding or in which sow turnover is high, clinical disease can be widespread. Infection of susceptible pigs occurs in weaner pools in fattening units, particularly when pigs from different sources are mixed, and the subclinical form of the disease occurs.

Diagnosis

The clinical signs of severe sneezing and tear staining in piglets suggest that *B.bronchiseptica* infection is present. When it is present alone, growth depression in non-immune pigs and some transient changes in the bones of the nasal cavity may be seen. Tear staining is common and pneumonic changes such as coughing, dyspnoea and some mortality may also occur.

When outbreaks of sneezing occur in piglets or older weaned animals, isolation of *B.bronchiseptica* from nasal swabs (cotton tip, not alginate) may be of use in confirmation. Selective medium containing penicillin, furaltadone, gentamycin and bromthymol blue may be used as may cephalothin media. Isolation may be made on simple blood agar or MacConkey medium at post mortem examination by culturing the turbinates, the sinus epithelium or the tracheal or bronchial epithelium. 48 hours incubation is necessary.

Sneezing should be differentiated from that of inclusion body rhinitis (earlier in non-immune herds and not responsive to antimicrobial therapy) and the pneumonic form from other causes of pneumonia such as enzootic pneumonia, pleuropneumonia and pasteurellosis. If Progressive Atrophic Rhinitis is present, the presence of *B.bronchiseptica* infection in the herd may be assumed in most cases. Agglutination and ELISA tests for serum antibody using the 68K outer membrane protein as antigen can be carried out.

Treatment

B.bronchiseptica may be sensitive *in vitro* to a number of antimicrobials. These include tetracyclines, ampicillin, erythromycin, cloxacillin, enrofloxacin, streptomycin, sulphonamides such as sulphadimidine, and trimethoprim: sulphonamide. Parenteral treatment with any of these agents may be given to severely affected pigs and this should be followed by oral dosing with the same drug if in piglets or water medication in older pigs if possible. Treatment should be continued for at least 10 days and preferably for 2 weeks.

Control

Prophylactic medication

(a)   In the feed. Clinical signs can be suppressed by the medication of the feed with trimethoprim:sulphonamides (30 mg/kg daily), tetracycline, sulphonamides such as sulphadimidine or a proprietary mixture of sulphadimidine with another agent such as tylosin (Tylasul, Elanco). All of these products may be used to medicate the feed especially in recently weaned pigs. All pigs in the same airspace should be medicated.

(b)   By strategic therapy. Parenteral treatment with trimethoprim: sulphonamide given at 3 days, 10 days and 3 weeks of age may prevent clinical signs of the disease and reduce the shedding of *B.bronchiseptica*. Long acting tetracyclines may also produce a similar effect.

Vaccination

(a)   Killed vaccines. A number of formalin-killed, alum-adjuvanted vaccines have been produced. Most were originally used to control Progressive Atrophic Rhinitis and most have now been supplemented with *P.multocida* toxoid. The *B.bronchiseptica* component of these combined vaccines and the few remaining vaccines containing the organism alone are of the killed organism type. They are used to immunise sows 6 and 2 weeks prior to farrowing and protect piglets from bronchopneumonia and rhinitis by means of passive antibody transfer. Active immunity can be stimulated by vaccination of piglets at 7 and 28 days of age. Reduction in clinical signs occurs on a herd basis and the rate of carriage of the organism is reduced. Recent studies have shown that purified adhesive antigens may protect against colonisation.

(b)   Live vaccines. An attenuated live vaccine has been described. It is given by nasal instillation, establishes in the respiratory tract and is claimed to reduce the incidence of gross lesions. The vaccine strain may not colonise upon first administration because of maternal immunity and may be eliminated accidentally by treatment.
Modern developments with other *Bordetella sp.* have not yet been applied to either killed or live *B.bronchiseptica* vaccines for pigs which

remain traditional in nature whether produced alone or in combination with *P.multocida.*

Eradication

The medicated early-weaning technique in which sows are medicated with trimethoprim:sulphonamide prior to farrowing and the piglets dosed orally for 10 days, being weaned at 5 days, has been shown to eliminate *B.bronchiseptica* infection. Similar results have been achieved by medication of the drinking water with the drug at levels of 7 and 35 ppm of trimethoprim:sulphadiazine mixture for 28 days. The use of this treatment coupled with all in, all out husbandry can free fattening herds from the infection and control the disease in a breeding herd.

Husbandry measures

The use of an all-in, all-out housing policy and the provision of good ventilation will reduce the severity of the disease by reducing the weight of infection. On a herd basis, the purchase of animals from herds known to be free from infection, or the treatment of incoming animals may reduce the chance of introducing the disease to any uninfected herd. The use of more old sows as mothers may also reduce the incidence of clinical disease.

References

Cameron, R.D.A., Giles, C.J. and Smith, I.M. (1980). Vet.Rec. 107, 146-149. The prevalence of *Bordetella bronchiseptica* and turbinate (conchal) atrophy in English pig herds in 1978-1979.

Collings, L.A., Rutter, J.M. (1985). J.Med.Microbiol. 19, 247-255. Virulence of *Bordetella bronchiseptica* infection in the porcine respiratory tract.

Jong, M.F. de., (1987). Vet.Quarterly 9, 123-133. Prevention of Atrophic Rhinitis in piglets by means of intranasal administration of live non-AR pathogenic *Bordetella bronchiseptica* vaccine.

Jong, M.F. de., Borst, G.H.A. (1985). Vet.Rec. 116, 167. Selective medium for the isolation of *P.multocida* and *B.bronchiseptica.*

Magyar, T., Chanter, N., Lax, A.J., Rutter, J.M., Hall, G.A. (1988). Vet.Micro. 18, 135-146. The pathogenesis of turbinate atrophy in pigs caused by *B.bronchiseptica.*

Rutter, J.M., Collings, J.A. (1983). The virulence of *Bordetella bronchiseptica* in atrophic rhinitis of pigs. In Atrophic Rhinitis of pigs. Eds. Pedersen, K.B. & Nielsen, N.C. Luxembourg CEE. 77-83.

Silveira, D., Edington, N., Smith, I.M. (1982). Res. in Vet.Sci . 33, 37-42 . Ultrastructural changes in the nasal turbinate bones of pigs in early infection with *Bordetella bronchiseptica.*

Smith, I.M., and Baskerville, A.J. (1979). Res. in Sci. 27, 187. A selective medium facilitating the isolation and recognition of *Bordetella bronchiseptica* in pigs.

Smith, I.M., Giles, C.J., Baskerville, A.J. (1982) Vet.Rec. 110, 488-494. The immunisation of pigs against experimental infection with *Bordetella bronchiseptica.*

Underdahl, N.R., Socha, .E. and Doster, A.R. (1982). Am J.Vet.Res. 43, 622-625. Long-term effect of *Bordetella bronchiseptica* infection in neonatal pigs.

Progressive Atrophic Rhinitis

Definition

Infection of non-immune piglets with toxigenic *P.multocida* results in severe sneezing, later followed by atrophy of the turbinate bones and distortion of the nasal septum, sometimes accompanied by shortening and twisting of the upper jaw. Depression of the rate of weight gain may occur.

Incidence

Progressive Atrophic Rhinitis has been reported in most intensive pig-rearing countries. At present it probably occurs to some extent in 26% of pigs slaughtered in Britain and severe atrophy may be found in pigs from up to 10% of herds. In the United States the condition varies in reported incidence from place to place but appears to be present in at least 10% of herds and more in some areas. The incidence may range from 5% to 40% in other European countries. The recent widespread use of effective vaccines has reduced the numbers of affected pigs without reducing the number of affected herds. Eradication programmes have reduced the incidence of infection (to 1% in nucleus herds in the Netherlands).

Aetiology

Progressive Atrophic Rhinitis is caused by infection with toxigenic *P.multocida* usually of type D but occasionally of type A.

P.multocida is a Gram-negative coccobacillus 0.3-1.0 µm in diameter and 1.0-2.0 µm in length which shows bipolar staining in tissue smears. It forms grey non-haemolytic watery colonies 3-5 mm in diameter on blood agar and does not grow consistently on MacConkey Agar. Capsules are formed and types A,B and D are recorded in pigs. Strains capable of causing Progressive Atrophic Rhinitis secrete the heat and trypsin labile polypeptide toxin *P.multocida* Dermonecro toxin (DNT) of molecular weight 143,000 Da coded for by the Pm T tox A gene which may be associated with a prophage. The gene has been cloned and toxin may be produced in *E.coli*. Toxigenic *P.multocida* strains form colonies which are indistinguishable from those of non-toxigenic strains and which behave like other *P.multocidal* strains. They only occasionally produce fimbriae and are susceptible to drying and a wide range of disinfectants and antimicrobials including penicillins, tetracyclines, cephalosporins and fluorinated quinolones. Transferable antimicrobial resistance may occur.

Pathogenesis

Long lasting atrophy of the conchae can result from the intramuscular or intraperitoneal injection of as little as 250 ng/kg of toxin or the instillation of pure toxin into the nasal passages three times at 27 days of age. The changes produced are seen in the natural disease and include degeneration and necrosis of osteoblasts, accelerated osteoclastic osteolysis and initial stimulation of osteoclast activity to result in the replacement of the bony core of the concha by fibrous tissue. Injection of pure toxin can lead not only to atrophic rhinitis but also to growth retardation and, at high doses, to liver damage, icterus and mortality. In natural disease the changes described above are accompanied by those associated with phase I *B.bronchiseptica* which colonises non-immune pigs and appears to allow toxigenic *P.multocida* of type D and sometimes type A to reach the levels necessary for the production of clinical disease. Infection may occur as early as 3-4 days of age when *B.bronchiseptica* adheres to the cilia of the nasal epithelium. Some isolates of serotypes 3 and 12 *P.multocida* type D have also been shown to be adherent by means of fimbria-like structures, but most workers agree that adhesion to ciliated epithelium is poor in this species.

The changes in the turbinate mucosa in atrophic rhinitis itself include loss of cilia, hyperplasia and metaplasia of epithelial cells, neutrophil infiltration and the secretion of mucus. Toxigenic *P.multocida* colonises this mucus layer apparently adhering to a low molecular weight (<25 kDa) substance in the mucus and reaching high numbers (10^4-10^7/ml) and producing the toxin which can be absorbed from the nasal mucosa. Toxigenic *P.multocida* may persist in moderate numbers for long periods in the tonsil. Numbers in the nose are reduced in the presence of antibody to toxin but infection is not prevented.

The toxin has been shown to produce a number of effects. It appears to enter cells by endocytosis and affects the uptake of porcine growth hormone. Individual fibroblasts may proliferate and osteoclast precursors are stimulated to develop calcitonin receptors and become osteoclasts. It has systemic effects, and at low levels (0.1 µg) affects levels of hepatic glycogen. At high levels (2.8 or 5.6 µg) hepatocellular degeneration occurs accompanied by icterus, ataxia, blindness and death after five days. Gastric ulceration, polioencephalomalacia, effects on ureters and necrosis of the liver were all seen in addition to turbinate atrophy.

Within the nasal mucosa the osteoblastic formation of bone is affected with an increase in the number of osteoclasts and later, a fall in their numbers. Disruption of osteoid synthesis is accompanied by a fibrous hyperplasia and eventually the bony core of the turbinate decreases in size. Secondary atrophy of the mucosa occurs and the whole turbinate may disappear within two weeks especially if the changes occur at the period of maximum growth between 2 and 4 weeks. They are more severe in the ventral conchae.

Sneezing may result from local irritation, the action of toxins and infection with secondary agents such as *Mycoplasma hyorhinis* to cause bleeding from the nose and blockage of the airways for short periods of time. Some degree of resolution may occur before slaughter but this is unlikely in severely affected animals from which the infections have not been eradicated. The severity of conchal changes may be associated to some extent with breed and growth rate. The absence of turbinates may be reflected in an increased incidence of lower respiratory tract disease but it is not clear whether the absence of conchae *per se* is the cause through reduction in the filtering and warming capacity of the nasal chamber or whether lower respiratory tract disease associated with the two causal agents is directly responsible. Toxigenic *P.multocida* type D appears to colonise the lung only poorly but can cause pneumonia.

Clinical signs

Outbreaks of sneezing occur in baby pigs aged between 1 and 8 weeks of age and are accompanied by blockage of the lachrymal ducts tear staining or even epistaxis. As the disease progresses, signs of deviation or shortening of the upper jaw may appear with corrugation of the skin of the snout and under shooting of the lower jaw. Signs of pneumonia or stunting may also be noted. In some animals or affected farms, sneezing may be transitory and little outward effect may be seen although turbinate atrophy may be found at slaughter. This form is most common where infection does not occur until after weaning and or where immunity is present.

Severely affected animals may have difficulty in eating and the nasal changes may be seen in pigs of all ages in affected pigs. Rates of daily liveweight gain may be depressed and there may be some mortality amongst piglets. The nasal changes may affect the value of weaners produced for sale. Economic effects on growth rate associated with the bony changes have been estimated at 0.5%, (growth depression of 25-40g/day) or nil, depending upon the study.

Humane slaughter is indicated in young piglets with severe nose bleeding and loss of condition which cannot feed. Infection can normally be reduced by treatment.

Pathological findings

Pigs may be in poor condition with grossly twisted snouts and tear staining. There may be pronounced corrugation of the skin of the snout and nasal discharge may be present.

Atrophy of the turbinates, distortion of the nasal septum and shortening or deflection of the snout are the most prominent findings. The nasal changes are most easily seen in snout cross-sections at the first premolar (level with the corner of the mouth).

The changes may be graded 1-5 in order of severity:-

Grade 1 = slight deviation from normal.
Grade 2 = slight atrophy.
Grade 3 = more severe atrophy.
Grade 4 = loss of at least 1 turbinate.
Grade 5 = loss of all turbinates.

Alternative grading systems include taking prints of the snout or photographing the cavity and recording the Total Perimeter Ratio (TPR normal pigs 1.3-1.5, abnormal 0.4-0.1) and the Turbinate Area Ratio (TAR, normal pigs 0.38-0.4, abnormal 0.16-0.17).

'Swastika' forms or spurs of bone growth out of line with the smooth curve of normal conchae may indicate resolution of pre-existing lesions. The degree of shortening of the upper jaw may also be measured between the upper and lower incisors as an indication of the severity of the changes. A purulent rhinitis may be present and the mucosa may be pale if affected animals are examined early in the disease. The mucosa is normally denuded of its epithelium and heavily infiltrated with inflammatory cells and a catarrhal exudate may be present at the surface. In chronic cases, metaplasia of the epithelium with loss of goblet cells occurs.

B.bronchiseptica and toxigenic P.multocida type D may be demonstrated in early cases although in older animals they may be difficult to isolate

Epidemiology

Infection is transmitted between pigs by aerosol or contact. In aerosols 69% of organisms survive for at least 5 minutes in 79% relative humidity at 37°C and survival is better at lower ambient temperatures. The organism can be recovered from clean water for up to 14 days, slurry for 6 days and from lung washings for 4 days. It may be demonstrated in up to 44% slaughter pigs, 57% young sows but may still be demonstrable in 17% of 3-year old sows.

Transmission between farms is principally by the movement of infected pigs but aerosol transmission and transmission on clothing may be possible over short distances. Toxigenic *P.multocida* from man has been shown to cause disease in pigs but contact with infected rabbits did not. Other species also carry the organism.

Atrophic rhinitis occurs most frequently in herds in which the toxigenic Pasteurella is present with the almost ubiquitous *B.bronchiseptica* and where the system of management is such that piglets born to non-immune mothers are exposed to heavy infection early in life. In herds composed of gilts obtained from a number of sources and farrowed continuously, the disease is likely to be severe. In herds which are closed and have a substantial number of older sows, early infection is less severe as are the nasal changes. Changes may also be severe on such farms when piglets of varying immune status are weaned early and kept in large groups.

Gross changes may develop in weaners purchased by fattening units but this is unusual. Within an affected unit the syndrome may rise and fall in prevalence because of changes in housing, prophylaxis, treatment and composition of the sow population. Infection can be introduced by animals which do not have clinical conchal atrophy or other nasal or facial changes. The introduction of new strains of *P.multocida* to herds with immunity to their existing strain may trigger new outbreaks. Restriction endonuclease analysis and ribotyping suggest that up to 4 REA types or ribotypes may occur in a single herd and that the majority of infections are due to a single type at any one time.

Diagnosis

1.   Clinical Diagnosis

Progressive Atrophic Rhinitis may be suspected when outbreaks of paroxymal sneezing occur in piglets and when the changes in the snout appear as the piglets age. Measurements of malocclusion of the upper and lower incisors may provide an early indication of severe disease as may biopsy of the nasal mucosa. Turbinate atrophy may also be detected in life by endoscopy, X-ray examination of computer tomography. Atrophy of the conchae and displacement of the nasal septum may be demonstrable.

2.   Pathological Diagnosis

Progressive Atrophic Rhinitis is often suspected first at post mortem or slaughter on transverse section of the snout at the level of the first premolar tooth. Recent studies suggest that additional sections anterior to this may also detect the changes in the tips of the turbinates. The changes can be graded according to the schemes described above. Within the nasal cavity evidence of active rhinitis may also be present and staining with phloxine-alcian blue may demonstrate metaplastic epithelium in longitudinal snout sections. The severity of the problem in a herd can be assessed by a computerised atrophic rhinitis monitoring scheme (A.R.M.S.) based scores obtained at slaughter but this is only of retrospective value and can only detect changes which have taken place 4-5 months previously. Regular clinical examination and post-mortem examination of piglets found dead is probably a more effective measure of the active disease situation.

In young pigs the condition should be differentiated from cleft lip (cheiloschisis), absence of lower jaw (agnathia) and craniofacial asymmetry (all present before birth), paranasal abscess or bullnose (bacterial infection from tooth-clipping or fighting in unweaned pigs) which occur in individual animals only. In pigs 1-6 months of age, osteodystrophia fibrosa of nutritional of unknown or hormonal origin may occur but spongy bone is present; brachygnathia superior or short snouts may occur especially in Large Whites and, formerly, Middle White Pigs (a breed character) and mandibular malalignment may occur especially in adults due to bone remodelling and protrusion of lower jaw which develops in association with the vice of bar biting.

3.   Demonstration of toxigenic *P.multocida*

This confirms clinical or pathological identification of Progressive Atrophic Rhinitis. The organism is isolated from nasal washings, cotton-tipped swabs from the posterior nares, tonsillar swabs or from the cut surface of crypts of the tonsils at slaughter.

P.multocida can be isolated directly on blood agar, but contamination is common and selective media containing clindamycin 75 mg, gentamycin 75 mg, vancomycin 4 mg and amphotericin 5 mg/L may be of value. Colonies may be identified at 24 and 48 hours or growth harvested at 24 hours for identification. Toxin is usually detected using commercially available ELISAs or occasionally by neutralisation assay on cell cultures. The gene for the toxin may be detected by PCR using oligonucleotide primers. PCR may be used on suspensions of nasal material as well as on early culture material.

4.   Demonstration of immunity

Intradermal setting of toxin produces lesions in non-immune pigs but no lesions in immune pigs. Neutralising antibody may be detected in serum in cell culture assays but antibody to the toxin is difficult to demonstrate by ELISAs in natural infections. It is readily detectable following vaccination.

Treatment

Acute disease in sucking piglets may be treated with trimethoprim sulphonamide, ampicillin, tetracyclines, ceftofur or enrofloxacin given by injection or oral doser as appropriate. A single dose may be sufficient for clinical cure or a short course may be required. Animals should be supported with additional food and electrolyte if they cannot suck. Where the *B.bronchiseptica* component is important, trimethoprim sulphonamide may be the drug of choice.

Disease in weaned pigs can be treated by injection or in drinking water using antimicrobials listed above with the addition of tylosin and penicillin (by injection). Feed medication is considered below under 'Control'.

Control

a) Antimicrobials

Progressive Atrophic Rhinitis may be controlled by the strategic medication of young pigs at 3 days, 10 days and 21 days of age using the antimicrobials listed above, but primarily trimethoprim sulphonamide. Weaned pigs at risk may be treated continuously with antimicrobial in feed or water at therapeutic levels. Feed medication can be given at this stage and may include combination products such as penicillin:sulphonamide:chlortetracycline as well as the agents listed above. Medication of groups of animals entering an airspace in an all-in, all-out system is the most efficient method.

The development of antimicrobial resistance may make re-assessment of antimicrobial control necessary from time to time and it should be regarded as short-term or appropriate only to systems such as finishers where vaccinated stock cannot be obtained.

b) Vaccination

Killed vaccines containing *P.multocida* toxoid alone, or with killed *B.bronchiseptica* antigens, are given to sows 5 and 2 weeks prior to farrowing and protect the piglets with passive immunity to the toxin. Protection may last up to 8 weeks and prevents the bony changes and improves growth rates. Improvements of up to 120g/day have been recorded. Protection depends upon the ingestion of colostrum but does not prevent infection. Piglets may be vaccinated at 7 days and 21 days to provide active immunity.

c) All-in, all-out systems

Progressive Atrophic Rhinitis and infection may be prevented by a combination of vaccination and isolated farrowing coupled with all-in, all-out rearing with or without medication of animals at entry. The isowean system may also be used.

d) Eradication

Infection has been eradicated consistently by depopulation and restocking with uninfected pigs from clean herds produced by hysterectomy, medicated early weaning (using trimethoprim sulphonamide) or testing and confirmation of freedom.
Testing sows for infection, slaughter of continued carriers coupled with treatment of sows into clean accommodation and batch farrowing and rearing has been shown to eradicate the organism from lightly affected herds (~20% infected sows).

e) Monitoring for infection

Primarily by culture of nasal swabs followed by ELISA or PCR for toxigenic *P.multocida*. Additional monitoring by clinical, and particularly post-mortem examination.

References

Chanter, N., Goodwin, R.F.W., Rutter, J.M. (1989). Res.Vet.Sci. 47, 355-358. Comparison of methods for the sampling and isolation of toxigenic *P.multocida* from the nasal cavity of the pig.

Chanter, N., Magyar, T., Rutter, J.M. (1989). Res.Vet.Sci. 47, 48-53. Interaction between *B.bronchiseptica* and toxigenic *P.multocida*, in atrophic rhinitis of pigs.

Donnio, P.Y., Avril, J.L., Andre, P.M., Vaucel, J. (1991). J.Med.Micro. 34, 333-337. Dermonecrotoxic toxin production by strains of *P.multocida* isolated from man.

Foged, N.T., Nielsen, J.P., Jorsal, S.E. (1989). Vet.Rec. 125, 7-11. Protection against Progressive Atrophic Rhinitis by vaccination with *P.multocida* toxin purified by monoclonal antibody.

Geiger, J.O. and 7 others (1992). Proc. IPVS 12, 166. Elimination of atrophic rhinitis using Isowean 3 site production.

Jolie, R., Thacker, B. (1990). Proc. IPVS 11, 53. Comparison of atrophic rhinitis morphometric measurements and macroscopic grades of nasal cross sections on computerised tomography scans of pigs.

Jong, M.F. de., Nielsen, J.P. (1990). Vet.Rec. 126, 93. Definition of Progressive Atrophic Rhinitis.

Robertson, J.F., Wilson, D., Smith, W.J. (1990). Animal Production 50, 173-182. Atrophic rhinitis, influence of the aerial environment.

Rutter, J.M. (1989). In Practice 11, 74-80. Atrophic Rhinitis.

Voets, M.T., Klaasen, C.H.L., Charlier, P., Wiseman, A., Descamps, J. (1992). Vet.Rec. 130, 549-553. Evaluation of an AR vaccine under controlled conditions.

Wallgren, P. and 5 others (1994). Proc. IPVS 13, 122. Age distribution of pigs carrying *P.multocida* in herds affected with rhinitis.

Pneumonic Pasteurellosis

Definition

Pneumonic pasteurellosis results from the colonisation of existing lung lesions with *P.multocida* to increase their severity and give rise to fever, respiratory distress and death in some cases. Growth may be depressed in chronically-affected animals.

Aetiology

P.multocida subsp. *multocida* of capsular type A, serotype 3 is most commonly isolated from lesions. It forms large, mucoid colonies 3-5 mm on blood agar, is rarely toxigenic and some isolates produce fimbriae. Toxigenic strains of type A and, occasionally of type D, have also been recovered from lesions.

Pathogenesis

P.multocida pneumonia is difficult to reproduce experimentally. Pure cultures have only rarely been successful in producing pneumonic lesions when given alone by the intranasal or aerosol routes. Pneumonia can be produced repeatably when pure cultures of non-toxigenic type A strains are given

186

following lung damage caused by large volumes of saline, *A.pleuropneumoniae* toxin and infection with *Mycoplasma hyopneumoniae* in enzootic pneumonia. The mechanism by which pneumonia results is not clear. Colonisation of the tracheal mucus may occur (as with toxigenic type D strains in the nose) and some isolates produce fimbriae and may adhere to epithelium. Toxigenic strains of type A and type D cause pneumonia but toxigenic type D strains are cleared faster.

Serum antibodies develop to the somatic antigens on *P.multocida* and can be demonstrated within 12 days of infection. They do not appear to be protective. Antibodies to the toxin can be demonstrated in some cases.

Clinical signs

In acute pasteurellosis affected animals may be lethargic and show dyspnoea, with laboured abdominal type breathing, coughing, slight nasal discharge and fever of 40-41.5°C, 104°-106°F. Mouth breathing and cyanosis of extremities may be seen. Lung sounds are often loud. The clinical signs usually last for 5-10 days and may end in recovery or death but may continue for 3-5 weeks. Recovered animals often remain thin.

Less severe degrees of pneumonia associated with coughing and fever may occur and last for 3-5 weeks. Humane slaughter should be carried out on animals which have collapsed, are lethargic and severely congested with white froth on the lips and low rectal temperatures. Animals which are thin with severe respiratory distress may also be destroyed.

Post-mortem findings

Lesions of enzootic pneumonia are almost always present and lesions of an exudative pneumonia are superimposed on these. Greyish-pink consolidation with reddish atelectic areas is found in the anterior lobes and, in severe cases, in the diaphragmatic lobes as well. Lesions often have a yellowish outline and a fibrinous pleurisy is often present. Congestion of the carcase is frequently seen and froth is commonly present in the trachea. Oedema of the cut lung tissue is evident. In more chronic cases of pasteurella pneumonia the cut surface has a granular whitish or greyish appearance.

Histological sections show oedema, congestion and haemorrhage with bronchiolar exudate containing bacteria, macrophages and neutrophils which are also present in the alveoli. The bronchi may be blocked by this material and by desquamated epithelial cells.

Aerobic culture of heart blood and lung lesions usually gives a pure culture of *P.multocida*. Anaerobic cultures may yield *Bacteroides* spp in addition. Examination for *Haemophilus* spp may also yield these organisms.

Epidemiology

Pasteurellosis is transmitted by aerosol by contact and by ingestion and usually occurs in fattening pigs or breeding stock in herds in which enzootic pneumonia is also present and it is commonest under poor husbandry conditions, e.g. overcrowding, dusty ammoniacal atmosphere, etc. Clinical signs may occur after mixing, weighing, transport or some other stress. *P.multocida* is readily killed by heating to 60°C and survives for less than an hour in aerosols at low humidity but survives for longer at high humidity and low temperatures. Organisms survive for up to 14 days in water, 6 days in slurry and for up to 7 weeks in nasal washings at room temperatures. Transmission between farms is by carrier pigs but restriction endonuclease analysis and ribotyping suggest that introduced types may not persist in the face of a prevalent herd type, usually A3. The role of rodent and bird carriage of *P.multocida* has not been evaluated for pneumonia using modern techniques.

Diagnosis

The clinical signs of fever, dyspnoea, and cyanosis without enteric involvement suggest the acute pneumonic or septicaemic condition and this can be confirmed by the post-mortem examination of dead animals when both gross and microscopic lesions provide further evidence. The presence of chronic coughing, reduced daily weight gain and fever may suggest that chronic infection is complicating enzootic pneumonia. The isolation of *P.multocida* in culture confirms its presence. In the absence of other respiratory pathogens such as viruses, *H.parasuis*, *A.pleuropneumoniae*, *B.bronchiseptica* or enzootic pneumonia, a diagnosis of uncomplicated pasteurella pneumonia may be made.

Treatment

Severely affected animals should be treated parenterally with an antimicrobial such as ceftiofur, penicillin, streptomycin, tetracycline, trimethoprim sulphonamide, ampicillin, amoxycillin, spiramycin, spectinomycin for 3-5 days. Parenteral treatment may be supplemented by medication of the drinking water of the affected batch with water soluble derivatives of the above injectable compounds. Long-acting oxytetracycline injections may also be used. All pigs in the same air-space should be treated and the space filled on an all in, all out basis. Antibiotic resistance may occur.

Control

Batches of animals may be treated in feed upon entry to an air space. Control is most efficient if all-in, all-out husbandry is practised. Reduction in predisposing diseases such s enzootic pneumonia by medicating with tiamulin at 40 ppm in feed or by vaccination, may reduce the prevalence and severity of disease.

Whole cell killed vaccines are still available and may prevent severe disease from occurring, particularly in older finishing pigs. Vaccination with toxoid vaccines has been shown to reduce the severity of pneumonic pasteurellosis and may be economic.

Husbandry conditions should be improved and dust and ammoniacal levels reduced.

References

Andrews, J.J., Lucas, T.E., Johnson, I. (1988). Agri Practice 9, 33-38. Prevention and control of experimentally induced *P.multocida* in swine by the use of chlortetracycline in feed.

Chung, W.B., Backstrom, L.R., Collins, M.T. (1994). Can.J.Vet.Res. 58, 25-30. Experimental model of swine pneumonic pasteurellosis using crude *A.pleuropneumoniae* cytotoxin and *P.multocida* given endobronchially.

Done, S.H. (1991). Vet.Rec. 128, 582-586. Environmental factors affecting the severity of pneumonia in pigs.

Kobisch, M., Pennings, A. (1989). Vet.Rec. 124, 57-61. An evaluation of NobiVac AR and an experimental atrophic rhinitis vaccine containing *P.multocida* DNT toxoid and *B.bronchiseptica*.

Mackie, J.T., Barton, M., Kettlewell, J. (1992). Aust.Vet.J. 69, 227-228. *P.multocida* septicaemia in pigs.

Ose, E.E., Tomkinson, L.V. (1990). Proc. IPVS 11, 94. Effect of pneumonic pasteurellosis on lung lesions and mortality in *M.hyopneumoniae* infected pigs.

Pijoan, C., Morrison, R.B. and Hilley, H.D. (1983). J.Clin.Microbiol. 17, 1074-1076. Serotyping of *P.multocida* isolated from swine lungs collected at slaughter.

Zhao, G., Pijoan, C., Murtaugh, M.P., Molitor, T.W. (1992). Inf. and Immunity 60, 1401-1405. Use of restriction endonuclease analysis and ribotyping to study the epidemiology of *P.multocida* in closed herds.

Infection with NAD-dependent *P.multocida*

V-dependent *P.multocida* of taxa D, E and F have been isolated from nasal swabs, lungs and joints.

Pasteurella haemolytica infections

P.haemolytica has been isolated from septicaemia in piglets and from localised areas of fibrinous pleurisy or pleuropneumonia in pigs. Infection in pigs may originate from sheep contact and be *P.trehalosi* (untypable) or of bovine origin and affect bovine leucocytes. Other strains resemble taxon 15 of *A.pleuropneumoniae* closely and should be distinguished from it and from *A.suis*. Infection in piglets may be inapparent.

Local lung lesions, 1 to 2 cm, red with fibrinous pleurisy and petechiation of the affected area are seen in acute cases and these become necrotic, greyish-red, and encapsulated with fibrous adhesions. No clinical signs have been associated with this condition and the local lesions are small and scarce, mostly near the bronchi in any lobe of the lung.

A septicaemic form may occur in piglets particularly when housed in the same airspace as sheep. Fever to 41°C, 106°F and death can occur. Localisation in the joints may result. Carcases of dead piglets resemble those which have died of *Actinobacillus suis* infections but have lung lesions of *P.haemolytica* infection (see above) and may have enteritis. Treatment and control may be necessary and should be as for *A.pleuropneumoniae* or *P.multocida*. Vaccines to many *P.haemolytica* serotypes are available should a problem persist and could be used.

Pleuropneumonia (Actinobacillus pleuropneumoniae infection).

Definition

A highly contagious, often fatal, respiratory disease of weaned growing finishing pigs in which infection of the lungs with *Actinobacillus pleuropneumoniae* causes fibrinous pleurisy, a pneumonia with characteristic infarcts and depression of growth rate in chronically affected pigs.

Incidence

A major problem in much of Europe, the USA., Canada and Eastern Asia *Actinobacillus pleuropneumoniae* is present in Britain and the disease was initially described here in 1957 but extensive outbreaks of the type so common elsewhere have only been seen since 1980. Control measures may suppress clinical disease but reports from many countries suggest that 30-50% of all pigs are infected.

Aetiology

The disease is caused by *A.pleuropneumoniae* which forms small translucent mucoid ß-haemolytic colonies on sheep blood agar with staphylococcal streaks. Freshly-isolated cultures may have colonies firmly adherent to the agar. The organism requires NAD (V factor) (Biotype 1).but some strains do not (Biotype 2). It is urease positive, reduces nitrate ferments D-xylose and ribitol and is indole, citrate, methyl red and VP negative.

The organism produces fine fimbriae, capsules and secretes toxins. Twelve major serotypes of Biotype 1 and at least three of Biotype 2 have been distinguished based on capsular antigens.

Three main toxins are produced. Apx 1 has a M.W. of 105-110 kDa, is haemolytic and cytotoxic and is produced by serotypes 1, 5a, 5b, 9, 10 and 11. Apx II has a M.W. of 103-105 kDa, is weakly haemolytic, moderately cytotoxic and occurs in all serotypes except 10. Apx III has a M.W. of 120 kDa, is non-haemolytic, strongly cytotoxic and occurs in serotypes. A CAMP factor of MW 29 kD which aids haemolysis, is also produced. The genes for all these toxic factors have been cloned, sequenced and recombinant proteins produced.

A.pleuropneumoniae is fairly delicate but can survive for 5 days at 18°C particularly in mucopurulent nasal discharge. It is sensitive to drying and may disappear from dry swabs within a few hours. Protection for organisms on swabs requires the use of a transport medium preferably including yeast extract and nicotinamide. The organism survives periods up to 30 days in clean water at 4°C. It is killed by formaldehyde, glutaraldehyde, ethanol, isopropyl alcohol and chlorhexidine.

A.pleuropneumoniae is sensitive *in vitro* to a number of antimicrobials but resistant strains occur. It is sensitive in most cases to penicillin and ampicillin, tetracycline, tiamulin, ceftiofur, cephalexin, chloramphenicol enrofloxacin, ciprofloxacin and trimethoprim sulphonamide.

Pathogenesis

Infection is by aerosol or by contact, enters the upper respiratory tract or oral cavity where it adheres only to the tonsillar epithelium. Experimental studies suggest that the caudal lobes, diaphragmatic and accessory, receive the bulk of aerosolised organisms. Here they attach to the alveolar epithelium possibly by means of fimbriae until the disease process disrupts the lung (1-3 hours). The exact cause of the lesions is not yet completely clear, but the production of transposon mutants lacking Apx I and studies with the infusion of toxins suggest that many of the changes described below are caused by toxins. The toxins (principally Apx I and Apx III) kill macrophages within 30-60 minutes of exposure and reduce the phagocyte efficacy of neutrophils. The presence of capsules reduces the efficacy of phagocytosis further and protects organisms against the effects of complement. Bacterial numbers increase and they may be found in microcolonies in the lung and in tracheal mucus and mucopus. Toxins are produced during the log phase of bacterial growth and cause the following changes.

The earliest lesions of the peracute form may be present at 3 hours post-infection and may be pronounced by 6 hours post-infection.

Capillary congestion of the alveolar wall with oedema of both it and the interstitial septum are marked. Lymphatics become dilated with oedema fluid, fibrin and inflammatory cells. Platelet aggregation and neutrophil accumulation exacerbate the alveolar wall damage and this necrosis is followed by pulmonary artery thrombosis. At any stage from 9 hours onwards *A.pleuropneumoniae* may be found in the blood. Microcolonies of organisms may be seen in affected lung. By 4 days post-infection the lesions, now filled with macrophages and lymphocytes, are clearly demarcated from normal lung. Later, fibrosis occurs and the centre of the lesion becomes greyish and necrotic. Bacteria are common in the lesion at this stage.

A.pleuropneumoniae induces antibodies to its capsule, lipopolysaccharide toxins, outer membrane proteins especially one of 42 kDa and enzymes such as superoxide dismutase and to the iron binding proteins. These antibodies occur in the respiratory secretions as IgA antibodies and in serum as IgG with some IgA. IgM does not appear in high concentration. The antibody neutralises the toxins and allows the successful phagocytosis and killing of organisms. Passive antibody protects against infection and can be demonstrated until 4 weeks of age. Active immunity can first be demonstrated 5-10 days after infection and appears to peak 3-4 weeks after infection. Immunity to the homologous serotype appears to be lifelong but disease may occur following challenge with a different serotype. Serotype 2 infections may give rise to protection against other serotypes.

Clinical signs

Acute disease occurs in a non-immune herd or individuals which have not received passive immunity. 15-30% of pigs may suffer depression, anorexia, high fever (41.5°C, 107°F), or laboured respiration, especially after rising to drink or after disturbance. Cyanosis, subnormal rectal temperature and death may follow within 4-6 hours of the onset of clinical signs. Blood stained froth may be seen at the mouth. Some pigs may be found dead and mortality may reach 30-50% of those affected. In the sub-acute form groups of pigs may be affected and are anorexic and show respiratory distress and coughing. Variable mortality occurs. Recovering animals may cough, and show respiratory distress particularly when disturbed. Exercise intolerance may continue for days and affected animals may have reduced appetites, appear gaunt and hairy, be depressed and show reduced rates of liveweight gain. Non-immune animals of all ages may be affected and abortion may occur in affected gilts or sows. Where infection is enzootic the condition is most common amongst pigs of 6-12 weeks of age. Medication can alter the clinical signs and mortality.

Humane slaughter should be carried out when blood-stained froth appears at the lips of acutely affected pigs with cyanosis of the extremities and sub-normal rectal temperatures. Chronically-affected animals with very poor bodily condition, continued exercise intolerance and respiratory distress may be killed.

Pathological findings

In most acute cases, the lesions are limited to the thoracic cavity. The nasal cavity and trachea may be filled with blood stained froth and the lungs are congested and oedematous with oedema of the interlobular septae (3-12 hours after onset). Later (12-24 hours) yellowish or blood stained fibrinous exudate appears on the pleural surface over pneumonic areas. Blood tinged fluid may be present in the pleural cavity. Firm, dark red irregular shaped, raised areas may be seen scattered throughout the lung but particularly in the caudal (diaphragmatic) lobes 14-30 hours after onset of clinical signs. These areas may be necrotic in severe cases by 48 hours after onset and occupy about 50% of the lung in fatal cases. In chronic cases, these lesions become encapsulated and greyish in colour. They may be felt as firm nodules at post-mortem or slaughter and allow the presence of the disease to be suspected. The severe fibrinous pleurisy becomes fibrous, and persists until slaughter and may lead to stripping of the pleura. Fibrinous pericarditis and inflammation and haemorrhage of the bronchial lymph nodes occur. Infarcts and alveolar haemorrhages re seen histologically with bronchopneumonia. Infarcts are often surrounded by a prominent ring of dead phagocytes. Micro colonies of the organism are often visible in the alveoli and the organism may be isolated from and demonstrated in the lesions (see Diagnosis).

Epidemiology

The organism spreads from animal to animal by contact, particularly during the oral contact associated with fighting after mixing and by aerosol when 10^4 organisms/ml are needed. It does not survive long in aerosols unless humidity is high and ambient temperature low. More than one serotype may occur in an animal and up to six serotypes have been identified in a single herd. Disease may be more prolonged and severe where more than one serotype is present and where infection with other agents such as PRRS and PRCV occur.

The organism survives for long periods in water (30 days at 4^oC), for hours in aerosols, appears to be rapidly killed on drying and to survive for up to four days in lung tissue and discharges at room temperature and for up to one year in frozen lung. It is rapidly killed by disinfectants in the absence of protein. The organism survives in pigs in lung lesions for weeks, and in tonsils for 4-6 months or more. Tonsillar and lung isolates have the same restriction endonuclease analysis pattern.

Spread between farms is mainly by the movement of carrier pigs, followed by transmission on fomites. Aerosol transmission is rare or non-existent. No vectors are known on farm although mice can be infected experimentally.

Different serotypes exist in each country. UK isolates are 27.3% 2, 22.2% 8, 13.1% 3, 14.1% 6, 16.2% 7 with 5, 9, 10 and 12 occurring rarely and 1 and 4 absent. Prevalent serotypes in Great Britain are 3, 6 and 8 while in Ireland 2 is common and 6 absent. Similar pictures exist in the US with 1 and 5 being relatively common. International trade in pigs results in spread of different serotypes.

Diagnosis

The clinical signs of acute and fatal respiratory disease are suggestive. Influenza rarely causes mortality and affects pigs of all ages, while enzootic pneumonia is more chronic. The post-mortem findings of massive pleurisy and pericarditis are suggestive and the firm lung infarcts are characteristic of this disease. Fibrous pleurisy and pericarditis at slaughter with firm nodules representing residual infarcts suggest the past presence of the disease.

Confirmation of the diagnosis is by demonstration of the agent or its products. Culture can be carried out on sheepblood agar with a streak of ß-toxin-producing staphylococcus across the inoculated area. Satellite ß-haemolytic colonies develop. It may be grown on chocolate (altered blood) agar and on selective media containing crystal violet 1 µg, lincomycin 1 µg, spectinomycin 8 µg and bacitracin 128 µg/ml. Isolates may be identified presumptively by possession of urease and CAMP factor and confirmed biochemically. They may be serotyped by slide agglutination using antibody to capsules, by coagglutination, latex particle agglutination, labelled DNA probes, PCR and restriction endonuclease.

Antigens may be identified and serotyped in lung tissue by coagglutination tests on extracts, indirect immunofluorescence and immunoperoxidase in tissues and DNA may be identified by PCR. Antigen ELISAs have also been described.

Chronically affected or carrier pigs may be identified by culture of tonsillar swabs or by the presence of antibody in saliva, nasal secretions or, more usually, serum. Most current antibody tests use ELISAs with capsular antigen but the Complement Fixation Test, radioimmunoassay, latex agglutination tests and 2-mercaptoethanol tube agglutination tests are still used. A wide variety of other tests have been described. Positive titres in agglutination tests may be >1:20, CFT >1:20 and in some ELISAs >1:160. ELISAs using toxins may require confirmation of neutralising ability as antibody to *A.suis* and *P.haemolytica* may occur. Most tests are serotype specific.

Treatment and control

The rapid onset of the lesions and clinical signs mean that treatment of clinically-affected animals may eliminate the organism but may not allow complete resolution of the damage. Both pneumonic damage and fibrinous pleurisy or fibrous pleurisy may persist to affect performance for the remainder of the finishing period and such animals may have persistent exercise intolerance and low average daily gain. Lesions may be colonised by organisms such as *Pasteurella* spp. and these may persist after *A.pleuropneumoniae* has been eliminated.

Clinically-affected animals should be treated parenterally with an antimicrobial likely to be effective. Water and food consumption is reduced by infection making medication of feed and water largely ineffective.

The agents which can be used include penicillin, cephalexin, ampicillin, amoxycillin, oxytetracycline, trimethoprim sulphonamide, tiamulin and chloramphenicol (not UK). Recently enrofloxacin has been used at 5 mg/kg as have ceftiofur 3-5 mg/kg and lincospectin. Parenteral treatment may need to be repeated for 3 days. Affected pigs may have to be given water by stomach tube. The remainder of the group can be treated in water or feed with the antimicrobials listed above.

Resistance to antimicrobials varies with their use. In the UK fewer than 10 per cent of isolates were penicillin and tetracycline-resistant in one survey in 1988, but elsewhere resistance has been recorded more frequently. Levels may reach 90% to tetracyclines in countries such as US and Denmark.

(a)   Treatment

Therapeutic levels of appropriate antimicrobials in feed given at entry to a house may prevent any further disease when used with all-in, all-out stocking of single airspaces or sites. Pulse dosing by treatment for a single day on introduction of new animals to an existing continuous flow system may also reduce or prevent disease. Treatment alone has not been shown to eliminate infection.

(b)   Vaccination

Deaths from pleuropneumonia can be prevented by current vaccines and the extent of lung lesions can be reduced by at least 50% and often more. They may improve days to slaughter by at least 5.5 and daily liveweight gain by up to 100 g. Current vaccines are made from killed whole cultures harvested young to obtain extracellular products and containing up to 4 serotypes chosen to reflect those present in the herd or country concerned. Oil adjuvants have been described but modern products contain less irritant adjuvants such as alum suitable for use in young piglets. The vaccine currently available (1995) UK (Suvaxyn HPP, Solvay Duphar) contains serotypes 3, 6 and 8 and is given as two injections two weeks apart to non-pregnant animals no younger than six weeks of age. Vaccine programmes often require the vaccination of the sow to give passive   protection and subsequent vaccination of the piglets. Where passive immunity is present (from enzootic infection or vaccinated sows) best results are obtained by vaccinating piglets after the disappearance of maternal immunity. This usually occurs from 4-6 weeks of age and weaners can be given the first injection at this stage. The most appropriate time for vaccination in any herd can be identified by serological monitoring to produce a serum profile for the disease.   These can vary from building to building on the same farm. Vaccination prior to entry to a finishing unit can be particularly effective.
Experimental studies have shown that a number of *A.pleuropneumoniae* antigens protect completely against the disease to some degree and a combination of Apx I, Apx III and the 42 kDa outer membrane protein OMP protects against other serotypes. Parenteral, aerosol and intraperitoneal routes and a number of adjuvants have been used.

(c)   Isolation; treatment; vaccination combinations

Isolation using all-in, all-out systems within a farm reduces infection but does not prevent it. The use of vaccination or treatment prior to or at the move increases the degree of control. Isowean (PIC) technology using separate site isolation for each stage also minimises disease.

(d)   Eradication

Hysterectomy-derived herds are free of *A.pleuropneumoniae* infection and may be maintained free by isolation. They form a source of disease-free stock for repopulation.
Depopulation of farms, cleaning, disinfection and repopulation with disease-free animals can be carried out. Antimicrobial treatment alone has not been successful in eradication but combinations with vaccination, partial depopulation and removal of serological and tonsillar carriers has been successful.

194

References

Bosch, J.F., van den, Jongenelen, I.M.C.A., Pubben, A.N.B., Vugt, F.G.A van, Segers, R.P.A.M. (1992). Proc. IPVS 12, 194. Protection induced by a trivalent *A.pleuropneumoniae* subunit vaccine.

Bosse, J.T., Gardner, I.A., Sheldrake, R.F., Rosendal, S. and Johnson, S.P. (1990). Proc. IPVS 11, 28. Monitoring of antibody levels to *A.pleuropneumoniae* serotype 7 in pigs between 1 and 6 months of age by ELISA.

Brandreth, S., Smith, I.M. (1985). Vet.Rec. 117, 143-147. Prevalence of pig herds affected by pleuropneumonia in Eastern England.

Frey, J. and 21 others (1993). J.Gen.Microbiol. 139, 1723-1728. *A.pleuropneumoniae* RTX toxins: uniform designation of haemolysin, cytolysins pleurotoxins and their genes.

Gutterez, C.B., Rodnguez Barbosa, J.I., Tuscon, R.I., Rodnguez Ferri, E.F. (1994). Proc. IPVS. 13, 180. Efficacies of several disinfectants against *A.pleuropneumoniae* serotype 1.

Liggett, A.D., Harrison, L.R. and Farell, R.L. (1987). Res.Vet.Sci. 42, 204-212. Sequential study of lesions development in experimental *Haemophilus pleuropneumoniae*.

Loftager, M.K., Eriksen, L., Aasted, B., Nielsen, R. (1993). Res.Vet.Sci. 55, 281-286. Protective immunity following immunisation of pigs with aerosol of *A.pleuropneumoniae* serotype 2.

Nicolet, J. (1988). Can.Vet.J. 29, 578-580. Taxonomy and serological identification of *A.pleuropneumoniae*.

Pijpers, A., Vernooys, J.A.C.M., Leengood, L.A.M.G. van, Verheiden, J.H.M. (1990). Proc. IPVS 11, 39. Feed and water consumption in pigs following *A.pleuropneumoniae* challenge.

Rycroft, A.N., Cullen, J.M. (1990). J.Vet.Res. 51, 1449-1453. Complement resistance in *A(H) pleuropneumoniae* infection.

Utrera, V., Pijoan, C. (1991). Vet.Rec. 128, 357-358. Fimbriae in *A.pleuropneumoniae* strains isolated from pig respiratory tracts.

Glasser's Disease

Definition

An infectious, sometimes fatal, polyarthritis, polyserositis and meningitis of young pigs caused by *Haemophilus parasuis*. Bronchitis and other syndromes may occur in older animals in non-immune herds.

Incidence

Infection occurs in all pig herds worldwide with the exception of a few primary SPF units. Clinical disease is sporadic in herds with enzootic infection but has become more important since the appearance of PRRS.

Aetiology

Glasser's Disease is caused by the infection of non-immune pigs with some serotypes of *Haemophilus parasuis*. *H.parasuis* is a Gram-negative coccobacillus which requires V factor but not X factor. It is not haemolytic.

Growth only occurs on blood agar in the presence of a staphylococcal streak. Small translucent I mm colonies develop adjacent to the streak within 48 hours. The organisms produce fimbriae and capsules. The species is currently (1995) divided into 15 serovars 1-12. Serovars 1, 5, 10, 12, 13, 14 are virulent, 4 and 15 less so and 3, 6, 7, 8, 9 and 11 appear to be avirulent. Pathogenic organisms appear to possess a 39 kDa outer membrane protein. A cytotoxin has been described but not defined.

Pathogenesis.

Most studies of Glasser's Disease have been carried out by intravenous or intraperitoneal infection which reproduces disease reliably. Aerosol and intranasal infection is less reproducable. As few as 10^2 colony forming units are capable of causing disease with serotype 5 and in SPF pigs.

The incubation period may be as little as 12 hours and septicaemia results in polyserositis, polyarthritis and a purulent meningitis. Aerosol or intratracheal infection can give rise to bronchopneumonia. Organisms appear to colonise the tracheal mucus rather than the cilia. Many H.parasuis pneumonias follow damage such as that caused by swine influenza.

Immunity to infection develops and is complete to the homologous serovar. Little protection occurs against other serovars.

Clinical signs

Outbreaks of the disease occur in young pigs 3-6 weeks of age. A sudden onset with fever (40-41°C, 104-107°F) complete anorexia, shallow, dyspnoeic breathing and extension of the head occurs. Coughing may occur. Lung sounds and pericardial rubbing can be heard by auscultation. Animals become lame and shuffle. All joints are swollen, warm and painful. There may be swelling of the face and one or both ears. Most cases die within 2-5 days of the onset of the disease and show a red to blue skin discolouration before death. Survivors may develop chronic arthritis, pericarditis and congestive cardiac failure, meningitis or intestinal obstruction after adhesions. Animals of any age may be affected in non-immune herds. Coughing, bronchitis and meningitis may occur in gilts or older fatteners and sudden death has been recorded in this age group.

Some animals may be infected and the clinical signs may be overlooked until signs of chronic disease appear. Animals unable to rise with arthritis, those paralysed following meningitis and animals with chronic cardiac failure or strangulated hernias should be humanely destroyed.

Pathological findings

Fibrinous pleurisy, pericarditis and peritonitis are always seen and bronchopneumonia may also occur. Thrombi may be present in these lesions. The spleen and liver may be enlarged and petechial haemorrhages may be seen on the kidneys. There is inflammation of the joints and the joint fluid is turbid and yellowish-green fibrin deposits may be present in the joint cavities. A purulent meningitis is often present. In animals which have died from chronic disease fibrous adhesions are present. Fibrous pericarditis is frequently present and is accompanied by signs of chronic congestive cardiac failure, enlarged heart, pulmonary oedema, enlarged liver and enlarged spleen with excess straw-coloured peritoneal fluid. Pure cultures of H.parasuis may be isolated from the joint fluids, heart blood or, if meningitis is present, from the tracheabronchial tree. Organisms cannot be isolated from the lesions of chronic systemic disease.

Epidemiology

Spread within units is primarily by contact or aerosol. Only a small number of organisms (10^2 - 10^4) is required to initiate infection. Maternal immunity declines after 2-4 weeks and infection commonly occurs at this stage. More than one serotype may occur in a herd and avirulent serovars may be present in the nose and in systemic infections. Spread between units is by the movement of carrier pigs. The organisms are delicate and are easily killed by drying.

Diagnosis

The clinical signs may be distinguished from those of streptococcal joint ill in young pigs and from polyserositis and arthritis cause by *Mycoplasma* spp. in older animals (much milder). The occurrence of fever and the death of the affected animal is often suggestive of Glasser's Disease. When death occurs following meningitis, *Streptococcus suis* Type II should be considered as should Oedema Disease, Talfan and Aujeszky's disease. Post-mortem findings of massive amounts of fibrinous pleurisy pericarditis and, especially peritonitis are particularly suggestive. Confirmation of diagnosis in the acute disease depends upon the isolation of the organism from the lesions. Serotyping as one of the virulent serovars is final proof. This is particularly important in respiratory tract infections. These may require selective media (chocolate altered blood agar with 10 units bacitracin/ml). Fresh specimens are essential and swabs should be submitted in transport medium. The presence of complement-fixing antibodies to the serovar responsible at titres greater than 1:80 is a useful indicator of herd infection.

Treatment and control

Parenteral penicillin, ampicillin, tetracycline, ceftiofur, chloramphenicol, (not UK).enrofloxacin and sulphonamide:trimethoprim may all be used to treat early cases with success. Spread to other animals at risk may be prevented and treatment continued by water medication with one of the above drugs for the appropriate treatment period. Feed medication over the period of risk may prevent disease. Killed vaccines have been produced and may be used to vaccinate sows or piglets. Studies with restriction endonuclease analysis have shown that vaccine failure is associated with infection with different serovars and successful protection depends upon inclusion of appropriate serovars in the vaccine. Vaccines made from the herd's own organisms are most effective.

References

Kielstein, P., Rapp Gabrielson, V.J. (1992). J.Clin.Microbiol. 30, 862-865. Designation of 15 serovars of *H.parasuis* on the basis of immunodiffusion using heat stable antigen extracts.
Smart, N.L., Hurnik, D., MacInnes, J.J. (1993). Can.Vet.J. 34, 387-490. An investigation of enzootic Glasser's disease in a specific pathogen-free grower finisher facility using restriction endonuclease analysis.

Smart, N.L., Miniats, O.P. (1989). Can.J.Vet.Res. 53, 390-393. Preliminary assessment of a *H.parasuis* bacterin for use in specific pathogen-free swine.

Tuberculosis

Definition

Tuberculosis rarely causes clinical disease but is a cause for the condemnation of carcases at slaughter when gross lesions are detected and is a potential risk to human health.

Incidence

The incidence has fallen in most developed countries, 0.7% US, 1989 and is now generally so low that single infected farms can cause an appreciable rise in cases. Where *M.bovis* and *M.tuberculosis* are controlled in cattle and human populations (UK, US) the incidence of infection is very low.

Aetiology

A wide range of mycobacteria has been associated with tuberculosis in pigs. Most important for zoonotic reasons are infections with the *M.tuberculosis:bovis* group and the infections with *M.avium*, its subspecies and *M.intracellulare*. All can now be identified to species by their DNA sequences and it is expected that new species will be identified in the pig. The organisms are acid alcohol fast, waxy bacteria which can be demonstrated easily in tissue and can be cultured.

Pathogenesis

Infection is generally oral and lesions may first be detected histologically in mesenteric and submandibular lymph nodes after 14 days. More often they require 6-10 weeks or even 90-115 days (some *M.avium* strains) Antibodies are produced early in infection but immunity to infection is cell-mediated.

Clinical signs

These are usually only seen in generalised tuberculosis and usually result from infection with mammalian tuberculosis infections such as *M.bovis*. The incubation period is at least 6-12 weeks after which loss of weight, chronic pneumonia or local sinus formation may be seen. Chronic diarrhoea has been recorded in enteric infections. Most infections are only detected at slaughter.

Humane slaughter is indicated when chronic wasting is identified, but infected animals are often destroyed for legislative reasons if detected in life.

Pathology

External changes such as sinuses may be obvious, but the principal findings are whitish or yellowish granulomatous lesions which may be calcified. They may be generalised in submandibular, bronchial and mesenteric lymph nodes, lungs, liver, spleen and kidney and may reach 1-2 cm in diameter, sometimes becoming calcified or necrotic centrally. *M.bovis* and *M.intracellulare* are mainly associated with this type of distribution.

Localised tuberculosis usually occurs only in the pharyngeal, cervical and mesenteric lymph nodes. The lesions vary between small yellowish-white caseous lesions and generalised enlargement of the node. Granulomata are often fleshy and are rarely calcified. Experimental infections with *M.avium* suggest that infection often occurs at about 8 weeks of age to produce the type of lesions seen at slaughter. 6-10 weeks after infection multinucleate giant cells are the most prominent feature of lesions from twelve weeks onwards. Diffuse infiltrations of epithelioid cells predominate with some caseation and by 18 weeks, encapsulation, necrosis fibrosis and caseation are common. Acid-fast organisms may be seen but may be sparse in some cases.

Epidemiology

Infections with avian bacteria usually originate from infected poultry infections or from contamination of feeders, etc. with bird droppings containing the bacilli. Gross lesions may take at least 85 days to develop. *M.intracellulare* infections appear to have originated in sawdust in some outbreaks and are not readily transmitted from pig to pig. In some cases these infections take place in the farrowing house and may also be associated with peat given to piglets. Water may be infected on some farms.

M.bovis infections arise from contact with tuberculous cattle or access to infected milk and may spread from pig to pig. Infection in wild boar has been identified in several parts of Europe and this poses a risk to outdoor pigs. *M.avium paratuberculosis* infection has been associated with contact with cattle.

Diagnosis

Tuberculosis is usually detected at slaughter or the post-mortem examination of wasted pigs. Lesions suspected of being tuberculous (granulomas, chronic pneumonia) can be confirmed as such by demonstration of the organism in smears by Ziehl Neelsen staining. Histological examination confirms the granulomatous nature of the lesions and acid-fast (ZN+ve) organisms may be seen. The organism may be demonstrated by culture in specialist laboratories. Mycobacteria are Category 3 pathogens in the EU and may only be grown in registered laboratories and identified to species. These laboratories can now use the polymerase chain reaction (PCR) to identify mycobacterial DNA in tissue or clinical and environmental samples and DNA probes to identify mycobacteria in histological sections. Tuberculosis must be notified to the veterinary authorities in most countries as it is a zoonosis (UK under the Tuberculosis Order).

ELISA tests have been developed to detect serum antibodies to recombinant mycobacterial proteins but are not yet widely used. Intradermal tuberculin testing may be used on a herd basis with either mammalian or avian tuberculins given intradermally on the ear. Pigs may be negative 6 weeks after infection but positive at 12 weeks.

Treatment

Treatment is technically possible for valuable individuals (e.g. rifampicin) but is not practised commercially.

Control

Remove source of infective material e.g. sawdust or prevent access by birds. Affected carcases may still be found at slaughter until unexposed stock reach slaughter age. Where *M.bovis* is involved, skin or ELISA testing may reveal infected animals which may be culled. Carcases for human consumption may be heat treated.

References

Acland, H.M. and Whitlock, R.H. (1986). J.Comparative Pathology 96, 247-266. *M.avium* serotype 4 infection of swine: The attempted transmission by contact and the sequence of morphological changes in inoculated pigs.
Charette, R., Martineau, G.P., Pigeon, C., Turcotte, C., Higgins, R. (1989). Can.Vet.J. 30, 675-678. An outbreak of granulomatous lymphadenitis due to *M.avium* in swine.
Dey, B.P., Parham, G.L. (1993). J.Am.Vet.Med.Ass. 203, 516-519. Incidence and economics of tuberculosis in swine slaughtered from 1976-1988.
Lysons, R.L. (1992). Pig Vet.J. 29, 193-197. Pigs, peat and avian tuberculosis.
Windsor, R.S., Durrant, D.S. and Burn, K. (1984). Vet.Rec. 114, 497-500. Avian tuberculosis in pigs: *M.intracellulare* infection in a breeding herd.

Exudative epidermitis (Greasy Pig Disease)

Definition

An acute generalised dermatitis of piglets characterised by the sudden onset of excess sebaceous secretion and exudation from the skin without pruritis, leading to dehydration, growth depression and death. Infected skin lesions occur in adults.

Incidence

Sporadic but can cause appreciable losses in non-immune herds (35% during the period of the outbreak, 9% over the year in one outbreak). Infection is probably world wide and has been reported from many countries.

Aetiology

Caused by a Gram-positive coccus, *Staphylococcus hyicus* subsp. *hyicus*, which forms non-haemolytic white 2 mm colonies on blood agar, pink colonies on MacConkey agar, is coagulase-negative but DNAase positive. It produces capsules, Protein A and an exfoliative toxin of M.W. 29-30 kDa. At least 6 serotypes and a large number of phage types exist. The organism is resistant to drying but does not form spores and is readily inactivated by heat. It is sensitive *in vitro* to many antibiotics including penicillins, aminoglycosides and cephalosporins. Resistance can occur.

Pathogenesis

Infection with S.hyicus often follows abrasions produced by scratches, bites or rough bedding, e.g. sawdust or rough concrete flooring. Fodder or mange mites may act as irritating agents in the development of the disease. Application of cultures to the skin of gnotobiotic or SPF piglets results in infection and similar lesions can be produced by the subcutaneous injection of culture filtrates containing the toxin. Pathogenic strains are encapsulated and resist phagocytosis.

Rounding of epithelial cells occurs within 12 hours of infection and lesions progress with exfoliation (bedding) of epithelial cells, crust formation, exocytosis i.e. neutrophil accumulation in the epidermis, formation of vesicles, formation of pustules and acanthosis. The gross changes of skin reddening are associated with inflammation and excess sebaceous secretion. Microcolonies of *S.hyicus* are present in the skin and a neutrophil response occurs followed by erosion down to the stratum germinativum in some areas. Affected piglets die from dehydration and sometimes loss of protein. Immunity (either passive or active) protecst against the homologous phage type or serotype.

Clinical signs

The disease commonly occurs in piglets of between 7 days and 5 weeks of age. The clinical signs begin with listlessness, a dulling of the skin and the appearance of thin, pale brown flecks or scales on the skin surface. There is often scabbing of the cheeks or knees due to fighting or kneeling on rough floors. Within 3-5 days the scabs become darker in colour and extend over much of the back and discolour the abdomen and axillae. The skin surface becomes covered with exudate which gives it a greasy texture and which matts the hair. There is no pruritis. Bacterial multiplication and dirt caught in the scabs soon give the skin a black colour. Affected animals lose weight rapidly and eventually die, often with a grossly thickened, wrinkled skin. Death normally occurs within 5-10 days. Recovery occurs by healing of the scabs, but takes at least 10 days. Fever is usually absent. Exudative epidermitis usually only affects a few litters on a farm and may not affect all the animals in any one litter. The disease affects younger pigs most severely and up to 90% of those affected may die. When affected piglets are weaned into flat decks with rough surfaces or humid atmospheres, infection may occur and persist in successive batches. Localised lesions may occasionally be seen on older pigs such as gilts or sows as 1-2 cm patches of greasy exudate or areas of ulceration usually on the back or rump. The organism has been incriminated with trauma and a streptococcus in ear necrosis.

Humane slaughter is only indicated in young pigs. Piglets with extensive chronic lesions and loss of condition should be destroyed, particularly if they cannot suck.

Pathological findings

At post-mortem examination, pigs are found to be dehydrated and emaciated and the superficial lymph nodes are normally oedematous and swollen. There is usually no food present in the bowel and a white or yellowish-white precipitate may be found in the pelvis of the kidney. Hypertrophy of the sebaceous glands and inflammatory changes are seen in histological sections of the skin. Rete pegs are prominent and microabscesses can be seen in the keratinised layers. Bacteriological examination of the skin usually yields a profuse growth of the staphylococcus and it may also be recovered from the enlarged lymph nodes. Non-specific organisms may be present in the parenchymatous organs and organisms such as *Pseudomonas aeruginosa* occur in older skin lesions. *Dermatophilus* spp. have been recovered from some lesions.

Epidemiology

The disease is introduced to clean herds by infected carriers and first occurs in litters in contact with those carrier sows. The latter remain unaffected. Infection may persist in improperly cleaned farrowing pens and may even persist in local lesions on older pigs caused by mange or harvest mites. In improperly ventilated flat decks the disease may spread from mildly affected animals and infection may remain on fittings. The progeny of non immune recently purchased gilts are susceptible in a herd where the disease is enzootic. Outbreaks are normally self-limiting lasting 2-3 months but may persist for 12-18 months. *S.hyicus* has been identified on a number of species such as cattle and horses but their role, as sources of disease for pigs, is as yet unknown.

Diagnosis

Diagnosis is normally made on the basis of the clinical signs, and this condition in piglets must be distinguished from parakeratosis (age), swine pox (discrete scabby lesions), dermatosis vegetans (Landrace pigs only) and from mange and other mite infestations (no pruritis). The location of the lesions, their non-circular nature and the age incidence differentiate them from ringworm. Post-mortem and bacteriological findings may provide confirmation. Staphylococci isolated from the lesions may be identified as *S.hyicus hyicus* by biochemical tests (such as the API staph system) but virulence and phage typing is only experimental at present. In older animals ringworm may resemble the lesions, as may bites, injections, abscesses and abrasions.

Treatment

Early cases may be treated successfully using tylosin (8 mg/kg) or amoxycillin, ampicillin, trimethoprim sulphonamide, erythromycin. Lincomycin has been shown to be particularly effective. Affected piglets should be given access to fluid such as Lectade (Beecham) and washed in a solution of cetrimide (Hibitane, I.C.I.) or other mild disinfectant. Injections may need to be repeated daily for 2-3 days. Antimicrobial resistance can arise, particularly after prolonged treatment if the wrong strains have been tested.

Control

The disease may be controlled by clipping the teeth of litters at risk, by providing soft bedding, e.g. chaffed straw and removing wood shavings if present. Hygiene, washing of sows into farrowing houses and local treatment of lesions on sows may all reduce infection. Segregation of infected animals before placing in flat decks prevents outbreaks in that type of accommodation. Thorough cleaning and disinfection of accommodation should be carried out between farrowings. Emergency vaccines (autogenous bacterins) have been used to reduce the duration of outbreaks in piglets by sow vaccination and by the vaccination of piglets when infection occurs at weaning. Vaccines made from one strain may cease to work if another virulent strain (serotype or phage type) is present in the herd or colonises it. Vaccines only protect against the homologous strain.

Reference

Sato, H., Tanabe, T., Kuramoto, M., Tanaka, K., Hashimoto, T., Saito, H. (1991). Vet.Micro. 27, 263-275. Isolation of exfoliative toxin from *S.hyicus* subsp. *hyicus* and its exfoliative activity in the piglet.

Other Staphylococci

S.aureus is the most common other pathogenic staphylococcus to be isolated from pigs and can be distinguished from *S.hyicus* biochemically. *S.aureus* can be isolated from umbilical abscesses, vegetative endocarditis, subcutaneous abscesses, foot lesions, arthritis, mastitis, metritis and from enteritis. *S.aureus* strains are known to produce enterotoxin but clinically it has not yet been associated with any specific type of enteritis. Apart from the presence of creamy pus there are few distinguishing features other than bacterial isolation. *S.aureus* is often sensitive to penicillin, streptomycin, trimethoprim sulphonamide but may be resistant to any of these. A wide variety of other staphylococci have been recorded in pigs but *S.hyicus* is the most important in the pig.

Spirochaetal granuloma

Localised areas of ulceration with a blackened weeping crust may occur on the lower margin and tips of the ears and on the neck nearby. Spirochaetes may be seen in smears made from the lesions. Parenteral or local treatment with tetracycline is usually effective.

Swine Erysipelas

Definition

An infectious condition of pigs caused by *Erysipelothrix rhusiopathiae* and characterised clinically by sudden death, fever associated with characteristic diamond skin lesions, arthritis or vegetative endocarditis and by abortion in pregnant sows.

Incidence

Clinical disease is commonly seen in pigs in extensive conditions and strawyards but is less common in housed animals. It is found worldwide.

Aetiology

E.rhusiopathiae is a slender, slightly curved aerobic Gram-positive rod forming I mm greyish translucent non haemolytic colonies on blood agar after 24-48 hours incubation. Different colonial types of *E.rhusiopathiae* may be distinguished and at least 28 different antigenic types exist. In general, strains forming smooth colonies and those of antigenic types 1 and 2 are most commonly isolated from the septicaemic form of the disease. "Rough" strains are generally considered to be less virulent. Virulent strains produce a capsule which resists phagocytosis and some produce neuraminidase. Recently the species has been subdivided by DNA relatedness into 2 new species which reflect biochemical and serological characters. *E.rhusiopathiae* comprises serotypes 1, 2, 4, 5, 6, 8, 9, 11, 12, 15, 16, 17, 19, 21 and N and *E.tonsillarum* comprises serotypes 3, 7, 10, 14, 20, 22 and 23 with serotypes 13 and 18 intermediate between them. The organism can live for months or years in animal tissue at +4°C, in frozen materials and is relatively resistant to drying and 0.2% phenol but is sensitive to penicillin, some other antimicrobials and to heat (15 minutes at 60°C).

Pathogenesis

E.rhusiopathiae is present in soil contaminated with faeces and urine from affected or carrier animals and is present on the tonsils of normal animals. Invasion of the susceptible pig by E.rhusiopathiae may occur in certain circumstances, especially during hot, muggy weather or in particular fields or buildings. Entry may be through the tonsils, gastrointestinal tract or through minute skin abrasions. In experimental transmission studies, clinical disease has followed the inoculation of scarified skin more repeatably than intravenous or subcutaneous inoculation with pure cultures.

Once invasion has taken place, multiplication proceeds and results in a septicaemia within 1-7 days of infection. Septicaemia may be sufficiently severe to cause acute clinical signs or even death, but usually results in fever with subsequent localisation of the organism in the skin, joints or the muscle or valves of the heart to give rise to the chronic form of the disease. The joint lesions begin with an acute synovitis and progress through a fibrinous exudation to a fibrosis. Synovial villous hypertrophy is severe and polypoid, there is diffuse erosion of articular cartilage and the draining lymph node is often enlarged. In the later stages antigen may still be demonstrable but cultivation is difficult. Heart lesions also begin with early inflammatory changes. Abortion appears to be due to fever but the organism has been isolated from foetuses and congenital erysipelas has been recorded. The organism produces a neuraminidase which may be responsible for these changes. Antibody develops to the sero type of organism involved but cannot penetrate the arthritic joint or the valvular endocarditis lesions.

Clinical signs

Hyperacute, acute and chronic forms of the disease occur.

Hyperacute form. Sudden death may occur or affected pigs of 55-80 kg. liveweight may be found to be dull, collapsed with a high temperature (41.1-42.8°C, 106-109°F) and often show a scarlet flush on the skin. This form is uncommon in adults.

Acute form. The signs of acute erysipelas vary with the age and the immune status of the animal. In younger pigs such as gilts, fattening pigs and young boars, anorexia, high fever of 41.1-42.2°C, 106-108°F is common and there may be flushing or blotching of the skin and ears. Affected animals may die within 12-48 hours with cyanosis of the ears and body and with dyspnoea. In older pigs, anorexia and thirst are most commonly noted and a high temperature is found. Affected animals may be dull and may be reluctant to move.

The pathognomonic diamond skin lesions appear within 24-48 hours of the onset of clinical sings. At first they can only be palpated as raised patches along the back or neck but, later, in white pigs, they take on an angry, purplish-red colour. Abortion may occur at this stage in pregnant sows, temporary infertility may develop in boars (possibly a temperature effect) and sows may return to service.

Chronic form. Affected animals may recover completely, but the skin lesions may become necrotic, turn black and slough. The tips of the ears may also be lost. Localisation of the bacteria in the joints may occur and the elbow, hip, back, stifle and knee joints may be affected. Affected joints become hot and painful to the touch but become swollen and firm after 2-3 weeks and may stiffen. Affected pigs become lame and may lose condition.

Valvular lesions may develop in the heart and give rise to a murmur. Sudden death or signs of congestive heart failure, cyanosis, tachycardia, tachypnoea and murmur may occur later, the latter occurring commonly at farrowing in older sows.

Humane destruction is not indicated in acute cases due to the excellent response to treatment but is indicated where chronic arthritis causes severe lameness or ataxia and in chronic congestive heart failure with cyonosis and a subnormal temperature.

Pathological findings

Gross lesions

a.   Hyperacute, Congestion of the carcase and discolouration of the skin may be seen but no specific lesions are present.

b.   Acute. The skin may show purplish discolouration and the ears may be cyanosed. Diamond skin lesions may present. Congestion of the carcase is common and there may be enlargement of the spleen. Lymph nodes may be haemorrhagic and swollen, and ecchymoses may be present under the kidney capsule, pleura, peritoneum and on the heart.

c.   Chronic. Affected pigs may have necrotic skin lesions or enlarged joints. A non-suppurative proliferative arthritis may be found in the limb and intervertebral joints in which thickening of the joint capsule and tags of granulation tissue may be seen. These changes are preceded by inflammatory synovitis and may be followed by erosion of the articular cartilage and ankylosis. Lesions of an embolic nature may be found in other organs and large granular vegetations may occur on the heart valves.

Specific histological features are absent. The vegetations on the heart valves are composed of granulation tissue and connective tissue. The synovial lesions are filled with macrophages and lymphocytes with proliferation of the synovial membrane.

E.rhusiopathiae may be seen as a short, fine Gram-positive bacillus in smears made from heart blood. It can usually be cultured from heart blood, spleen or bone marrow (a long bone is best) in hyperacute and acute cases. Examination of local lesions, e.g. synovial fluid or vegetations may be necessary in chronic cases, but E.rhusiopathiae cannot always be isolated from these. Freezing the organ and thawing may improve the isolation rate as may homogenising in serum broth with neomycin, kanamycin and vancomycin. Fluorescent antibody may be used to identify the organism in tissue and may demonstrate *E.rhusiopathiae* antigen in sites such as joints from which the organism cannot be isolated.

Epidemiology

E.rhusiopathiae is commonly recovered from the tonsils of clinically normal pigs and from other parts of their bodies. It may also be recovered from the ground on farms where clinical disease has occurred. The association with hot weather, viral infection, fatigue, pregnancy and vaccination may be circumstantial. It is now thought that immunity to the local strain of organism is present and that the introduction of susceptible pigs to a contaminated environment, e.g. newly purchased gilts or the introduction of a new strain - with pigs or in fish meal in which *E.rhusiopathiae* is common may be the cause of outbreaks.

Affected pigs shed the organism in faeces and urine and it can survive on the ground for long periods although there is as yet no evidence for its multiplication in soil. It appears to survive for about 7 days in slurry when distributed on soil. As many birds and mammals may be infected with this organism they provide a reservoir of infection for the pig population.

Outbreaks of disease are most common amongst pigs kept in poor conditions, in yarded sows, fatteners in irregularly cleaned pens and in batches of recently purchased gilts, especially in hot weather. Recovered animals retain lifelong immunity to the local strain, but remain carriers of *E.rhusiopathiae* for life. Vaccination may not protect against all 24 serotypes and disease may therefore occasionally occur in vaccinates, especially with vaccines from types 1 or 2 which do not protect against serotypes 10 and 20 (*E.tonsillarum*).

E.rhusiopathiae commonly (20-50%) contaminates pork and infections in slaughtermen, veterinarians, abattoir workers and butchers are common. The disease in man is known as *erysipeloid* and is usually localised as inflammation and swelling of a finger.

Diagnosis

Erysipelas should be considered if a high fever of 41.1°C, 106°F or more is found in any fattening or adult pig which has gone off its feed and shows no respiratory signs. The development of the pathognomonic skin lesions in one of an affected group of animals is sufficient to confirm the diagnosis, and erysipelas should be considered in cases where lameness and fever occur together. Sows in difficulties and with fever at farrowing may also be affected.

If post-mortem examination is necessary, a reliable diagnosis can only be made after bacteriological examination in the absence of the pathognomonic skin lesions. Spleen, kidney and a long bone should be submitted for examination. Serological tests for infection in recovered animals are unreliable although a rising titre in an agglutination test using the homologous serotypes and performed with suitable controls is diagnostic. The complement fixation test has recently been shown to be reliable. An ELISA has been developed but also requires appropriate antigens.

Treatment

Penicillin is the drug of choice and the response to treatment is normally rapid. It is advisable to give 2 or 3 daily injections to prevent relapse or the persistence of the organism to give chronic infection. Hyperimmune serum is commercially available for treatment in some countries, but is more expensive than doses of antibiotic. If used, it should be given intraperitoneally or intravenously at the stated dose.

Control

As *E.rhusiopathiae* is widespread in the environment and is carried by clinically normal pigs, its total elimination is not practicable. However, it is advisable to clean out and disinfect the pens of affected animals as high concentrations of virulent bacteria may be present.

Control is normally exercised by prophylaxis and this takes the form of preventing the spread of outbreaks to other susceptible or in contact animals by prophylactic injections of penicillin (short term protection) or hyperimmune serum (medium term protection, about 6 weeks). The latter is of particular value in preventing disease in finishing pigs which will soon be marketed, but the product is no longer available in the UK.

Vaccination is commonly employed to prevent clinical swine erysipelas in breeding stock and in young fattening pigs over 12 weeks of age on farms which have an erysipelas problem. Most commercially available vaccines are formolised whole cultures and include an adjuvant. Vaccination is normally practised in recently weaned pigs (fattener protection) and in gilts or sows before service or, to prevent conception problems soon after farrowing. Immunity lasts for 6 months and regular re-vaccination should be practised. The vaccination of pregnant animals is not recommended with some dead vaccines and all live ones. All boars should be vaccinated at 6 month intervals. Vaccine breakdowns may occur if a serotype with sufficient antigenic divergence from the vaccine is encountered. Vaccines prepared from serotypes 1 and 2 (those most common in acute disease and belonging to *E.rhusiopathiae*) do not protect against serotypes 10 or 20 (*E.tonsillarum*).

Vaccines containing serotypes 2 and 10 protect against both *E.rhusiopathiae* and *E.tonsillarum*. Recent studies suggest that a 64-66 kDa protein antigen produced during log phase protects against both species but it has not been marketed commercially.

References

Johnston, K.M. Doige, C.E. and Osborne, A.D. (1987). Can.Vet.J. 28, 174-180. An evaluation of non-suppurative joint disease in slaughter pigs.
Molen, G., Soderlind, O., Ursing, J., Norring, V., Ternstrom, A., Lowenhiels, C. (1989). J.Appl.Bact. 67, 347-352. Occurrence of *E.rhusiopathiae* on pork and in pig slurry and the distribution of specific antibodies in abattoir workers.
Takahashi, T., Fujisawa T., Tamura, Y., Suzuki, S., Muramatsu, M., Sawada, T., Mitsuoka, T. (1992). Int.J.Syst.Bact. 42, 469-473. DNA relatedness among *E.rhusiopathiae* strains representing all 23 serovars and *E.tonsillarum*.
Timoney, J.F., Groschup, M.M. (1993). Vet.Micro. 37, 381-387. Properties of a protective protein of *E.rhusiopathiae*

Streptococcus suis infections

Infections with *Streptococcus suis* cause septicaemia, arthritis (joint ill) and meningitis in sucking piglets and similar syndromes in recently weaned growing and finishing pigs and occur in bronchopneumonia

Streptococcal infection of young pigs (Joint III)

Definition

A condition of young piglets 7-14 days of age in which septicaemia may cause death or local infections such as meningitis, arthritis or endocarditis.

Incidence

Worldwide.

Aetiology

Most infections are associated with *S.suis* serotype I but infection with *S.suis* type 2 may also occur. *S.suis* is described below in detail.

Pathogenesis

Infection is by aerosol, ingestion or contact and invasion may take place through the tonsils (see *S.suis* type 2 below). Bacteraemia may lead to septicaemia or localisation in joints, meninges or heart valves. Animals recover but may remain chronically infected.

Clinical signs

The disease is seen in piglets of 10-14 days of age. Affected animals cease to thrive, become rough-coated and may die. Fever (40.6-41.1°C, 105-106°F) may be present. Later, enlarged, hot, painful joint swellings may be seen or the animals may appear stiff and may be blind or show muscular tremors ending in ataxia or death. Sudden death may occur in endocarditis due to streptococcal infection. Typically, up to 2/3rd of the litter may be affected with one or another form of the disease. Affected pigs rarely recover completely.

Affected piglets respond to treatment, so humane destruction should be carried out on those with paralysis or ataxia after meningitis following treatment and on chronically stunted animals.

Post mortem findings

Few lesions are seen in the septicaemic phase, but a purulent meningitis may be seen where brain involvement occurs and in arthritis there is inflammation around the joint with mucoid joint fluid. In endocarditis, the organisms are a major feature of the histological lesion on the valves. They may be demonstrated in culture and in smears.

Epidemiology

Infection may arise from carrier sows, infected animals within the same airspace (by contact, ingestion or aerosol) and by transfer on needles used for routine injections. Infection may remain in uncleaned accommodation.

Diagnosis

The characteristic spectrum of clinical signs and the age of the affected pigs (10-21 days) is normally sufficient. Bacteriological examination of joint fluid, blood or post-mortem specimens will confirm and distinguish the condition from *H.parasuis* infections.

Treatment and control

Parenteral antibiotic such as penicillin or trimethoprim: sulphonamide for 3-5 days is most satisfactory. Animals with advanced septicaemia, meningitis and arthritis rarely respond and must be nursed by giving milk supplement and water by stomach tube.

Control may be possible in herds where the disease occurs by farrowing sows in isolation and by fumigating the accommodation between animals. Where arthritis is associated with knee damage on floors, additional bedding may prevent the development of the condition. Injection of piglets at birth with long-acting penicillin may prevent. Inactivated vaccines have been prepared and used on sows to provide passive immunity to piglets but are often effective only against the homologous strain.

Epidemic streptococcal meningitis

An epidemic disease of weaned and fattening pigs which occurs after mixing and moving, resulting in sudden death, fever, nervous signs or, in younger pigs, arthritis. Bronchopneumonia is being identified increasingly.

Incidence

Present in all countries of Western Europe, the United States, Canada, Australasia and the Far East.

Aetiology

S. suis is a weakly ß-haemolytic streptococcus which forms clear greyish mucoid colonies 1-2 mm in diameter on blood agar. The cells may appear boat-shaped and produce a polysaccharide capsule and have fimbriae. The capsule has been used to separate isolates into at least 29 serotypes. Virulent strains of *S.suis* type 2 appear to produce two specific proteins, the muramidase related protein MRP of 136 kDa and the extracellular factor (EF) of 110 kDa. The capsular types appear to be related to DNA structure and 1-8 can be distinguished by restriction endonuclease analysis. It survives in distilled water at 4°C for 1-2 weeks, in nutrient medium at 4°C for 9 months, is relatively resistant to heating, being destroyed only after 2 hours by heating to 50°C and after 10 minutes after heating at 60°C. It is sensitive to a wide range of antimicrobials but least so to aminoglycosides. Resistance has been reported.

Type 1 is consistently associated with piglet infections and type 2 is responsible for about 50% of all invasive infections in older pigs.

Pathogenesis.

S.suis type 2 infects pigs by aerosol or contact within 5-25 days after mixing with carrier animals and can infect in the presence of antibody. The organism multiplies in the tonsillar crypts and enters the circulation in some cases to give rise to a bacteraemia. It is taken up by both neutrophils and macrophages. The organism is protected from phagocytosis in macrophages by its polysaccharide capsule and multiplies to give a septicaemia within a few hours. This may kill the animal directly or organisms carried by macrophages may localise in the brain, joints or other areas to produce local lesions. In the brain these take the form of a purulent meningitis which is frequently fatal. Immunity develops and includes opsonising antibody to the capsular polysaccharide antigen. Antigens which may be important include ones of 94, 86 and 44 Kd, but recent studies suggest that MRP (136 kDa and EF (110 kDa) are protective.

The organism may survive after clinical recovery in the tonsillar crypts or nose for up to 512 days.

Restriction endonuclease analysis suggests that organisms isolated from meningitis and bronchopneumonia belong to different REA types.

Clinical signs

The incubation period varies from 24 hours to 2 weeks or more. The first signs of an outbreak may be the death of a pig in a good condition. If the pig is seen alive, fever of 40.6-41.7°C, 105-107°F and evidence of septicaemia may be seen. Nervous signs such as incoordination, tremor, paralysis, paddling, opisthotonus and tetanic spasms may be seen in that order before death which may occur within 4 hours of the onset of the clinical signs. Arthritis may occur in younger pigs and some untreated animals with meningitis may not die. Animals developing the meningitis may be detected early in the condition by the glassy stare, flushed skin and their unsteady gait. Head tilt is sometimes present.

In Canada, a syndrome has been reported in which neonatal disease is followed by death within 24 hours of birth. The clinical signs of bronchopneumonia are not distinctive but include fever, raised respiratory rate and bronchial sounds. Disease may occur in animals of any age in susceptible herds but is most common in the 3-12 week age group in herds where the infection is enzootic but may occur not uncommonly in animals up to 6 months of age. Mortality varies from 1-50% in any batch of pigs and in enzootic herds may be 0.5% with morbidity of 1%.

Decisions about humane slaughter are commonly required in this condition. Affected pigs should be treated and their condition assessed after 3 days' treatment and nursing. Those unable to stand or feed themselves as a result of meningitis should be humanely destroyed as should chronically stunted animals and those with severe chronic polyarthritis. Blind animals and those with head tilt can be left if properly managed.

Pathology

The skin and the carcase may be reddened, lymph nodes are often enlarged and congested and congestion of the parenchymatous organs is common. Fine strands of fibrin may be seen in the peritoneal and pleural cavities. Lung lesions are common in some outbreaks, varying from severe localised pleurisy to pneumonia with congestion and oedema of the interlobular septae. Gross oedema and congestion of the brain may be visible and the cerebrospinal fluid may be cloudy. Purulent arthritis may be present in young pigs. Histological features of the meningitis include a polymorphonuclear leucocyte infiltration in the meninges and sometimes the ventricles. Cortical necrosis and spongiform changes in cerebellum and brain stem have been recorded. Neuritis of cranial nerves may occur. In treated pigs, the predominant cells in meningitis may be lymphocytes. The organisms may be seen in sections and isolated from the brain and from most organs in untreated animals.

In animals with enzootic pneumonia, *S.suis* type 2 may be isolated from a suppurative bronchopneumonia.

<u>Epidemiology</u>

S.suis infection is spread by contact and to a lesser extent by aerosol and ingestion. Most pigs become infected, but not all develop the disease. Lack of specific immunity is important, but intercurrent disease and environment are also important in the initiation of disease.

Overcrowding, poor ventilation and mixing of pigs from different litters appear to be predisposing features in a herd. There may be some increase in cases in Autumn and Winter. Although carrier sows may pass on infection to their litters, restriction endonuclease analysis confirms that spread is horizontal within a herd.

S.suis can survive in faeces for 104 days at 0°C, 10 days at 9°C and 8 days at 22-25°C and in dust for 54 days at 0°C, 25 days at 9°C and for less than 24 hours at room temperature. Survival for 6 weeks at 4°C and 12 days at 22-25°C has been recorded in carcases. It is killed in less than a minute by recommended dilutions of most farm disinfectants. It survives on plastic and rubber both directly and in manure and in porcine body fluids. Fomites may contribute to the spread between pens.

Spread between farms is by means of carrier pigs although fomites such as clothing and hypodermic needles may also introduce the disease. *S.suis* has been isolated from other species but these have neither been confirmed as vectors nor as reservoir hosts.

S.suis persists in the tonsils and may be present in the carcases of slaughter pigs. Infection occurs in veterinarians, farmers, abattoir workers and butchers and, occasionally in housewives in whom it may cause a fatal meningitis or septicaemia. Antibody and carriage are more common than disease in the exposed human population.

<u>Diagnosis</u>

The clinical signs and post-mortem findings, particularly of a meningitis are sufficiently distinctive for *S.suis* infection to be considered, along with *H.parasuis* infection. The organism can be demonstrated in smears of heart blood, C.S.F. or brain tissue and joint fluid by Gram stain or, more specifically, by immunofluorescence or immunoperoxidase and can be isolated from these sites in recently dead untreated animals. When sought from the tonsils a gag should be used and the tonsillar crypts swabbed. The material from tonsillar and nasal swabs should be plated on supplemented with 5% horse serum, a selective medium for streptococci (Oxoid SR74, sodium azide, nalidixic acid colestin and crystal violet). and specific hyperimmune serum to the polysaccharide. Halos of precipitate occur around *S.suis* colonies.

Isolates may be identified as *S.suis* biochemically with API strep strips or using starch containing media flooded with iodine to detect amylase Colonies may be identified serologically using coagglutination and then serotyped by capsular typing. Restriction endonuclease analysis patterns may also be used. More than 1 serotype may be present in a herd.

Serum antibody may be detected using ELISAs with antigens such as capsular polysaccharide but not all pigs are seropositive.

Treatment

Penicillin is the drug of choice in the parenteral treatment of the condition although amoxycillin, ampicillin, cephalosporins, lincomycin and other antimicrobials except for aminoglycosides such as streptomycin may be used. Treatment should be repeated more than once and supportive therapy given. Affected pigs should be removed to a quiet pen and given water and food, manually if necessary. Paralysed animals rapidly become dehydrated and should be rehydrated using saline given per rectum. Recovery may be faster in a cooler, dryer environment. Other pigs in affected pens may be injected individually or given water or feed medication as described below.

Penicillin resistance has been described but resistance to ampicillin is less common.

Control

This may be achieved by:-

1. Medication

    This may be strategic by means of long-acting penicillin given at birth and 10 days post weaning or at entry to the weaner housing or 7 days before the expected peak of the disease. Water medication should be given for 7 days before the expected peak and should be with ampicillin, cloxacillin or the tetracyclines although resistance to these is widespread.

    In-feed medication should be carried out with penicillin. The most effective penicillin and that which survives pelleting best may be phenoxymethylpenicillin at 75-100 g/tonne although procaine penicillin at 200-300 g/tonne may be as good. Freshly medicated feeds should be used. Penicillin, tetracycline, sulphonamide preparations have also been used.

2. Vaccination

    Inactivated vaccines are still under investigation and are not yet (1995) marketed in the UK. All are killed and adjuvanted and may at times protect completely against the homologous strain. Restriction endonuclease analysis has shown that a single REA type persists in a herd for 6-12 months when it is replaced by another. Failure of vaccine appears to be due to the use of an incorrect strain or serotype of the organism. The MRP and EF proteins appear to be capable of producing protective immunity which is effective against heterologous strains.

3.   Husbandry measures

Continuous production systems should be avoided, all-in all-out policies followed, mixing batches as little as possible and putting animals into clean, dry pens with a low slurry level and low humidity.

4.   Eradication

Treatment of herds and removal of carriers and internal isolation are not effective.

5.   Slaughter and restocking

Slaughter and farm disinfection to eliminate residual infection in faeces and dust followed by restocking with meningitis-free pigs is practicable. These can be produced by hysterectomy, by medicated early weaning or by purchase from clean herds.

References

Clifton-Hadley, F.A. and Alexander, T.J.L. (1980). Vet. Rec . 107, 40-41 The carrier site and carrier rate of S.suis type 2 in pigs.
Clifton-Hadley, F.A., Alexander, T.J.L., Upton, I. and Duffus, W.P.H. (1984). Vet.Rec. 114, 513-518. Further studies on the subclinical carrier state of S.suis type 2 in pigs.
Clifton-Hadley, F.A. and Enright, M.R. (1984). Vet.Rec. 114, 584-586. Factors affecting the survival of S.suis type 2.
Johnston, P.L., Henry, N., Boer, R. de., Braidwood, J.C. (1991). Vet.Rec. 130, 138-139. Phenoxymethyl penicillin potassium as an in-feed medication for pigs with streptococcal meningitis.
McKellar, Q.A., Baxter, P., Taylor, D.J. and Bogan, J.A. (1987). Vet.Rec. 121. 347-350. Penicillin therapy of spontaneous streptococcal meningitis in pigs.
Mogollon, J.D., Pijoan, C., Murtaugh, M., Collins, J.E. (1990). Proc. IPVS 11, 168. Use of genetic markers in the study of the epidemiology of S.suis in a swine herd.
Sanford, S.E. (1987). Can.J.Vet.Res. 51, 481-485, 486-489. Gross and histopathological findings in universal lesions caused by S.suis in pigs I and II.
Sanford, S.E. and Tilker, A.M.E. (1982). J.Am.Vet.Med.Assn. 181, 673-676. S.suis associated diseases in swine. Observations of a 1-year study.
Walsh, B., Williams, A.E., Satsangi, J. (1992). Reviews in Med.Micro. 3, 65-71. S.suis type 2: pathogenesis and clinical disease.
Williams, D.M., Lawson, G.H.K., Rowland, A.C. (1973). Res.Vet.Sci. 15, 352-362. Streptococcal infections in piglets. The palatine tonsil as a portal of entry for S.suis.
Windsor, R.S. (1977). Vet.Rec. 101, 378-379. Meningitis in pigs caused by Streptococcus suis Type II.
Vecht, U., Wissenlink, H.J., Jellema, M.L., Smith, H.E. (1991). Inf. & Immun. 59, 3156-3162. Identification of two proteins associated with virulence of S.suis type 2.

Lancefield's Group *E streptococci* (S.porcinus, Streptococcal abscess

These cause abscesses particularly in the cervical lymph nodes of pigs in the US. The organisms have been identified in other countries but do not seen to cause the same lesions. Group E. streptococci occur in at least 8 serotypes and infection is transmitted by contact, in drinking water, by scarification or by the ingestion of food contaminated by abscess discharge or infected faeces. Infection appears to cause disease most consistently in pigs aged 28 days or more. The incidence in the US is declining due to medication of feed and the use of inactivated alum adjuvanted vaccines.

References

Miller, R.B. and Olson, L.D. (1983). Am.J.Vet.Res. 44, 937-944. Distribution of abscesses and shedder state in swine inoculated with Group E streptococci via routes other than oral.
Miller, R.B. and Olson, L.D. (1983). Am.J.Vet.Res. 44, 945-948. Frequency of jowl abscesses in feeder and market swine exposed to Group E streptococcus as nursing pigs.
Wood, R.L. and Wessman, G.E. (1984). Am.J.Vet.Res. 45, 1933-1936. Immune response of swine vaccinated with a Group E streptococcus whole culture bacterin.

Lancefield's Group C, and other ß-haemolytic streptococci.

ß-haemolytic streptococci of these groups and especially *S.equi* subsp. *equisimilis* (Group C) are commonly isolated from the upper respiratory tract, pharynx, retropharyngeal lymph nodes and genital tract of carrier pigs. They are associated with vaginitis in sows and neonatal septicaemia in newborn piglet, may be isolated from arthritis and vegetative endocarditis in older animals and may be isolated from septicaemia and pneumonic lesions in older, fattening pigs. The bacteria are best isolated in anaerobic conditions and carrier animals may be detected not only by culture but by the demonstration of serum antistreptolysin O antibody.

They may be controlled in the same way as the other streptococci if they appear to give rise to problems on a farm. *S.equi* subsp. *zooepidemicus epidemicus* has also been recorded.

Enterococcus (Streptococcus) *durans* infection

E.durans (Lancefield Gp.D) has been isolated from the intestines and faeces of 3-5 day old piglets with loose watery faeces and has been demonstrated adhering to the villous epithelium. Villous atrophy in the small intestine and epithelial shedding occur in the large intestine. The condition should be considered when faecal culture or smears demonstrate that the faecal flora is almost entirely streptococcal.

Reference

Drolet, R., Higgins, R., Jacques, M. (1990). Med.Vet.du Quebec 20, 114-115, 118. L'enteropathie associee a *Enterococcus* (Streptococcus) *durans* chez le porcelet.

Anthrax

Caused by *Bacillus anthracis* and rare in pigs. Affected animals may die suddenly, pass bloody faeces or die after swelling of the neck. Recovery may occur. Transmissible to man.

Incidence

Worldwide, rare and sporadic in UK, more common in Southern USA, tropics.

Aetiology

B.anthracis is a large Gram-positive toxin-producing encapsulated rod which grows rapidly to produce large granular medusa-head colonies on a wide variety of media. It forms spores which are resistant to boiling and which persist for long periods (>50 years) in the soil. Sensitive to penicillin and other antimicrobials and to disinfectants such as formaldehyde and glutaraldehyde which kill the spores.

Pathogenesis

Infection is by ingestion and rarely by direct entry through abrasions or by aerosol. Infection in the pig may remain localised near the portals of entry (pharyngeal region and draining lymph nodes and intestine) or become generalised to give bacteraemia and septicaemia. Organisms resist phagocytosis by means of the polyglutamic acid capsule and affect tissue by means of the 3 toxins. Organisms may be shed in urine and faeces and in discharges/blood in dead animals. Recovery and solid immunity may occur but local skin necrosis may remain.

Clinical signs

Septicaemia, pharyngeal and intestinal forms of the disease occur, most commonly as a result of entry of the organism through the tonsils or pharyngeal mucosa.

Pharyngeal form. Oedema and swelling of the neck region associated with dyspnoea and, usually, a fever of up to 42°C, 107°F are the commonest signs noted. Depression, vomiting and inappetence may occur. Death usually follows with a day of the onset of cervical oedema. Blackening and necrosis of the skin over the affected area may occur during recovery.

Septicaemic form. This form is characterised by sudden death and may occur more frequently in young pigs. It is relatively uncommon.

Intestinal form. In some cases, the infection localises in the intestine and digestive disturbance, loss of appetite and the passage of bloody faeces may be seen. Death is uncommon in this form.

A proportion of animals may develop transient fever and then recover. Severely affected animals should be killed for humane reasons where massive pharyngeal swelling leads to respiratory distress and when collapsed. Chronically affected animals with large areas of necrotic skin should also be destroyed. The disease can be treated but animals are often killed for regulatory reasons.

Post-mortem findings

If anthrax is suspected, the animal should only be opened in order to obtain material for the confirmation of diagnosis and the outbreak should be reported in the usual way. Samples of oedema fluid may be taken with a long needle. However, as the clinical signs of anthrax may be indistinct, and as the disease is an uncommon cause of sudden death in the pig, it may sometimes only be recognised at post-mortem.

Pharyngeal form. Oedema of the cervical region may be obvious when the trachea is exposed at post-mortem. Bloody or clear fluid may be present or the tissues may appear gelatinous. The mandibular and retropharyngeal lymph nodes are usually swollen and reddish in colour. Inflammatory changes of the pharyngeal mucosa may be seen.

Intestinal form. The intestinal mucosa may be covered in diptheritic membrane and the walls may be thickened with fibrinous adhesions on the serous surface and swelling of the lymph nodes. Copious peritoneal fluid and peritoneal oedema may be present. There may be splenic infarcts.

Septicaemic form. The spleen may be enlarged, but little change may be evident. The carcase is congested and the kidney may be spotted with petechiae and may be pale in colour. The lymph nodes may be engorged.

In animals killed for diagnostic purposes or at slaughter, the changes may be less obvious and petechiation of the kidney, oedematous submandibular lymph nodes or excess blood stained peritoneal fluid may be the only findings.

Epidemiology

Anthrax is relatively rare in pigs, and is normally associated with the ingestion of contaminated feed containing meat or bone meals. Outbreaks may occur where pipeline feeding is practised, as the organism may multiply in the feed. Recovered animals may remain as carriers, and pig to pig transmission may occur. The organism dies out in an unopened carcase within a few days but if allowed to sporulate (air, 22°C) persist. Spores persist in slurry, contaminated pens and on clothing and implements and can form a reservoir of infection. Other species may also be affected. Anthrax may affect and kill man. It primarily affects those cutting carcases and less frequently affects workers in contact or consumers of meat.

Diagnosis

Anthrax may be suspected in life where the pharyngeal form or the haemorrhagic diarrhoea and fever occur. When a case is examined post-mortem, the pathological features described above should suggest anthrax. In known cases the carcase should not be opened and direct smears should be made from blood, but, if negative, any swelling of the neck should be incised and the cut surface of an affected lymph node used to make an impression smear. In the peritoneal cavity, the surface of organs e.g. kidney should be used especially if perirenal oedema is present.

Smears should be heat fixed and stained with polychrome methylene blue. The square ended bacilli will be surrounded by a purple-staining capsule. At this stage the Ministry of Agriculture should be informed and any further samples will be handled by the State Veterinary Service. The isolation of the 3-5 mm greyish medusa head colonies from swabs or tissue confirms. Handling *B.arthracis* is permitted in the UK only in registered laboratories as it is a Category 3 pathogen.

Treatment

Anthrax responds to penicillin treatment and tetracyclines have been used parenterally and in feed and water.

Control

a) Technical

The disease may be controlled by vaccination of animals at risk using the Anthrax spore vaccine coupled with medication of affected animals, disinfection with formaldehyde and burning or deep burial of the carcases of affected animals. Slurry should also be disinfected and disposed of safely.

b) Legal obligations

The disease is Notifiable in the UK and in the EU and is controlled by National legislation (Anthrax Orders, 1991, UK). Restrictions of movement and a supervised disposal and disinfection programme will be carried out. This may or may not require the slaughter of the herd.

c) Commercial requirements

Modern abattoirs are unlikely to accept animals from affected farms and, with no slaughter outlet, the animals may have to be slaughtered after which whole farm disinfection can occur.

Reference

Edgington, A.B. (1990). Vet.Rec. 127, 321-324. An outbreak of anthrax in pigs : a practitioner's account.

Cystitis in sows

A group of syndromes associated with a number of different bacteria can be distinguished. One syndrome is, however, particularly striking and will be described separately.

Actinomyces (Eubacterium, Corynebacterium) suis Cystitis and Pyelonephritis

Definition

A syndrome in which a small group of sows or gilts pass bloody purulent urine, often soon after service. They rapidly lose condition and die.

Incidence

Present in all major pig-rearing countries, infection is widespread in Britain (60-90% boars and hog pigs) but outbreaks of the disease are sporadic

Aetiology

Caused by Actinomyces (formerly Eubacterium and Corynebacterium) suis, a large Gram-positive rod which occurs in pathological material in characteristic clumps and palisades. Cells bear 2 types of pili. The organism can be cultured anaerobically on blood agar on which it forms dry colonies 2-3 mm in diameter after 3 days' incubation. It can however, be grown aerobically on urea-enriched medium. It is urease positive, liquefies gelatine and ferments maltose, xylose and starch.

Pathogenesis

The organism is widespread in the prepuce of boars and is introduced to the vagina at service but dies out within an hour in most cases. It does not appear capable of colonising the intact urinary bladder of the sow and infection disappears within 3 days of experimental infection in 30% cases. The organism can be isolated from clinically normal sow urine in a small number of cases. Colonisation of the bladder is most successful and leads to disease most consistently when pre-existing lesions or infections with organisms such as E.coli are present. A.suis adheres to the bladder epithelium by means of pili and splits urea to produce ammonia.

Inflammation of the bladder wall results with loss of epithelium and colonisation by goblet cells. Infection ascends the ureters and causes a pyelonephritis, tubule damage and uraemia. Circulating antibody can be detected from 3 weeks after infection and lasts 4-9 months.

Clinical signs

In a typical outbreak, a small group of sows or gilts may die suddenly or be found ill, depressed, thirsty with hunched backs and passing blood stained, purulent urine with or without a vulval discharge. Clinical signs may be noted 2-3 weeks after service by a particular boar or may be delayed until farrowing. Affected sows frequently die. Mild cases may occur in which inappetence and vulval discharge is the only obvious sign. Animals with pyelonephritis can be identified by the presence of uraemia.

Humane slaughter should be carried out on chronically-affected animals in poor bodily condition and those which have not responded to treatment.

218

Pathology

At post-mortem examination the kidneys are haemorrhagic with pus, excess mucus and blood in the pelvices. The ureters are dilated and filled with pus. The bladder wall is grossly thickened and the mucosa is inflamed and covered with excess mucus. *A.suis* may be demonstrated in Gram-stained smears and on culture of pus from the lesions. Other bacteria may also be present.

Epidemiology

Young boars are infected from 9-10 weeks of age onwards, frequently from pen floor contamination but infection has been recorded as young as 20 days. Semen is frequently contaminated, but antimicrobials used prevent its spread by A.I. Infection frequently follows the use of a particular boar.

The organism persists on flooring and can be transmitted to clean areas on footwear. It is sensitive to most disinfectants at recommended dilutions. Predisposing factors include multiparity and low water intake.

Diagnosis

This is based on the clinical signs and the history of recent service and is confirmed by the presence of large Gram-positive bacilli in Gram-stained smears of the pus by immunofluorescence or by the isolation of *A.suis* on urea containing medium or blood agar with 50 µg/ml polymyxin or on nalidixic acid: metronidazole blood agar. Immunofluorescence and culture have similar sensitivity and specificity. Indirect immunofluorescence may be used to detect serum antibody.

Treatment and control

Affected animals may be treated parenterally with penicillin and this may be effective in the early stages. Recovered sows should be culled. In the later stages, treatment is rarely effective. Other sows served by the same boar and the boar itself should be treated parenterally with penicillin and penicillin injections after service should continue for 2-3 weeks after the outbreak has subsided. It is of advantage to wash out the preputial diverticulum with antimicrobial, but neither this practice nor parenteral or oral medication with tetracyclines or enrofloxacin eliminate the agent completely from sow or boar. Disinfection of contaminated areas and the use of clean boars on gilts may prevent further outbreaks.

References

Dagnall, G.J.R. and Jones, J.E.T. (1982). Res.Vet.Sci. 32, 389-390. A selective medium for the isolation of *C.suis*.
Larsen, J.L., Hogh, P. and Hovind Hougen, K. (1986). Acta Vet.Scand. 27, 520-530. Haemagglutinating and hydrophobic properties of *C.(E) suis*.
Ludwig, W., Kirchhof, G., Weizenegger, M., Weiss, N. (1992). Int.J.Syst.Bact. 42, 161-165. Phylogenic evidence for the transfer of *E.suis* to the genus *Actinomyces* as *A.suis* comb nov

Wendt, M., Langfeldt, N., Amstberg, G. (1990). Proc. IPVS. 11, 177. Comparison of different methods of detection of *C.suis* infection in sows and boars.

Pyelonephritis and cystitis caused by *E.coli* and other bacteria

Definition

Cystitis and pyelonephritis occurs in sows particularly when tethered as a result of ascending infection particularly when stalled or tethered and leads to loss of condition, increased frequency of urination and the presence of blood or pus in the urine. It may be fatal.

Incidence

Worldwide and in some situations may be responsible for up to 25% of sow culls.

Aetiology

A wide variety of bacteria have been isolated. 50% are *E.coli* with *Proteus* spp *Pseudomonas aeruginosa*, streptococci and staphylococci in the remaining cases.

Pathogenesis

Infection is ascending with faecal contamination of the vulva often responsible in dry sows and endometritis contributing in recently farrowed sows. Low water intake, reduced frequency of nutrition in fat sows or those with leg problems, short sow places with a solid back panel, solid floor or inadequate slats which lead to increased faecal build-up all contribute to the condition. In the last third of gestation, mild prolapse of the vagina may occur where the sow place slopes too much.

Clinical signs

An increased frequency of urination and the presence of blood and or pus in the urine are seen. There may be mucoid discharge of vesicular origin or the vulva. The appetite is depressed and the rectal temperature occasionally raised. When pyelonephritis is present temperatures may fall and blood urea rise. Death may occur. Asymptomatic infection may also occur.

Humane slaughter should be carried out when rectal temperatures fall or at blood urea levels above 15 mmoles/l and when sick animals cannot be nursed.

Pathology

Thickening and inflammation of the bladder mucosa is seen at post-mortem and both the ureters and kidneys may be involved. The bladder contains cloudy purulent urine of which may be of neutral or alkaline pH when opened.

Diagnosis

The clinical signs are sufficiently distinctive to enable a diagnosis of urinary tract infection to be reached. The only confusing condition is the presence of phosphate crystals in the urine, occasionally seen and causing no clinical signs. Crystal deposits as a white crust maybe seen on the vulva. Pus of vaginal origin may cloud the urine in recently farrowed sows.

The organism concerned can often be identified and the presence of *A.suis* should be ruled out. The use of dip slides to enumerate bacteria may be misleading as endometritis may contribute bacteria to the urine and *A.suis* may not be identified.

Treatment

Daily parenteral treatment with tetracyclines, ampicillin, enrofloxacin, other broad-spectrum antimicrobials and with streptomycin may all be of value. Affected sows should be encouraged to drink by placing meal on water in front of them or ion replacers in the water which should be presented in a trough.

Prevention

The stalls should be cleaned of faeces and water intake encouraged by increasing the salt concentration of the ration to 1% in the presence of water *ad libidum*. The design of sow places should be considered in relation to the size of the animal and sows should be maintained in fair but not fat condition. Sows should be encouraged to rise by feeding twice daily and ensuring that drinkers are in good working order and delivering water at the correct pressure. AI should be considered, and service and farrowing hygiene improved.

References

Carr, J., Walton, J.R. (1993). Vet.Rec. 132, 575-577. Bacterial flora of the urinary tract of pigs.

Carr, J., Walton, J.R. (1991). Pig Vet.J. 27, 122-141. Cystitis and pyelonephritis in pigs.

Madec, F. (1984). Pig News and Information 5, 89-93. Urinary disorders in intensive pig herds.

Smith, W.J. (1983). Pig News and Information 4, 279-281. Cystitis in sows.

Miscellaneous bacteria

Aeromonas hydrophila

A.hydrophila has been isolated from cases of enteritis and from lymph nodes. It appears to be associated with an enterotoxin-type watery diarrhoea, especially in young or recently-weaned pigs. Isolates from pig faeces contain virulence factors and *A.caviae* and *A.sobria* are also present

Acinetobacter calcoaceticans

Recovered in profuse culture from some cases of rhinitis in piglets and from the trachea in tracheitis.

221

Actinomyces pyogenes

A.pyogenes is a small Gram-positive coccobacillus which produces an exotoxin and proteolytic enzymes. It is found, with other bacteria, such as *Bacteroides* spp. in abscesses in many parts of the carcase, particularly following foot damage and tail biting. It is chiefly responsible for the abscesses found in the vertebral bodies which collapse and cause the paralysis in spinal abscesses.

It complicates chronic pneumonic lesions and is found in vaginal discharge, metritis and abortion. Invasion of the foetus does not appear to occur, but it can enter via the umbilicus to cause umbilical abscess in 7-10 day old pigs.

A.pyogenes attaches to eggs and may destroy them. *A.pyogenes* may be found in enlarged, caseous head lymph nodes.

A.pyogenes can be demonstrated in Gram-stained smears or isolated as 1mm ß-haemolytic colonies after 48 hours' incubation on horse blood agar. Other species are currently being identified from the reproductive tract (currently and incorrectly called "*A.suis*") but their significance is not yet certain.

Antibody may be detected by indirect ELISA to the 25 kDa protease of *A.pyogenes*. Penicillin or tetracycline may be used to treat infections. Severe abscessation may not respond readily to treatment.

Reference

Hommez, J., Devriese, L.A., Miry, C., Castryck, F. (1991). J.Vet.Med. Series B 38, 575-580. Characterisation of 2 groups of Actinomyces-like bacteria isolated from purulent lesions in pigs.

Bacteroides and diarrhoea

Bacteroides fragilis is a strictly anaerobic Gram-negative rod found in the large intestine. Enterotoxigenic strains have been isolated from diarrhoea in piglets both before and after weaning and have been shown to cause diarrhoea when fed to pigs.

Other species such as *B.vulgatus and Bacteroides, now Prevotella melaninogenicus* have been found in enteritis.

Experimental disease in piglets occurs 2-3 days after inoculation as a watery diarrhoea which lasts 4-6 days and is accompanied by anorexia and dehydration. Natural disease in weaned pigs can only be distinguished bacteriologically but lasts 3-6 days, presenting as a soft faeces and diarrhoea accompanied by loss of condition. Pathological findings in piglets include epithelial cell swelling and vacuolation, crypt hyperplasia in the distal small intestine and large intestine and an exfoliative colitis and occur, with *B.fragilis* in abscesses, pleurisy and consolidated pneumonic lesions. Treatment with nitroimidazoles is usually effective as they penetrate the pus

Reference

Duimstra, J.R., Myers, L.L., Collins, W.C. (1991). Vet.Path. 28, 514-518. Enterovirulence of enterotoxigenic *B.fragilis* in gnotobiotic pigs.

Chlamydial infection

Definition

Chlamydial infection is associated with pneumonia, pleurisy, pericarditis, polyarthritis, infertility or the birth of weak piglets. It has been demonstrated in enteritis and conjunctivitis.

Incidence

Rarely isolated but it is widespread in birds and occurs in many mammalian species. Antibody may be widespread (23% slaughter pigs 1966 UK), 46.7% diarrhoeic faeces samples and 72.7% pneumonic lung samples were positive in West Germany. The infection is rarely diagnosed or considered in the UK, the US and many other countries, but if Central European figures and UK serology are guides, infection is widespread.

Aetiology

Most publications refer to *C.psittaci* as the cause of chlamydial infections in pigs, but studies with newly available gene sequences and immunoperoxidase reagents have demonstrated that *C.trachomatis* or variants of it are present in keratoconjunctivitis and enteritis in pigs.

Pathogenesis

Experimental infection of the respiratory tract results in an acute exudative or interstitial pneumonia within 4-8 days of infection. Raised pale red lesions are present in the diaphragmatic lobes and become paler with age. An arthritis may occur at the same time. Venereal infection can lead to persistent infection in sows and orchitis with semen infection in boars. Stillborn piglets and vaginal discharge have also been associated with infection. Chlamydial infection of the intestine may complicate and exacerbate other enteric diseases. Infection has been associated with PRRS in the UK.

Clinical signs

Mucopurulent keratoconjunctivitis in piglets and sows has been recorded. Reproductive disturbances such as an increase in premature farrowings, and abortions, pigs born dead and a rise in piglet mortality to weaning have all been recorded. Weak piglets may have diarrhoea. Respiratory distress in weaned pigs and an increase in coughing have been recorded.

Animals with severe respiratory distress or arthritis may require humane destruction.

Pathology

Lesions from which chlamydia may be isolated include pericarditis, pleurisy, enlarged spleens, synovitis, orchitis and dead foetuses and mummified piglets. The most recognisable lesions are probably those in the lung. These occur largely in the posterior lobes as pale red raised areas of consolidation extending deep into the lung. Enzootic pneumonia-like lesions may be produced in the anterior lobes. Oedema, a suppurative necrotising alveolitis and bronchiolitis have been described with penbronchiolar accumulations of plasma cells, lymphocytes and macrophages. In the gut there may be a pseudomembranous colitis.

C.psittaci may be demonstrated as clumps of red dots in Kosters-stained smears, isolated in McCoy cells or demonstrated by immunofluorescence or immunoperoxidase.

C.psittaci is a Category 3 pathogen and isolation should only be attempted in a registered laboratory.

Epidemiology

Pigs of all ages may be infected and antibody is widespread in affected herds. Infection can be by aerosol, contact, ingestion or by the venereal route as the agent can be demonstrated in semen. Outside the host the agent is relatively resistant to drying and may survive months in that state. Birds, and to a lesser extent, other mammals, may represent sources of infection.

C.psittaci and *C.trachomatis* infect man and pig strains appear to be the cause of chlamydeal antibody in pig keepers.

Diagnosis

The clinical signs of reproductive failure, conjunctivitis and raised respiratory rate may suggest the condition. Isolation of the agent from, or its demonstration in the lesions will confirm. Serum antibody would confirm infection if rising titres occurred.

Treatment

Tetracyclines are the drugs of choice and should be given by the route most appropriate to the age of pig affected. The organism is not eliminated by treatment.

Disinfection and the exclusion of wild birds and rodents may help reduce contamination of the environment.

References

Harris, J.W., Hunter, A.R. and Martin, D.A. (1984). Comp.Immun.Microbiol.Inf.Dis. 7, 19-26. Experimental Chlamydial pneumonia in pigs.
Popischil, A., Wood, R.L. (1987). 24, 568-570. Interstinal Chlamydia in pigs.
Rogers, W.G., Andersen, A.A., Hogg, A., Nielson, D.L., Huebert, M.A. (1993). J.Am.Vet.Med.Ass. 203, 1321-1323. Conjunctivitis and keratoconjunctivitis associated with Chlamydia in swine.
Wilson, M.R. and Plummer, P.A. (1966). J.Comp.Path. 76, 427-433. A survey of pig sera for the presence of antibody to the PLV group of organisms.
Woollen, N., Daniels, E.K., Yeary, T., Leipold, H.W., Phillips, R.M. (1990). J.Am.Vet.Med.Ass. 197, 600-603. Chlamydial infection and perinatal infection in a swine herd.

Corynebacterium pseudotuberculosis

Recovered from the vaginas of healthy sows (Japan).

Coxiella burneti

Antibody has been demonstrated in pigs but no clinical signs have yet been reported. It is a zoonosis and may be fatal in man (Q fever).

Dermatophilus spp.

Dermatophilus spp. have been demonstrated in tonsillar material and found in lesions of exudative epidermitis. They are filamentous Gram-positive organisms which break up into coccal bodies and may be seen in Gram-stained smears or isolated on blood agar plates containing polymyxin B as haemolytic colonies after 48 hours' incubation. If suspected, penicillin treatment is of value.

Klebsiella

Klebsiella spp. are present in chronic respiratory tract disease, especially rhinitis, in enteritis and cause mastitis (*K.aerogenes*). Treat as *E.coli.* Often present in sawdust (*K.aerogenes*). Distinguished from *E.coli* by biochemical tests.

Legionella

Antibody to *L.pneumophila* has been demonstrated in the sera of pneumonic pigs in the UK and pneumonia and antibody have been recorded in China.

Melioidosis (*Burkholdaria* formerly *Pseudomonas pseudomallei*

B.pseudomallei is a cause of melioidosis in pigs in tropical and subtropical regions. Infection may be asymptomatic or result in fever, unsteady gait, weakness, nasal discharge and subcutaneous swelling of the limbs. Abscesses occur in lungs, bronchial lymph nodes, spleen and elsewhere in the carcase. The organism may be isolated from lesions in acute cases. Antibody may be detected by CFT and IHA tests. Infection may result from contaminated water or from consumption of infected swill. Tetracyclines or ampicillin may be of value in treatment and chlorination of water supplies may prevent. A zoonosis. Category 3 pathogen only to be handled in secure accommodation.

References

Ketterer, P.J. (1986). Aust.Vet.J. 63, 146-149. Melioidosis in intensive piggeries in South Eastern Queensland.
Webster, W.R., Shield, J., Arthur, R.J., Blackall, P.J, Thomas, A.D., Spinks, G.A., D'Arcy, T.L., Hoffman, D. (1990). J.Clin.Micro. 28, 1874-1875. Evaluation of a modified complement fixation test and an indirect haemagglutination test for the sero diagnosis of melioidosis in pigs.

Pseudomonas spp

Pseudomonas aeruginosa is often isolated from mastitis, vaginitis, cystitis, chronic pneumonia, enteritis and chronic skin disease such as complicated exudative epidermitis. Its presence cannot be recognised clinically but it should be suspected when chronic lesions fail to respond to antimicrobials. Its presence may be confirmed by isolation on a number of media on which it can be identified as 3-5 mm colonies with a characteristic smell and green pigment. It is resistant to many disinfectants and antimicrobials but is relatively sensitive to chlorine and to gentamycin, polymyxin, enrofloxacin and, sometimes, to streptomycin and chloramphenicol. Other pseudomonads may be isolated from the nasal passages and respiratory tract in chronic respiratory disease.

Rhodococcus equi

Present in submandibular nodes with granulomatous lesions. Experimental infections with the organism resulted in severe consolidation and pneumonia of the anteroventral lobes at 7-10 days p.i. which gradually resolved. *R.sputi* has been isolated from mesenteric lymph nodes in Japan.

Reference

Zuik, M.C. and Yager, J.~A. (1987). Can.J.Vet.Res. 51, 290-296. Experimental infection of piglets by aerosols of *Rhodococcus equi*.

FUNGAL CONDITIONS

Ringworm

Definition

Ringworm or dermatomycosis is uncommon in the pig and often causes little effect on productivity but is a source of infection for man.

Incidence

Sporadic worldwide but some species e.g. *Microsporum nanum* do not occur in Britain.

Aetiology and pathogenesis.

Microsporum nanum is involved in other countries such as Australia. Most infections in the UK. are caused by *Trichophyton mentagrophytes* but *T.verrucosum*, *M.gypseum* and *M.canis* may also occur. Infection may occur in piglets but only become apparent later.

Clinical signs

T.mentagrophytes infections present as circular areas of brown discolouration on the back or behind the ears. The lesions enlarge gradually and may be greasy in texture. There may be little or no alopecia, skin thickening or inflammation but hairs plucked from the lesion may appear reddish brown or orange along most of their length. The lesions are often seen in weaners and older pigs but may be detected in piglets from affected farms by close inspection.

M.nanum infections often occur behind the ear as expanding rings or circles of reddish or light brown scabs which may be raised above the surrounding skin but are not common on the belly. As in *T.mentagrophytes* infections there is little alopecia or irritation.

Humane slaughter is unnecessary.

Epidemiology

Infected weaner producers may spread infection to fattening farms. Infection may be transferred from pig to pig or from pig to man. Infection in the form of resistant spores may remain for months on wooden or other pen fittings. Rats and other species may also carry the infection and be a source of it for pigs. Cattle are the commonest source of *T.verrucosum*.

Diagnosis

The clinical signs are extremely suggestive. The presence of fungus in hairs plucked from the lesion may be confirmed by microscopic examination and scrapings and hairs may be cultured and the organism responsible identified. Common conditions with which ringworm may be confused include pityriasis rosea in which expanding rings of reddish-brown dermatitis are found usually on the skin of the belly and thighs of young pigs. Swine pox lesions on the skin of the belly may also resemble ringworm lesions in their early stages. Exudative epidermitis lesions in older pigs must also be distinguished.

Treatment

If found, topical treatment with enilconazole, sodium benzuldazate, undecylinic acid preparations, copper salts, or natamycin may be adequate. Topical treatments may be ineffective unless greasy lesions are cleaned first with a disinfectant such as cetrimide, or better still, hexetidine. Systemic treatment with griseofulvin will certainly be effective at 10 mg/kg griseofulvin daily for 7 days. Disinfection of buildings with formaldehyde, hypochlorite or detergents should be carried out. Steam and phenolic disinfectants have also been used. If rats are suspected of introducing infection, they should be controlled.

Reference

Wilkinson, J.D. (1985). Proc.Pig Vet.Soc. 12, 103-107. Ringworm in pigs.

Yeast infections

Infections with *Candida albicans* occur in chronic gastroenteritis in piglets 5-14 days of age and are often secondary. Piglets may be dull, may vomit and have a chronic diarrhoea which has failed to respond to antimicrobial treatment. Some may die. 2-5 mm circular whitish lesions may be seen on the tongue and hard palate. A chronic enteritis may be seen and yeasts may be demonstrated in histological sections and by culture. In cutaneous candidiasis, a moist grey exudate may appear on the surface of the skin of the abdomen and legs with eventual skin thickening and hair loss. Cleaning of skin with detergent or hexetidine-based shampoos may remove the lesions. Nystatin, miconazole and amphotericin B may be used to reduce clinical signs. Other yeasts may be involved. The skin yeast *Malassezia pachydermatis* (*Pityrosporum canis*) has been recorded from pig skin.

Other systemic mycoses

Mucormycosis may occur in piglets and be a cause of chronic enteritis and gastritis in piglets and Cryptococcus infections may cause pneumonia in areas where the organism is present (Not UK. Zygomycetes infections have been identified in the USA in antibiotic unresponsive diarrhoeas in piglets aged 10-28 days. Catarrhal to fibronecrotic gastroenteritis with histological evidence of the invading fungi was recorded.

Reference

Reed, W.M., Hanika, C., Mehdi, N.A.Q. and Shackelford, C. (1987). Am.Vet.Med.Asoc. 191, 549-550. Gastrointestinal zygomycosis in sucking pigs.

Mycotoxicoses
Mycotoxicosis of pigs occurs as a result of fungal growth on damp feed or the inclusion of affected grain etc. in the ration. A number of moulds have been incriminated but the following toxins produce the most clearly defined syndromes.

Zearalenone Poisoning (*Vulvo vaginitis* in sows)

Definition

The ingestion by sows in late pregnancy of zearalenone (Fusarium F2 toxin) present in spoiled barley in feed may result in the birth of small litters, stillborn and weak, splay-legged piglets. Vulval enlargement may occur in the sow and other female stock on the same ration. The subsequent breeding behaviour of such females may be affected.

Aetiology

Barley or other grains harvested or stored under moist conditions or treated with propionic acid may be contaminated with fungi of the genus Fusarium (e.g. *F.culmorum, F.graminearum*). These produce a number of toxins including the oestrogenic toxin zearalenone and deoxynivalenol (vomitoxin).

Pathogenesis

Zearalenone is absorbed from the ration where some may be in the form of zearalenone glycosides and is detectable in the plasma for 5 days after last administration either as zearalenone or as α-zearalenol. It is excreted in the urine for up to 5 days after last administration bound to glucuronic acids and is passed out in faeces where bacteria may break it down. It has an effect on reproductive functions, may reduce the activity of 3 α-hydroxysteroid dehydrogenase and depress plasma LH levels. Experimental studies have shown effects on non-pregnant gilts, on embryonic mortality after service and on sows in the last two weeks of pregnancy. Effects appear to depend upon levels of pure compound. They are summarised below.

Age	Threshold level of Zearalenone	Effect
Prepubertal gilts gilts >3 weeks old	1-3 ppm 3-5 ppm	Mammary enlargement, vulval swelling, ovarian and uterine swelling and uterine oedema
cycling gilts	3-5 ppm	Enlargement and oedema of uterus, retention of corpora lutea, anoestrus for up to 50 days. Lengthening of cycles. Spontaneous return to oestrus 45 days after removal of zearalenone.
Sows 2-15d. post service	5-30 ppm 60 ppm+	No effect on embryos. Complete embryonic failure
Mid-term	3-5 ppm	Some reduction in weight of uterus and foetuses
14 days prior to farrowing	3-5 ppm	Birth of weak and splay-legged piglets, vulval enlargement in piglets.
Lactating sows	3-5 ppm	Weaning: Service interval extended.

| Boars | 3-5 ppm | No effect on semen quality or slight rise in abnormal sperm. |

Clinical signs

Enlargement of the vulva with eventual prolapse and some development of oedema around the teats may be seen in gilts and sows within 14 days of changing to contaminated feed. In addition to vulval swelling, small litters may be produced and conception rate may be reduced with extension of weaning to service intervals. Sows in the last third of gestation may come into milk early and may give birth to substandard litters composed of fresh, stillborn piglets and a mixture of weak and splay-legged piglets. The weak or splay-legged piglets grow weaker as the toxin is secreted in the milk and they may die of starvation. Any survivors may be normal by 10-14 days of age. In some accounts, rectal swelling and oedema of the prepuce have been described in males. Spermatogenesis has been said to be affected but this effect appears not to be permanent. In females an increase in returns to service and other reproductive changes has been reported. The weaning to service interval is extended, but puberty in the gilt and subsequent fertility does not appear to be affected provided that zearalenone is withdrawn 14 days before service. There is no effect on growth rate.

Splay legged or weak or wasting piglets may be destroyed humanely as may animals with irreparable vulval damage after prolapse.

Pathology

Affected females may have enlarged vulvas, sometimes with prolapse and there may be mammary enlargement most obvious at slaughter. The uterus is heavy and may be turgid and in served gilts or sows corpora lutea of pregnancy may be present with degenerating blastocysts from 14-35 days post-service.

Diagnosis

The presence of vulval enlargement and oedema of mammary tissue and the presence of mouldy grain in the ration indicate that an outbreak of stillbirths and splay leg may be caused by this toxin. The absence of virus antibody and the demonstration of toxin in the feed, milk, plasma or faeces (by feeding trials in 8-10 week gilts, thin layer chromatographic analysis, direct competitive ELISA or by cell culture assay) would confirm.

Treatment

The vulval enlargement and the piglet mortality soon disappear if a normal, clean ration is fed. All clinical signs have normally disappeared 3-4 weeks after mouldy feed is discontinued. Recent studies have shown that antibody to zearalenone can be produced and vaccination can increase the rate of zearalenone excretion. None of the feed treatments appear to inactivate the toxin in feed. Safe levels of presence of zearalenone may be as low as 10 ppb but are generally regarded as much higher (see table).

230

References

Diekman, M.A., Long, G.G. (1989). Am.J.Vet.Res. 50, 1224-1227. Blastocyst development on days 10 or 14 after consumption of zearalenone on days 7-10 after breeding.
Edwards, S., Cantley, T.C., Rottinghaus, G.E., Osweiler, G.D., Day, B.N. (1987). Theriogenology, 28, 43-49. The effect of zearalenone on reproduction in Swine I.
Edwards, S., Cantley, T.C., Day, B.N. (1987). Theriogenology 28, 51-58. The effects of zearalenone on reproduction in swine II.
Etienne, M, Jemmali, M. (1982). J.Anim.Sci. 55, 1-10. Effects of zearalenone (F-2) on oestrus activity and reproduction in gilts.
Miller, J.K., Hacking, A., Gross, V.J. (1973). Vet.Rec. 93, 555-559. Stillbirths neonatal mortality and small litters in pigs associated with the ingestion of fusarium toxin in pregnant sows.
Pestka, J.J., Liu, M.T., Knudson, B.K., Hogberg, M.G. (1985). J.Food Protection 48, 953-957. Immunisation of pigs for production of antibody against zearalenone.

Vomitoxin

Ingestion of vomitoxin results is vomiting, feed refusal and growth depression. Vomitoxin (deoxynivalenol) may also be present in zearalenone-contaminated feeds and is a 12, 13 epoxytrichothecene. It has been recorded in feeds at concentrations of 0.1-42 ppm but levels rarely exceed 3-10 ppm. Up to 65% of deoxynivalenol present in the pig diet may be absorbed. At 1-2 ppm food refusal can occur initially although animals may become accustomed to it and growth become almost normal. At higher levels 12-20 ppm, vomitng occurs within 5-15 minutes and complete feed refusal follows. Growth depression is the major clinical finding and there are no effects on reproductive behaviour not attributable to reduced feed intake. Vomitoxin is rapidly absorbed, rapidly distributed to all tissues and rapidly excreted unchanged so that plasma is negative within 12-24 hours of withdrawal. It is excreted at very low levels in the milk. Residues may occur in kidneys for up to 3 weeks after withdrawal. Inactivation of deoxynivalenol by heating with aqueous sodium metabisulphite has been described.

References

Young, L.G., McGirr, L., Valli, V.E., Lumsden, J.H. and Lun, A.(1983). J.Anim.Sci. 57, 655-664. Vomitoxin in corn fed to young pigs.
Young, J.C. Trenholm, H.L., Friend, D.W., Prelusky, D.B. (1987). Agricultural & Food Chemistry 35, 259-261. Inactivation with sodium metabisulphite.
Veno, Y., Ed. Trichothecenes, chemical, biological and toxicological aspects. Elsevier (1983).

Aflatoxicosis

Definition

A syndrome in which reduced growth, weight loss and inappetence, jaundice and death results from liver damage caused by the ingestion of feed contaminated with *Aspergillus flavus* aflatoxin.

Incidence

Rarely diagnosed in the UK where import restrictions are placed on aflatoxin levels in feeds (Aflatoxin Orders)but more common in countries where maize and groundnut meal are common ingredients of the diet.

Aetiology and pathogenesis

Aspergillus flavus or *Aspergillus parasiticus* may contaminate feed components such as groundnut meal and the aflatoxin produced may be present at levels of 360-3422 ppb Aflatoxin B1 when clinical signs occur. Such levels produce liver damage such as fatty change, lobular necrosis with an increase in basophilic cells at the periphery of the lobule, bile duct proliferation and, in chronic cases, cirrhosis. The hepatocytes may be variable in size with increased staining of the nuclei. Death may occur in a few days following ingestion of more than 0.2 mg aflatoxin Bl per kg. The L.D.50 is 0.6 mg/kg and levels of 0.4 mg/kg almost always produce clinical signs. 0.1 mg/kg (100 ppb in feed) has been reported to be a 'no effect' level with a safe level of 0.05 mg/kg.

Aflatoxin is excreted in urine as B1, B2, M and G forms. There may be immunosuppression.

Clinical signs

These may appear within 6 weeks of a change to the contaminated ration and consist of depressed growth rate, inappetence, arched back and apathy. Jaundice, ataxia and convulsions may occur before death. Sows may lose their milk or abort. Mange and other diseases may be more common.

Humane slaughter is commonly required in field outbreaks and severely jaundiced or stunted animals should be destroyed.

Pathological findings

Jaundice of the carcase is prominent and the liver may be white, tan, or bright orange in colour. There may be oedema of the wall of the gall bladder in acute cases and the whole liver is friable with much blood in the sinusoids. The blood fails to clot and serous or bloody effusions may be present in the thoracic and abdominal cavities. In addition, bleeding into a number of other organs may occur and petechiae and ecchymoses may be present on serous or mucous surfaces. Liver changes including centrilobular necrosis, bile duct proliferation and fatty change may be seen, followed later by regeneration.

Epidemiology

Associated with groundnut meal or maize which has been spoiled in cobs in drought years or stored in moist conditions.

Diagnosis

A history of introduction to a particular feed or batch of feed is of value. It may be possible to confirm that aflatoxin is present in samples of the feed. The clinical signs, post-mortem and histological findings may suggest a diagnosis of aflatoxicosis. Levels of liver enzymes such as alkaline phosphatase serum aspirate transferase and serum glutamyl oxaloacetic transaminase may be raised. Creatine kinase levels are depressed. Aflatoxin levels should be measured in the feed where possible using ELISA, thin layer chromatography HPLC or cell culture toxicity methods.

Similar conditions include warfarin poisoning which is not accompanied by growth depression, phenol-type poisoning, leptospirosis and acute copper toxicity.

Treatment

None. Remove suspect ration. Feed a high protein, aflatoxin-free ration. Most ration components are screened for aflatoxicosis now and the importation of contaminated feed is now prohibited in the UK. Hydrated sodium calcium aluminium silicate added to feed can reduce the adverse effects and folic acid and lysine may also have an effect. None prevent absorption and growth depression entirely.

Reference

Cook, W.O., Alstine, W.G. van., Osweiler, G.D. (1989). J.Am.Vet.Med.Ass. 194, 554-558. Aflatoxicosis in Iowa swine: Eight cases (1983-1985).
Harvey, R.B., Huff, W.E., Kubena, L.F., Corrier, D.E., Phillips, T.D. (1988). Am.J.Vet.Res. 49, 482-487. Progression of aflatoxicosis in growing barrows.

Ergot Poisoning

Ergot (*Claviceps purpurea*) on grain or on pasture may be an uncommon cause of agalactia and the birth of small, weak, shortlived or dead piglets. There may be no enlargement of the teats and udder at parturition and repeat oestrus may occur in affected sows and gilts. On rare occasions, the gangrenous form may appear, and extremities such as the ears may become dry or gangrenous. In most cases, little or no abnormality may be seen in growing pigs other than some growth depression. Up to 2g ergot/kg may be fed without effect.

The agalactia does not respond to oxytocin treatment and the gangrenous lesions must be differentiated from those of swine fever, salmonellosis and erysipelothrix infection. Removal of the source of ergot in the feed leads to the resumption of milk flow within 48 hours in affected sows.

Humane slaughter may be indicated when gangrene has developed or if piglets cannot be nursed successfully.

Mycotoxic nephropathy (Ochratoxicosis)

Definition

A syndrome in which decreased rate of daily liveweight gain, tubular degeneration and interstitial fibrosis of the kidney result from the ingestion of mouldy rations containing Ochratoxin A and other mycotoxins. The lesions are normally only seen at slaughter but an acute syndrome, perirenal oedema, may occur in recently weaned pigs.

Incidence

First seen in Denmark in the kidneys of slaughter pigs, Ochratoxin A and the changes in pig kidney have now been identified in many countries including the U.K., Eire, U.S.A., Australia, Canada, Poland, Germany and Hungary. In 1000 sows surveyed in the U.K. in 1984 20% had demonstrable ochratoxin A but only one had levels above 24 ug/kg.

Aetiology and pathogenesis

Ochratoxin A, citrinin and oxalic acid are produced by *Penicillium viridicatum* in mouldy rye and barley and by fungi like *Aspergillus ochraceous* in maize. The levels necessary to cause disease differ betwen pure compound and levels in natural feed . In the latter levels of 200 ppb appear to cause disease but levels of 4000-7000 ppb have been reported. At 200 ppb or more clinical signs may appear within 3 weeks. Decreased glomerular filtration rate and impaired proximal tubular function result from the administration of Ochratoxin A. Urinary glucose and protein levels of the urine rise and the concentrating power of the kidney is lost. Ochratoxin is immunosuppressive.

Clinical signs

Few, other than reduction appetite and in the rate of daily liveweight gain, polydypsia and polyuria in fattening and adult pigs. In recently weaned pigs, subcutaneous oedema, ataxia, stiff arched back and distention of the lumbar part of the abdominal wall may be seen followed by death in 1 or 2 days. Mortality may reach 40-90% of affected batches. A possible decline in semen quality has been reported. Ataxic pigs should be slaughtered humanely. .

Pathology

In the chronic form, the kidneys are enlarged and pale with an uneven surface. There is degeneration of the proximal tubular epithelium and interstital fibrosis. Glomeruli may be hyalinised. The acute form is less clearly associated with ochratoxin as perirenal oedema and changes such as those described for the chronic form can result from poisoning by weeds in the U.S. Meat from affected pigs contains ochratoxin.

Epidemiology

Has been identified in Eire following feeding with wet-stored barley. In Denmark where the incidence is recorded, the rate per 100,000 seems to vary with the year, and clear associations between wet years, late harvests and organically grown grains and high feed levels have been found. Ochratoxin A is present in a wide range of pig-derived foods such as sausage, black pudding and liver products.

Diagnosis

The clinical signs of increased thirst and polyuria may suggest ochratoxicosis and the finding of enlarged pale kidneys may also suggest the presence of the condition. Reduced levels of renal phosphoenol pyruvate carboxykinase (70-80% reduction) and a similar reduction in gamma glutamyl transpeptidase have been shown to occur and can be used for diagnosis.
Confirmation is by the demonstration of Ochratoxin A in feed, plasma or tissues using ELISA or High Pressure Liquid Chromatography (HPLC) assays.

Levels in feed >200 ppb lead to growth depression and mild renal lesions. Those >1,000 ppb may lead to polydipsia and >4,000 ppb to full clinical disease. Levels in tissue vary and even in grossly affected kidneys may not be high. Levels of >2 ng/ml blood indicate potential ochratoxicosis in a herd and levels in excess of 45 ng/ml have been recorded. Levels up to 98 ppb in liver and to 89 ppb in kidney have been recorded. Safe levels for human consumption are considered to be <25 ppb (Denmark).

Treatment and control

Ochratoxin is cleared from the body within 3-4 weeks if contaminated feed is withdrawn. Supportive therapy can be given. Bin hygiene helps prevention but none of the feed treatments save 10% activated charcoal appears to reduce effective feed levels.

References

Holmberg, T., Breitholtz-Emanuelsson, A., Haggblom, P., Schwan, O, Hult, K. (1991). Mycopathologia 116, 169-176. *Penicillum verrucosum* in feed of Ochratoxin A positive swine herds.
Madsen. A. (1980) Pig News and Information 1, 335. Ochratoxin A - a mycotoxin in feeds and pigs.
Madsen, A., Mortensen, H.P., Hald,B. (1982) . Acta.Ag.Scand. 32, 225-239. Feeding experiments with Ochratoxin A contaminated barley for bacon pigs. I. Influence on pig performance and residues.

Fumonisin toxicity (Porcine pulmonary Oedema Syndrome

Fumonisin causes reduction of feed consumption, mild respiratory distress and death from pulmonary oedema at high levels.

Fumonisin is produced by *Fusarium moniliforme* growing on maize and acts to inhibit sphingosine and sphinganine N-acetyl transferase. At low levels <23 ppm in feed, liver damage develops and at higher levels of >175 ppm in feed, acute pulmonary oedema develops followed by death.

Fumonisin is excreted in urine (21%), and faeces (58%) of feed but enterohepatic circulation takes place. Excretion is virtually complete 3 days after withdrawal of contaminated feel.

Clinical signs begin about 5 days after the first ingestion of feed with a rapid decrease in feed intake. At low levels of fumonisin intake, the only clinical signs may be those of a progressive hepatic disease. At higher levels the reduction in feed intake is followed by mild respiratory distress, pulmonary oedema and death. Humane slaughter should be carried out when pulmonary oedema is first noted.

The major pathological findings are the presence of severe oedema of the lung and pleural effusions. The lungs are heavier than normal and hepatic changes are always present. Membranous material is present in the hepatic sinusoids, and there are multilamellar bodies in hepatocytes, Kupffer cells, pancreatic acinar cells and pulmonary macrophages.

Diagnosis is based on the clinical signs, the rise in liver enzymes and the tissue and serum sphinganine : sphingosine ratio. The gross and microscopic pathological findings support the diagnosis but confirmation depends upon the demonstration of fumonisin by HPLC in feed or in tissue.

There is no treatment and control depends upon screening feeds and the dilution of fumonisin-containing feed to safe levels.

235

References

Haschek, W.M., Motein, G., Ness, D.K., Harbin, K.S., Hall, W.F., Vesonder, R.F., Peterson, R.E., Beasley, V.R. (1992). Mycopathologia <u>117</u>, 83-96. Characterisation of fumonisin toxicity in orally and intravenously dosed swine.
Riley, R.T. and 10 others (1993). Toxicological and Applied Pharmacology <u>118</u>, 105-112. Alteration of tissue and serum sphinganine to sphingosine ratio: an early biomarker of exposure to fumonisin-containing feeds in pigs.

Mycotoxin control

1. Mycotoxin-free feed can be used to dilute contaminated feed down to the no effect levels.

2. High protein, activated charcoal, and high (2.5 ppm) selenium have been reported to protect.

3. Ammonia and sodium hydroxide treatments of feed have been described but have little effect in practice.

4. Prevention using mould inhibitors should be considered where mould damage may occur after harvesting. Calcium propionate, sorbic acid and propionic acid may all be used.

5. Routine bin hygiene.

PARASITIC DISEASE

Parasitic disease in the pig is caused by 3 main groups of organism: the helminth parasites (nematode worms and cestodes especially tapeworms or flukes); the protozoa, primarily coccidia but also including flagellates and trypanosomes and the arthropod ectoparasites. Only a few of the parasitic diseases of pigs are considered here. They are those important in large scale pig rearing and particularly those which occur in housed pigs. Porcine parasites may cause syndromes which are recognisable clinically or pathologically, but most require laboratory examinations such as microscopy to confirm the presence and identity of the agent concerned. Isolation and culture of the agent is rare. Parasitic infections are generally resistant to antimicrobials and this may be of value when an unknown syndrome develops.

1. ENDOPARASITES

Helminthiasis in the pig seldom appears as clinical disease in Britain where the majority of animals are kept on concrete for much of their lives. It is a potential problem in pigs housed outdoors and the current importance of extensive systems in the UK makes it more important. Its importance is chiefly economic with subclinical infections delaying the achievement of marketing weight and being responsible for poor food conversion rates.

Reference

Hale, O.M., Stewart, T.B. and Marti, O.G. (1986). Pig News and Information 7, 439-441. Endoparasite effects on performance of pigs.

Hyostrongylosis

Definition

Primarily a disease of sows and hardly ever found in growing pigs. It is characterised by anaemia, inappetence, and loss of weight and may contribute to the 'thin sow syndrome'.

Incidence

28% of sows were found to be infected in a recent survey but less than 1% of growing pigs.

Aetiology and life cycle

Hyostrongylus rubidus occurs in the stomach. The adults are less than 1 cm long, slender and reddish, and are found closely applied to the gastric mucosa. The eggs are thin shelled and typical of strongyles. They develop on the ground into infective L3 larvae in about 7 days. The remaining (parasitic) moults occur in the gastric glands following ingestion of the third-stage larva. The prepatent period is about 15 days to the first egg production with highest levels reached at 22 days post-infection.

Pathogenesis

The pathogenesis depends upon invasion of the gastric glands with resulting loss of parietal cell function. Macroscopically the mucosa has a cobble-stone or morocco leather appearance and a diptheritic membrane may form in heavy infections, with detachment of the mucosa and ulceration. Protein leakage from the gastric lesions and increases in plasma pepsinogen both occur.

Inhibition of larvae in the mucosa is a common phenomenon in this infection, and development of the inhibited stages with effects on the gastric mucosa occurs after farrowing. This resumption of development appears to have a hormonal basis, and to be related to lactation. It may also occur after therapy with an anthelmintic not effective against inhibited larvae.

Clinical signs

The clinical disease is seen predominantly in the lactating sow where marked weight loss is observed despite adequate feeding: this weight loss continues after the litter is weaned. In typical cases the sow is thin, shows pallor of visible mucous membranes and skin and, although diarrhoea is not present, the faeces may be intermittently dark. In chronic cases affected animals become dull, lethargic and may have a depraved appetite.

Experimental studies with moderate infections suggest that growth in weaners may be depressed by 8% compared with controls and that crude protein is less well utilised, that faecal nitrogen is greater and that a worse nitrogen balance occurs than in uninfected animals.

Infertility manifested by reduced fecundity and irregular returns to oestrus, especially after farrowing, have been reported in sows with high Hyostrongylus egg counts. Birth weights may be reduced by 15% and survival and weaning weights are also reduced.

Epidemiology

Hyostrongylosis often appears when sows and gilts have been turned on to permanent pig paddocks with the boar between litters. Studies with pasture in the South of England suggest that larvae can develop to the infective stage from May to October. These infective larvae survive best on herbage and may survive for 10 months. Eggs do not hatch and produce infective larvae at 4°C but do so between 10°C and 27°C. Drying kills eggs and developing larvae and frequent freezing and thawing also does so. In spite of this, overwintering can occur.

Diagnosis

Diagnosis is based on clinical signs of weight loss and a history of poor food conversion rates in sows and gilts which have previously grazed on permanent pasture. Faecal egg counts and plasma pepsinogen levels are useful aids to diagnosis.

Treatment and control

See below.

References

Connan, R.M. (1967). Vet.Rec. 80, 424-429. Observations on the epidemiology of parasitic gastroenteritis due to *Oesophagostomum spp.* and *H.rubidus* in the pig.
Davidson, J., Murray, M. and Sutherland, I.H. (1968). Vet.Rec. 83, 582-588. *H.rubidus: A* field study of its pathogenesis diagnosis and treatment.
Rose, J.H. and Small, A.J. (1982). Parasitology 85, 33-42. Observations on the development and survival of the free-living stages of *H.rubidus* both in their natural environments out of doors and under controlled conditions in the laboratory.
Stewart, T.B., Hale, D.M. and Martin, O.G. (1985). Vet. Parasitology 17, 219-227 Experimental infections with *H.rubidus* and the effects on the performance of growing pigs.

Oesophagostomiasis

Definition

Oesophagostomum infection may cause diarrhoea but is more frequently associated with poor weight gain, and, in sows, with reduced productivity.

Incidence

Oesophagostomum is the most common helminth in British pigs, (85% of sows, 45% of weaners in 1980), and similar figures have been recorded elsewhere. Recent surveys in Denmark suggest a much lower incidence because of the increasing numbers of SPF herds. It is seldom present in sufficient numbers to cause the clinical disease characterised by diarrhoea and weight loss.

Aetiology and pathogenesis

Two species of Oesophagostomum are involved, *O.dentatum* and *O.quadrispinatum.* The adult worms are about 1.5 cm long and occur in the colon and caecum. The life cycle is direct, infection occurring by ingestion of the third stage larvae which enter the mucosa of the caecum and proximal colon where they remain for at least 2 weeks. Here they moult to become fourth stage larvae which complete their development in the lumen, taking a further 3 weeks. The lesions seen and the diarrhoea appear to result from the tissue damage and the subsequent infection with bacteria such as campylobacters and spirochaetes.

Clinical signs

In heavy infections, which are comparatively rare in the U.K., the principal clinical sign is diarrhoea. The main effect of the parasite is a subclinical one, usually associated with reduction in weight gain and poor milk yields of sows (in conjunction with Hyostrongylus it is thought to contribute to the 'thin sow syndrome'). Performance of litters from infected dams is impaired as reflected by the litter size, birth weights, growth and food conversion. Growth may be depressed by 13% and feed conversion raised by 15%.

Pathology

All that may be seen at post-mortem examination may be a diffuse enteritis in the colon and caecum but the mucosal surface may bear nodules containing larvae. These should be distinguished from the enlarged lymphoid diverticulae present in normal animals and made prominent from the serosal surface by any inflammation. Larvae may be seen in histological sections of mucosa.

Epidemiology

The infective larvae do not survive on dry concrete and theoretically this disease can be prevented under conditions of good husbandry. However, despite the high proportion of pigs housed in ideal conditions, infections with Oesophagostomum remain common. Eggs require moisture and a minimum temperature of 15-17°C for infective larvae to develop. Outdoor development of infective larvae takes place largely between April and November with 3-10% of all eggs reaching the infective stage within 1-5 weeks. Indoors, where development occurs all the year round, 70-90% of eggs reach the infective stage within 1-2 weeks. All may survive for up to 20 weeks. Effective cleaning under most indoor regimes reduces transmission to a minimum.

The 'periparturient rise' in sows is an epidemiological phenomenon based primarily upon Oesophagostomum infection. During the first half of pregnancy, the burdens of adult worms are low, but in the second half, the egg count begins to rise, reaching a maximum during lactation. At weaning there is an abrupt drop to the low level of early pregnancy. The importance of the phenomenon is that piglets are born into a highly infective environment. It has been shown that the rise can be eliminated by the application of a single dose of anthelmintic one week before farrowing (see control section). Wild boar and rats may be infected.

Diagnosis

Based on identification of the eggs from faeces and the recovery of adults from the intestinal contents.

Treatment and control

See below.

References

Barutzki, D. (1990). Proc. IPVS 11, 310. On the development of O.quadrispinulatum in pigs.
Connan, R.M. (1967). Vet.Rec. 80, 424-429..Observations on the epidemiology of parastic gastroenteritis due to Oesophagostomum spp. and Hyostrongylus rubidus in the pig.
Kendall, S.B., Small, A.J. Phipps, L.P. (1977). J.Comp.Path. 87, 223-229. Oesophagostomum sp. in pigs in England.
Pattison, H., Thomas, R.J., Smith, W.C. (1980). Anim.Prod. 30, 285-294. The effect of subclinical nematode parasitism on digestion and performance in pigs.
Pattison, H., Thomas, R.J. and Smith, W.C. (1980). Vet.Rec. 107, 415-418. UK. A survey of gastrointestinal parasitism in pigs.
Thomas, R.J. and Ferber, M. (1985). Proc.Pig Vet.Soc. 12, 50-55. The epidemiology of helminthiasis in pigs.

Ascariasis

Definition

Infection with *A.suum* is widespread but causes few clinical signs. The main importance of ascariasis is as a cause of condemnation of livers and 'plucks' (heart and lungs) due to the lesions produced by migrating larvae.

Incidence

A. suum occurs relatively commonly in growing pigs in all parts of the world.

Aetiology and pathogenesis

The adults occur in the small intestine and may be up to 40 cm long. The life cycle is direct with infection resulting from the ingestion of eggs containing second stage larvae. The development of the egg to the infective second larval stage depends on temperature (15°C minimum, 30-33°C optimum) and relative humidity (minimum 80%) and takes 2 months outdoors and 2-4 weeks indoors in the U.K. although this may be reduced indoors or in hotter climates. After ingestion, larvae hatch and migrate to the liver where they moult then migrate to the lungs, reaching them 5-8 days post-infection and then enter the tracheobronchial tree after a further moult to fourth stage larvae to be coughed up, swallowed and to mature in the small intestine. Transient lesions develop in lung and liver but resolve within 40 days. The pre-patent period is 40-53 days. Immunity can develop but may take some time. Both cellular and humoral immunity, including IgE has been demonstrated and is not dependent upon the presence of adult worms. In immune pigs larvae may be prevented from penetrating the gut wall or be stopped in the liver or lung. In some cases liver lesions may occur. Experimental studies suggest that damaged infective eggs, or ultrasonicated extracts of second stage larvae, larval cell walls and intestinal aminopeptidase from larvae may stimulate protection. When large numbers of eggs are ingested, fewer adults are found in the intestine than in infections with small numbers of eggs.

Clinical signs

Clinical signs of intestinal infection are rarely observed even in heavy infections. Growth rate may be reduced by 2-10% and food conversion by 5-13% following experimental infections and reduction in the digestibility of food has been demonstrated. Occasional animals may develop jaundice and some of these may die.

A moist cough, "heaves", may occur during the migration stage, about a week after infection. The role of ascarids in this cough is not clear, but it can be reproduced experimentally. Affected pigs appear hairy, may develop congested extremities and even die.

Humane slaughter is indicated in obstructive jaundice but even severely congested pigs with respiratory distress recover rapidly in the migration stage and should be given symptomatic treatment.

Pathology

Icteric pigs may be found to have bile ducts stuffed with adult ascarids. Normally, lesions are only incidental findings at post-mortem. They consist of the 'milk spot liver' in which whitish fibrous or fleshy lesions up to 1 cm in diameter occur on the liver surface and local petechial haemorrhages occur in the lung. The lung lesions occur during migration and resemble petechiae but consist of worm tracks filled with debris and the occasional larva. Mild hyperaemia of the small intestinal mucosa may be noted where adult worms are located. Occasionally large clusters of worms plug the intestinal lumen.

Epidemiology

In pigs at pasture in the UK infective eggs gradually rise in numbers developing only between June and September to give peak numbers in early autumn. Development occurs indoors from April to October but may extend beyond this in moist warm conditions or in heaps of warm damp material. Transmission rarely occurs between adults and offspring because of the time required for the development of the eggs. Their persistence in suitable conditions for up to 7 years means that weaner-weaner transmission can occur in uncleaned pens. Man and sheep may also become infected after eating infective eggs. Human infections with adult worms have been shown by mitochondrial DNA analysis to be *A.lumbricoides* where exposure to *A.suum* is also common.

Diagnosis

Clinical signs are variable and difficult to correlate with significant levels of infection. Transient coughing and, later a high egg count in pigs newly moved into contaminated pens, the presence of icteric pigs with no fever and post-mortem or slaughter findings of milk spot liver or ascarids in the intestine are indications for treatment or that treatments given have not been effective. The eggs of Ascaris suum are round, rough shelled and 45-85 um in diameter. They may be identified in faeces by flotation methods.

ELISAs for serum antibody have recently been described using L2/L3-ES (excretory fluid from cultured larvae) as antigen.

Control

Control is difficult because of the adhesive nature of the egg and its longevity on the ground (up to 5 years). In premises where ascariasis is a continuous problem, thorough cleaning of farrowing and fattening quarters with detergent or hot washing soda should be combined with anthelmintic treatment of the sow stock. The use of a horticultural flame gun has given good results in reducing the numbers of ascarid ova on concrete floors and thorough drying may also be of value. Pressure washing without drying may enhance survival. Composting of manure may destroy eggs but requires long periods (30 days at 37°C) or temperatures of 55-60°C and they may be killed by some proprietary disinfectants such as oocide (Antec International). Methods of treatment are given below.

References

Bernado, T.M., Dohoo, J.R., Ogilvie, I. (1990). Cn.J.Vet.Res. 54, 274-277. A critical assessment of abattoir surveillance as a screening test for swine ascariasis.
Lind, P., Eriksen, L., Nansen, P., Nilsson, O., Roepstorff A. (1993). Parasitological Research 79, 240-244. Response to repeated inoculations with *A.suum* eggs in pigs during the fattening period II: specific IgA and IgM determined by ELISA.

Nilsson, 0. (1982). Acta.Vet.Scand. Supplement 79, 108 pp. Ascariasis in the pig. An epizootiological and clinical study.
Stewart, T.B. and Guerrero, J. (1986). Proceedings I.P.V.S. 9, 371. The economic significance of pig endoparasites.
Urban, J.F., Alizadeh, H. and Romanowski, R. (1988). Experimental Parasitology 66, 66-77. *A.suum*, development of intestinal immunity to infective second stage larvae in swine.

Lungworm (Metastrongylosis)

Definition

Lungworm infection of the bronchioles of the lung may give rise to coughing, depression of growth and emphysematous lesions of the periphery of the diaphragmatic lobe of the lung in pigs housed outdoors.

Incidence

Present in all parts of the world. Rare in the UK. for many years, the recent increase in herds with access to pasture has led to its reappearance.

Aetiology and pathogenesis

Metastrongylus elongatus (*M.apri*) and *M.pudendotectus* are white in colour and measure up to 48 mm. The live in the bronchi or bronchioles of the posterior part of the diaphragmatic lobes of the lungs. Eggs measuring 40 x 50 um contain first stage larvae and are thick walled. They are coughed up, passed out in the faeces and ingested by earth worms in which they moult to produce the infective third stage larva (L3). Infected earth worms are ingested by pigs and the L3 larvae enter the host, move in lymphatics to the mesenteric lymph nodes where they form L4 and then to the lungs to form L5 and mature to produce patent infection after 20-24 days.

Following heavy experimental infection, severe cellular reaction to aspirated eggs may occur in the small bronchioles and marked lymphoid and muscular changes have been recorded. Some degree of immunity appears to result from infection.

M.salmi and *M.confusus* may occur in wild boar.

Clinical signs

Heavy infections are characterised by coughing and dyspnoea in weaned and growing pigs but adults are largely resistant and heavy infections are rare and cause only an intermittent husky cough.

Post-mortem findings

These are restricted to the lungs and consist of consist of scallop-shaped raised pale areas of emphysema on the edges of the caudal part of the diaphragmatic lobes. When these portions of the lung are cut off and squeezed gently the worms may be seen. There may be hypertrophy of the bronchial muscles, and the bronchi contain neutrophil eggs and adults when examined histologically. Bronchial lymph nodes may be enlarged and white spots 0.5-1 cm in diameter may be present on the liver.

Diagnosis

Infection may be suspected in outdoor pigs or wild boar on clinical grounds and confirmed by identifying the embryonated eggs in faeces or the characteristic lung lesions at slaughter.

Epidemiology

The earthworm vector is essential and infection is most common in pigs housed outdoors on pasture. Pigs with access to outdoor concrete yards may be infected by eating wandering earthworms. Breeding stock or finishers originally reared outdoors may also be infected. Infection may persist for 2-3 years in individual earthworms in a pasture.

Control

Heavily contaminated pasture may need to be cropped for 2 or 3 years and pigs may have to be housed or yarded to prevent re-infection after treatment. Treatment is described below.

Other Infections

Strongyloides ransomi infection occurs mainly in very young piglets and weaners. Though recognised as a pathogen in the United States and Europe, it has never been recognised in clinical disease in the UK. *A.ransomi* adult females 3.3-4.5 mm in length are found in the small intestine and pass thin shelled eggs containing larvae into the intestinal contents (45-55 by 26-35 µm) and faeces. Eggs hatch to first stage larvae which may develop into free living males and females or, within a day, into infective larvae. Larvae enter the host through the skin, the oral cavity via the colostrum and transplacentally. All but colostral larvae (which mature directly) enter tissue and migrate to the gut where they produce a patent infection within 4-8 days.

Anorexia, listlessness, anaemia and diarrhoea may be seen. The presence of larvae in the sows' colostrum or milk and of adults in the intestines of piglets 14 days of age can be used to confirm a diagnosis. Free living forms of this parasite exist and it is particularly associated with warm unhygienic conditions.

Reference

Murrell, K.D. and Urban, J.F. (1983). J.Parasitol. 69, 74-77. Induction of immunity to transcolostrally-passed *S.ransomi* larvae in neonatal pigs.

Trichuris suis is common in porkers and baconers in the U.K. (25% prevalence), but the numbers of worms present are usually low; it is uncommon in adult stock. In other countries, it is sometimes responsible for a severe ulcerative typhlitis. This has been shown to be associated in experimental infections with invasion of the damaged mucosa by small spirochaetes and other bacteria (see Spirochaetal Diarrhoea) and severe enteric disease has also been associated with *C.perfringens* type A. The epidemiology and transmission resemble those of ascaris as eggs containing second stage larvae are infective but remain infective for up to 6

244

years. First stage larvae enter large intestinal crypts and remain for 2 weeks, then
larvae mature in the lumen giving a prepatent period of 6-7 weeks.

Reference

Beer, R.J.S. (1973). Parasitology 67, 253-262. Studies on the biology of the life
cycle of Trichuris suis.
Rutter, J.M. and Beer, R.J.S. (1975). Infection and Immunity 11, 395. Bacteria and
worms in colitis.

Kidney worms (Stephanurus dentatus) do not occur in the UK but are
important causes of liver and kidney condemnation from the southern USA to
southern Brazil and in other subtropical areas. Eggs are passed in the urine, larvae
hatch in the soil and may persist there or in earthworms to be ingested. They
migrate to the liver and remain there to produce abscesses before migrating to the
ureters as adults 2-3 cm in length. Patency takes 9 months to 1 year. Clinical
signs are not seen in adult animals and diagnosis depends upon finding eggs in
urine or lesions in liver and kidney post-mortem. Infection in growing pigs may result
in depression of growth by up to 25% and of feed conversion by 9%. Worms and
larvae may be eliminated by single injections of ivermectin.

Trichinosis. An infection of porcine muscle with the larvae of Trichinella
spiralis (and some other species of Trichinella) which causes no clinical effects on
the pig but represents a major zoonotic hazard to those consuming under-cooked
pork or imperfectly cured products. Infection occurs in all European countries with
wild boar populations and in Asia, North and South America and Africa.

T.spiralis is considered to be absent from Northern Ireland and has rarely
been identified in Great Britain in spite of the examination of pig carcases for
export. Recent serological surveys (1994) suggest that it is absent. Infection can
be detected using trichinoscopy, muscle digestion or stomaching using diaphragm
and tongue and, more recently ELISA methods, using excretory antigen and
monoclonal antibodies on serum or tissue extracts. The most common method of
transmission is rat-pig-rat but cannibalism by pigs may maintain disease once
introduced. Transmission may also occur where uncooked pigmeat is fed back to
pigs and where home killing of pigs or the consumption of wild boar meat is
common. Albendazole has been shown to eliminate larvae at 10 mg/kg.

Ollulanus worms may be found in gastritis in pigs where the animals have
been in contact with cats. It has been recorded in continental Europe.

Fasciola hepatica can occur in grazing pigs and cause severe liver lesions,
particularly in young pigs.

Hepatitis cysticercosa is occasionally seen in the U.K. The condition results
from the ingestion of onchospheres of Taenia hydatigena, where there is mass
migration through the liver tissue toward the capsule. It usually occurs as single
cases.

Finally, the pig may be infected by Cysticercus cellulosae, which is both
important in public health. It is not of any clinical importance in the pig itself. The
latter has not been recorded in the UK for many years.

Anthelmintic Treatment and Control of Helminthiasis in the Pig

Treatment

A variety of compounds is available for treating helminth parasites in the pig. The spectrum of activity of each compound differs and the species of worm present should be determined before anything more than emergency treatment is attempted. The actual choice of compound used will depend upon:

1. The species of helminth present (multiple infections are common).

2. The spectrum of activity of the compound and whether active against both adults and larvae.

3. The presence of absence of resistance in the helminth population present.

4. The route of administration required by the farm management system.

5. The products available to fulfil (4). Different countries have registered or marketed different products.

6. Any side effects.

7. Any safety requirements and the capacity of the farm and its staff to meet them.

8. The withdrawal period.

9. The cost.

Anthelminthics may be given to pigs as pour-ons or as injections to individual pigs known to be heavily parasitised. In-feed formulations are usually either a powder, pellets or granules and palatability of the product is important. As with all in-feed drugs, the main problem is to ensure adequate uptake of medicated feed in *ad libitum* feeding systems. Continuous low level medication is sometimes practised to ensure an adequate uptake and compounds administered in this way may prevent economic loss and the establishment of patent infections but protection may cease when they are withdrawn.

At least 6 distinct compounds are registered for use in the U.K. Most are effective against the adult stages of the common helminths but some lack activity against individual species. Activity against larvae is less complete. The table given below lists the compounds which have been shown to be effective and indicates the form in which they can be administered. Their availability UK is indicated by product names for each class but withdrawal and exact doses recommended for each product are not given and can be found on data sheets and package inserts. The same applies to other countries. The Compendium of Data Sheets for Veterinary Products 1994-1995 was the source for the UK data. Where a product is known to be effective but is not registered for pigs, the cascade system should be employed. but is limited to products available for food animals only and 28 day withdrawals are required.

Sows and Gilts	Treat and wash prior to entering clean farrowing house and again at weaning. Possible mid gestation			
Compound	Effective against	Route	Single dose or course	Brands (UK)
Thiabendazole	Adult H,O,T,S Larval H,O.T.S Adult and Larval H,O	Feed	Continuous Single	
Ivermectin	Adult H,O,S,M,A Larval H,O,S,A	Injectable	Single	Ivomec injection for pigs MSD Ivomec Premix for pigs (to 100 kg) 100 µg/kg. 7 days and transfer to clear.
Cambendazole	Adult A,H,O	Feed	Single	None UK
Dichlorvos	Adult H,O,T,A L4 HO,T,A	Feed	Single	
Tetramisole	Adult H,O,A,M Larval H,O,A,M	Feed	Single	
Levamisole	Adult H,O,T,A,M Larval H,O,A.M	Injectable	Single	
Febantel	Adult H,O,T,S,A,M Larval H,O,T,S,A,M	Feed	5 days	Bayverm Pellets (Bayer)
Thiophanate	Adult H,O,T,A Larval H,O,T,A	Feed	14 days or single	Nemafax 14 6-7 mg/lg
Flu-bendazole	Adult H,O,T,S,A,M Larval H,O,T,A,M	Feed	Single or 5-10 days	Premix Flubenol (Janssen)
Fenbendazole	Adult H,O,T,A,M Larval H,O,T,A,M	Feed	Single course Divided 7d.	Panacur pellets (Hoechst) powder power 5 mg/kg.
Oxibendazole	Adult H,O,A Larval	Feed	10-day course	Loditac Pellets, Powder (SKB) 1.6 mg/kg.
Piperazine	Adult A,O	Feed	Single	
Pyrantel tartrate	Adult H,O,A	Feed	Single	22 mg/kg

H = Hyostrongylus, O = Oesophagostomum, T = Trichuris
S = Strongyloides, A = Ascaris, M = Metastrongylus
Growers   Treat on purchase or on entry to growing house.
Finishers   On entering finishing house and after 8 weeks.
Boars   Every 6 months.

Control

The treatments given above may be used in control programmes. These are based upon the ability of the compounds concerned to eliminate most, if not all, of the helminth species present and their larvae. In indoor units with slatted floors, no straw and a regular programme of cleaning and disinfections operating all-in all-out housing policies helminths may be reduced or even eradicated.

In all programmes treatment schedules must take account of the possibility that some adults or larvae may survive and that the environment may be contaminated with eggs or larvae. The basic interval between treatments must take into account the prepatent period and be based upon the movement of animals into clean accommodation or uninfected pasture.

If routine therapy is practised, it is usual to carry out a programme which includes regular treatment of the breeding stock as well as the growers. A popular control programme is as follows:

Outdoor sows should be treated as above but may require treatment before entering clean paddocks in rotation and monthly between July and October in UK. A sample treatment programme for controlling helminths in pigs at pasture in the UK is to dose in December and repeat the dose 3 weeks later. In June treatment is carried out on 3 occasions and again in October 2 weeks prior to a move to fresh pasture and 1 week after it. This schedule eliminates adult Hyostrongylus and Oesophagostomum and helps keep larval levels to a minimum.

Specific treatment regimes

To prevent milk spot liver in *Ascaris* contaminated accommodation it may be necessary to combine monthly treatment with rigorous hygiene. Eradication may not be achieved for several years.

Trichuris may require special treatment e.g., with flubendazole it may be necessary to divide the dose over 7 days.

Metastrongylus may require the use of fenbendazole or ivermectin.

References

Barth, D. and Preston, J.M. (1985). Vet.Rec. 116, 366-367. Ivermectin against somatic *S.ransomi* larvae.
Rose, J.H. and Small, A.J. (1983). J.Helminthology 57, 1-8. Observations on the effect of anthelmintic treatment on the transmission of *H.rubidus* and Oesophagostomum spp. among sows at pasture.
Taffs, L.F. (1969). Br.Vet.J. 125, 304-310. Helminths of the pig: pathogenicity diagnosis and control.

Coccidiosis

Definition

Coccidiosis is most important in the 5-15 day old sucking piglet in which diarrhoea and subsequent growth depression may be accompanied by mortality of up to 20%.

Enteric infections with a number of coccidial species may occur in pigs kept in unhygienic conditions.

Incidence

The incidence of clinical coccidiosis in neonates in the UK is not known but it is present in herds in all parts of the country. It is also present in most pig-rearing countries worldwide and figures from the US and Canada suggest that it may cause disease in 30-60% piglets.

Coccidial infections in older pigs has been recorded from domestic pigs on all continents and in wild boar wherever they occur.

Aetiology

Isospora suis causes coccidiosis in young piglets worldwide. Coccidiosis in older pigs is associated with Eimeria species, *E.debliecki, E.suis, E.perminuta, E.neodebliecki, E.spinosa, E.porci, E.polita, E.scabra* and local species such as *E.szechuanensis.* Most of these species e.g. *E.debliecki* do not occur in, or are of very low pathogenicity for neonates.

Pathogenesis

Infection with *I.suis* is entirely enteric. Infective sporulated *I.suis* oocysts are ingested by piglets from infected faeces and contaminated pen fittings and food. After ingestion the oocysts give rise to sporozoites which infect epithelial cells in the cranial third of the jejunum within 24 hours of infection and produce a first asexual generation of 2-7 merozoites at about 48 hours post-infection. They invade cells to give secondary meronts which give rise to 2-12 large merozoites at 3-4 days p.i. These become 3rd generation meronts which at 4-5 days post-infection give rise to 4-24 small crescent-shaped merozoites. These invade cells in the distal half of the small intestine to give rise to the sexual stages (micro and macro gamonts) which are mature at 5-6 days post-infection and give rise to multiple microgametes and single macrogametes which, after fusion with a microgamete, give rise to oocysts.

Oocysts may be seen in the faeces from 5 days onwards until days 8 or 9 and again from days 11-14 after infection. This second wave of oocysts appears to result from a reappearance of second generation meronts on days 8-9 post-infection and a further crop of sexual stages. Some evidence of extra intestinal infection has been identified. Oocysts sporulate within 48 hours at 24-27°C (farrowing house temperatures) and may remain infective for more than 10 months. From 1,000-400,000 oocysts per gram of faeces may be passed. Lesions of villous atrophy develop in affected portions of the small intestine by 5 days post-infection to resolve in the absence of other infectious agents by 10-14 days post-infection.

Other agents such as rotavirus infection may occur at the same time. *Eimeria* species have an essentially similar life cycle in older pigs.

Clinical signs

Faecal changes ranging from transient pasty diarrhoea or whitish faeces to profuse yellowish, watery diarrhoea occur in piglets of 5-15 days of age and are most common at 7-10 days of age. Affected piglets may be thinner than unaffected litter mates and remain gaunt and hairy for some weeks thereafter. Severely affected piglets may die. Mortality rates may reach 20%. The diarrhoea responds poorly to antimicrobial therapy and growth depression occurs in recovered animals. Recently, diarrhoea in the post-weaning period has been associated with *I.suis* infection. Mortality in most indoor units is normally reduced by the provision of electrolytes but may be 20% in outdoor units.

Wasting and diarrhoea have been recorded in gilts, finishing pigs and wild boar infected with *Eimeria* spp. Wasting and moribund piglets should be destroyed, particularly if they cannot be nursed.

Pathology

Carcases of affected piglets may be in poor condition and dehydrated. Gross lesions are restricted to the jejunum and ileum which appear turgid and thickened with a necrotic lining. The intestinal contents may be creamy or watery with flecks of milk and the villi are stunted and local bleeding points and fine fibrino-necrotic flakes may be seen using a dissecting microscope on the mucosa of freshly killed pigs. Histological changes include villous atrophy, increased mitotic activity in the crypt epithelium and the presence of large numbers of coccidial merozoites and male and female gametocytes within vacuoles in the epithelial cells. Oocysts can be demonstrated in colonic contents or faeces.

Epidemiology

Infection has been described both in extensive husbandry systems and indoors. Sows rarely pass *I.suis* oocysts in faeces and the major source of infection for piglets is the faeces of other piglets which contaminates farrowing and rearing accommodation. The high levels of oocysts passed by piglets and their ability to survive for months make environmental contamination important. Carrier sows may, however, be the means of introduction of the disease into clean buildings or farms. Less disease and oocyst shedding has been demonstrated on fully slatted cleaned floors. Eimeria species are carried by sows and may be passed to their offspring. *E.scabra* infections may occur from 4-8 weeks of age onwards but 96% of piglet infections are due to *I.suis*.

Diagnosis

The clinical signs, especially the age incidence and the failure to respond to antimicrobial therapy may suggest coccidiosis. The presence of coccidial oocysts in the faeces may be suggestive. Faeces from acutely affected pigs may contain few oocysts as the diarrhoea may precede oocyst production and faeces from less severely affected animals in the litter or 5-10 adjacent litters should also be examined. Other agents such as rotavirus may be present and *Clostridium perfringens* Type A or Type C infections may resemble coccidiosis. The presence of merozoites and sexual stages of coccidia in histological sections, and stained

2

50

smears of jejunal and ileal mucosa, the absence of Clostridia and the failure to respond to antimicrobial treatment confirm the diagnosis. Oocysts may be sporulated in potassium dichromate to identify the species involved. Cryptosporidia may also be present.

Treatment and control

Toltrazuril (Baycox Bayer) 20 mg/kg given as an oral suspension or by injection on day 3 prevents diarrhoea prevents oocyst shedding and can maintain piglet growth. Given as a treatment it stops diarrhoea and oocyst shedding, prevents mortality but growth rate in treated animals will depend upon the damage already caused but will be improved.

Until this product is registered (not UK 1995), less effective methods of treatment will have to be used. Trimethoprim sulphonamide may be given by injection or orally to affected piglets and should be supplemented by electrolyte.

The inclusion of an anticoccidial such as amprolium at 1 kg premix per tonne or monensin at 100g/tonne in sow feed for 7-10 days prior to farrowing and for 2 weeks afterwards will reduce the shedding of oocysts by sows. Similar inclusion rates will reduce shedding by other pigs. Amprolium may also be used to treat affected pigs at 10-20 mg/kg given orally for 4-5 days and reduces oocyst numbers but does not eliminate clinical signs. Treatment should include both clinically-affected pigs and their littermates. None of these products are registered for this use in pigs in the UK. All could be used for Eimeria infections. Scrupulous attention should be given to hygiene in control. Sows should be cleaned on entry to farrowing houses which should be disinfected or fumigated with methyl bromide or ammonia (final concentration 2%) to kill oocysts. Steam cleaning at 65°C for 15 minutes and flame guns (safety!) will also destroy oocysts. The disinfectant, oocide (Antec International) can also be used to destroy oocysts.

References

Harleman, J.H. and Meyer, R.C. (1984). Veterinary Parasitology 17, 27-39 Life cycle of I.suis in gnotobiotic and conventionalised piglets.
Harleman, J.H. and Meyer, R.C. (1985). Vet.Rec. 116, 561-565. Pathogenicity of I.suis in gnotobiotic and conventionalised piglets.
Jones, G.W., Parker, R.J., Parke, C.R. (1985). Aust.Vet.J. 62, 319. Coccidia associated with enteritis in grower pigs.
Koudela B., Vitovec, J. (1992). Int.J.Parasitol. 22, 651-666. Biology and Pathology of E.spinosa (Henry 1931) for experimentally infected pigs.
Lindsay, D.S., Blagburn, B.L., Boosinger, T.R. (1987). Vet . Parasitology 25, 39-45. Experimental E.debliecki infection in nursing and weaned pigs.
Lindsay, D.S., Current, W.L., Ernst, J.V. and Stuart, B.P. (1983). Vet.Med. S.A.C. 78, 89-95. Diagnosis of neonatal porcine coccidiosis caused by Isopora suis.
Lindsay, D.S., Ernst, J.V., Current, W.L., Stuart, B.P. and Stewart, T.B. (1984). J.Am.Vet.Med.Ass. 185, 419-421. Prevalence of oocysts of I.suis and Eimeria spp from sows on farms with and without a history of neonatal coccidiosis.
Madsen, P., Henriksen, A.A., Larsen, K. (1992). Proc.IPVS. 12, 366. Efficacy of Baycox on I.suis coccidiosis in piglets - a pilot study.
Martineau, G.P., Menard, J., Carabin, H., Villeneuve, A. and Dumas, G. (1994). Proc.IPVS. 13, 243. Strategic control of porcine coccidiosis with toltrazuril.
Nilsson, O. (1988). Vet.Rec. 122, 310-311. I.suis in pigs with post-weaning diarrhoea.

Nilsson, O., Martinsson, K. and Persson, E. (1984). Nord.vet.Med. 36, 103-110.
Epidemiology of porcine neonatal streatorrhoea in Sweden. 1. Prevalence and
clinical significance of coccidial and rotavirus infections.
Roberts, L., Walker, E.J., Snodgrass, D.R., Angus, K.W. (1980) Vet. Rec. 107,
156. Diarrhoea in unweaned piglets associated with rotavirus and coccidial
infections.
Stuart, B.P., Lindsay, D.S., Ernst J.V., Gosser, H.S. (1980) Vet. Path. 17, 84-93.
Isospora suis enteritis in piglets.

<h2 style="text-align:center">Cryptosporidium</h2>

Definition

Heavy enteric infections with this sporozoan parasite may cause diarrhoea
in young piglets but in older pigs infection may be common, clinically inapparent or
associated with diarrhoea.

Incidence

Worldwide with between 5 and 20% of pigs infected.

Aetiology and pathogenesis

Cryptosporidia are small coccidian parasites which attach to the brush
border of intestinal and respiratory tract epithelial cells and multiply there. The
oocysts and schizonts of *C.parvum* are 3-4 µm in length by 0.3 µm. Infection is oral
and multiplication on the brush borders of the jejunal and ileal epithelium appears to
reach a peak and initiate clinical signs in sucking pigs within 72 hours of infection.
The clinical signs appear to be due to the occupation of the absorptive brush
borders by large numbers of parasites and the associated inflammation, villous
atrophy and crypt hyperplasia. The oocysts are passed out in the faeces from 8-9
days post-infection and remain infective for at least 45 days. Immunity develops
and the numbers of organisms rapidly fall after the initial burst of multiplication,
persisting on individual cells in the ileum of recovered carrier pigs, particularly on
cells of villi adjacent to ileal lymphoid tissue and on the dome cells of the Peyer's
patches. In pigs aged 4-8 weeks they may be found throughout the gastrointestinal
tract but their role in the associated diarrhoea is not clear.

Clinical signs

These rarely appear before 3 days of age and are most commonly reported
in piglets at 10-21 days of age. Affected piglets are depressed and pass a watery,
sometimes brownish diarrhoea which may persist for 3-5 days. The organism can
be demonstrated in the faeces of diarrhoeic weaners. Affected weaned pigs are
often depressed and anorexic, in poor condition with a rough dirty coat and pasty
faeces. Chronically wasted animals should be killed.

Pathology

Gross changes of inflammation, villous atrophy and fusion and the presence
of diphtheresis on the mucosal surface may be seen in both jejunum and ileum.
Flattening and alteration of the large intestinal mucosa may also occur. The

contents may be watery or blood-stained and contain necrotic material. Cryptosporidia may be seen attached to the brush borders of epithelial cells and lying amongst neutrophils and dead epithelial cells in the exudate in slides made from freshly killed freshly fixed intestinal tissue. In chronically infected, clinically normal pigs they may be seen on eosinophilic cells of the mucosal epithelium particularly in the ileum.

Epidemiology

Cryptosporidial oocysts are resistant to drying and may persist for at least 45 days in pig faeces. The organism is present in many species including rats and mice and can infect man. In herds in which the infection is enzootic, oocysts may be found in the faeces of pigs of all ages including sows, but infection is most common in weaners and growers. Infected animals may be parasitised but shed few organisms in the faeces. Antibody can be demonstrated in colostrum and it may be that piglets are protected to some extent.

Diagnosis

The organism can be readily distinguished in formalin vapour-fixed faecal smears stained by Ziehl Neelsen's method using cold carbol fuchsin and 1% acid alcohol. Oocysts appear as 3-4 µm orange-red ovals or circles. In histological sections they are clearly visible on the brush borders of infected epithelial cells. Faecal smears may also be stained by auramine or by fluorescent antibody Antigen ELISAs and DNA probes have been developed by the water industry and techniques of filtration and demonstration n the environment are well developed.

The presence of cryptosporidia in an enteric syndrome does not confirm that it causes the syndrome and other pathogens such as rotavirus, epidemic diarrhoea, *E.coli,* and, especially, *C.perfringens* types A and C should be sought. It may contribute to enteritis when present in large numbers.

Treatment and Control

No treatment has yet been shown to affect the organism. The oocysts can be destroyed by ammonia and formalin treatment, by hydrogen peroxide and hypochlorite. The propietary disinfectant oocide (Antec International) can also be used.

References

Heine, J., Moon, H.W., Woodmansee, D.B. and Pohlenz, J.F.L. (1984). Vet.Parasitol. 17, 17-25. Experimental tracheal and conjunctival infections with *Cryptosporidium sp* in pigs.
Sanford, S.E. (1987). J.A.V.M.A. 190, 695-698. Enteric cryptosporidial infection in pigs: 184 cases (1981-85)
Vitovec, J., Koudela, B. (1992). Vet.Parasitol. 43, 25-36. Pathogenesis of intestinal cryptosporidiosis in conventional and gnotobiotic piglets.

Toxoplasmosis

Infection with *Toxoplasma gondii* is usually inapparent, but may result in abortion, stillbirths and the production of weak piglets. Older pigs may develop clinical signs. Toxoplasmosis is a zoonosis.

Incidence

Toxoplasmosis occurs worldwide with prevalences of 5% in finishers and 11% in sows and gilts (Iowa, USA) 2% (Netherlands) but higher rates of infection have been recorded.

Aetiology and pathogenesis

T.gondii is a coccidian parasite of cats which produce the oocysts in faeces. Ingestion of oocysts or tissue cysts by pigs results in the release of sporozoites or bradyzoites in the stomach which multiply rapidly in the intestinal epithelium as tachyzoites which spread to all parts of the body including the foetus and may be found in the milk. They encyst to produce tissue cysts. Antibody is produced.

Clinical signs

Infection may be inapparent but abortion may occur in sows infected between days 42 and 50 of gestation and mummified, stillborn and weak piglets may be born following later infections (70-90 days). Congenitally-infected piglets are weak, may develop diarrhoea and ataxia or incoordination. Clinical signs in older animals include anorexia, apathy, fever, cyanosis and hindlimb weakness. Severely affected comatose animals or those with serious incoordination or ataxia should be killed humanely.

Pathology

Affected piglets may have splenic enlargement, lymphadenopathy and there may be grey, white or reddish circumscribed lesions in lungs, liver and kidney. The carcase may be congested or multiple haemorrhages may be present. There is excess pleural and peritoneal fluid. Encephalitis, a catarrhal pneumonia and necrotic lesions in lymph nodes may be present and tissue cysts may be seen in histological sections.

Epidemiology

The prime source of oocysts is cat faeces but the ingestion of tissue cysts may result from the ingestion of raw meat, other animals such as mice and rats and cannibalism including tail biting (tissue cysts have been found in the tail). Transplacental transmission occurs. Tissue cysts are mature within 103 days of infection with oocysts and are still viable 875 days p.i. Tachyzoites in muscle are not infective for older animals as they cannot pass the stomach.

Diagnosis

Toxoplasmosis can be suspected as a cause of abortion in sows and of nervous signs in weak piglets, particularly where cats and their faeces are prominent. The pathology is suggestive and the identification of tissue cysts confirms the involvement of *T.gondii*. Cysts may be confirmed as those of *T.gondii* by immunoperoxidase, immunofluorescence ELISA and animal transmission. Antibody may be detected by the Sabin Feldman test, indirect haemagglutination, latex agglutination tests and principally by ELISA. Antibody is present in transudates from foetuses and confirms transplacental infection.

Treatment

Treatment is technically possible but not practised in pigs. Control relies upon the separation of cats from pigs, their pens and their feed, the prevention of cannibalism and control of rodents. Live attenuated vaccines have been tested but are not available UK. The sheep vaccine is not licensed for pigs.

Tissue cysts in meat remain viable at 5°C but are killed by freezing to -12°C, heating at 70°C or irradiation at 700 Greys.

References

Dubey, J.P. (1986). Veterinary Parasitol. 19, 181-223. A review of toxoplasmosis in pigs.
Dubey, J.P. (1988). Am.J.Vet.Res. 49, 910-913. Long-term persistence of *T.gondii* in tissues of pigs inoculated with *T.gondii* oocysts and effects of freezing on viability of tissue cysts.
Dubey, J.P. and Urban, J.F. (1990). Am.J.Vet.Res. 51, 1295-1299. Diagnosis of transplacentally-induced toxoplasmosis in pigs.
Dubey, J.P., Kotula, A.W., Sharar, A., Andrews C.D., Lindsay, D.S. (1990). J.Parasitol. 76, 201-204. Effect of high temperature on the infectivity of *T.gondii* tissue cysts in pork.
Jones, M.A., Hunter, D.H. (1979). Vet. Rec. 104, 529, Toxoplasma infection in a newborn piglet.

Pneumocystis carinii infection

Causes retarded growth and dyspnoea at 4-5 weeks of age lasting for 4-10 weeks with deaths amongst dyspnoeic pigs There is no response to antimicrobial. The lungs are enlarged and do not collapse easily and there are focal brownish areas of consolidation in the cranial lobes. There may be interstitial oedema. Lobular or diffuse interstitial pneumonia with foamy, acidophilic (honeycomb) material and macrophages filling the alveoli. The alveolar septae are thickened by lymphocytes, plasma cells and lymphocytes Toluidine blue O staining or immunoperoxidase reagents identify *P.carinii* as round or crescent-shaped cysts in the alveoli.

Infection has been identified in Japan and Denmark but occurs in man and other animal species in the UK. It appears to be secondary to other conditions.

Reference

Bille Hansen, V., Jorsal, S.E., Henriksen, S.A., Settnes O.P. (1990). Vet.Rec. 127, 407-408. *Pneumocystis carinii* pneumonia in Danish piglets.

Trypanosomiasis (NOT UK)

A wide variety of Trypanosoma species have been reported to infect the pig. Some infections are inapparent such as *T.cruzi* and *T.rangeli* infections in Venezuela. *T.evansi* is normally considered non-pathogenic in pigs in India but can cause death after fever, laboured breathing and necrosis of the extremities.

The African trypanosomes have been recorded as causing inapparent infections (*T.brucei, T.b.rhodesiense* in Uganda, *T.b.gambiense* and *T.congolense* in Congo and *T.b.brucei* infection in Liberia where both direct and delayed infection by *Glossinia palpalis gambiense* were demonstrated.

Infection with *T.b.brucei, T.congolense* and *T.simiae* can cause disease. *T.b.brucei* causes pyrexia, weight loss, and anaemia with nervous signs in some animals, particularly after relapse. The prepatent phase lasts 4-7 days and acute disease may occur 9-15 days after infection. Chronic infection follows with a fluctuating pyrexia 37.6-41.6°C. Petecchial haemorrhages and plaque-like lesions may develop. Infertility has been recorded in boars.

T.simiae infection is more severe and may cause dyspnoea, inappetence, pyrexia, dullness and abortion in pregnant sows. Death occurs 12-96 hours after the onset of clinical signs. The infections are spread by Glossina sp. principally *G.palpalis palpalis, G.pellicera pellicera, G.nigrofuscans nigrofuscans* and *G.brevipalpis* from wildlife reservoirs which include the warthog in which infection is largely subclinical. Diagnosis is based on the clinical signs and post-mortem findings of haemorrhages, the demonstration of trypanosomes in the blood and in the cerebral capillaries and C.S.F. Blood smears can be supplemented by the Testryp CATT card test, antigen detection ELISAs and the KIVI system of isolation. Multilocus enzyme electrophoresis may be used to identify species.

Treatment with isometidium chloride 1 mg/kg clears experimental *T.brucei* infections within 72 hours and maintains freedom for 8 weeks and 20 mg/kg diminazeneaceturate (Berenil) has been shown to treat *T.simiae* and to provide at least 17 days' relapse from parasitaemia. Affected pigs may not grow at the same rate as formerly. Prophylaxis with Berenil and Antrycide at 3-6 monthly intervals can prevent diease but pigs should be housed in insect-screened buildings.

References

Gill, B.S., Singh, J., Gill, J.S., Kwatra, M.S. (1987). Vet.Rec. 120, 92. *Trypanosome evansi* infection in pigs in India.
Onah, D.N., Uzoukwa, M. (1991). Tropical Animal Health and Production 23, 39-44. Porcine cerebral *T.brucei brucei* trypanosomiasis.
Truc, P. and 6 others (1992). Trans.Royal Society of Tropical Medicine and Hygiene 86, 627-629. Direct isolation *in vitro* of *T.brucei* from man and other animals and its potential value for the diagnosis of Gambian trypanosomiasis.

Other protozoa

Balantidium coli occurs in gut lesions but is probably a secondary invader. It multiplies on and may penetrate inflamed mucosa. Nitroimidazole drugs eliminate it.

Giardia lamblia has been identified in the duodenum, jejunum and ileum of recently-weaned pigs without causing clinical signs. The cysts are more common in pens with solid floors and piglets and weaners appear to be infected by the sow.

Sarcocystis infect pigs, cause little if any disease in natural cases but *S.suihominis. S.suicanis* and *S.miescheriana* may be noted at meat inspection. Experimental infections suggest that the ingestion of high numbers of cysts can lead to abortion in sows, fever and death in weaned pigs. Meat quality is not infected. Cysts of *S.mescheriana* took 63 days to become infective for dogs.

2. ECTOPARASITES

The most important ectoparasites of pigs in the UK are the sucking louse, *Haematopinus suis* and the mange mite *Sarcoptes scabei var suis.* Demodectic mange may also occur in debilitated pigs and biting by the stable fly, *Stomoxys calcitrans* may cause distress to young piglets, especially in hot weather.

Lice

Haematopinus suis is the only louse commonly found on pigs in the UK and is most common on the folds of skin of the neck or jowl around the base of the ears, inside the ears, on the insides of the legs and on the flanks. It is a large, yellowish-brown louse (5 mm) which moves about amongst hairs on the pig's skin and may be seen most readily on white pigs.

Life cycle

Eggs are laid on the bristles and appear as a yellow crust which is prominent in black pigs. The eggs hatch into nymphs in 12-20 days. Following two further nymphal stages, the life cycle is completed in 29-33 days. The lice can only live away from the host for 2-3 days. The pig is the only host.

Pathogenesis and clinical signs

In severe infestations, the constant irritation and itching results in scratching and rubbing against grates, rails, etc. and this may lead to damage to the skin. Localised ulceration is found inside the pinna of the ears where lice congregate to feed. Large numbers of lice may cause restlessness and a reduced growth rate. The pig louse may act as a vector for the swine pox virus and Eperythrozoon.

Epidemiology

Spread of infection is via pig to pig contact. Wild birds may eat lice on pigs outdoors.

Treatment and control

Treatment has been carried out using a wide variety of insecticides, but those most commonly used at present are ivermectin, amitraz and phosmet.

Ivermectin (Ivomec, MSD) at 330 µg/kg s/c or orally as the 2% premix for 7 days, amitraz (Taktic, Hoechst) spray and phosmet (Porcit, SKB) pour on can be used to eliminate lice from affected animals.

Control can be carried out by the routine treatment of all sows entering farrowing accommodation, boars every 4 weeks and weaners and growers at weaning and during the finishing period together with a mange programme.

Eradication is relatively straightforward and is the preferred option. A whole herd treatment by injection or in feed (ivermectin) should be followed by a second course 18-21 days later and then brought into the herd 7 days after the second treatment. Similar programmes can be carried out using the other agents.

Reference

Davis, D.P. and Williams, R.E. (1986). Vet.Parasitol. 307-314. Influence of hog lice *H.suis* on blood components, behaviour, weight gain and feed efficiency of pigs.

Mange

Definition

The most common form of mange in pigs is that caused by *Sarcoptes scabei* var *suis* which burrows in the skin and causes intense pruritis resulting in loss of condition and trauma to the skin, particularly in the region of the ears.

Incidence

A 1990 survey showed that 67% farms in GB were infected, 30% slaughter pigs, 26% boars and 17% sows. Similar figures from Canada (69% farms), France (56% pigs), Netherlands (5% pigs), Switzerland (10.4% pigs) and US 22-25% pigs suggest that the disease is common worldwide. Figures from Denmark differentiate between conventional herds (42.5% positive with 30% pigs positive) and SPF farms which were all free from infection.

Aetiology

Mange is caused by *S.scabei*, a small burrowing mite 0.5 mm in length which lives in galleries in the horny skin and feed on epidermal cells. They are circular and may be identified by the pattern of sucker-and-bristle-bearing legs. In the male this is sucker-sucker-bristle-sucker and in the female, sucker-sucker-bristle-bristle.

Up to 50 eggs are laid in the burrows before the female dies and they develop through larval and 2 nymphal stages to become ovigerous females, sometimes within as short a period as 10 days, although the normal life cycle usually takes 14-15 days. Multiplication can only occur on the host, although the mites may survive for up to 2-3 weeks in moist places in piggeries etc.

Pathogenesis

Lesions appear at least 3-4 weeks after initial infestation during which period the mites multiply and the host becomes sensitised. The burrowing and feeding activities of the mites cause intense pruritis which causes scratching which in turn results in the liberation of fluid from small vesicles near the burrows of the mites. The serum coagulates and dries on the skin to cause crusts which block the mite burrows 6-7 weeks after infection. Hyperkeratinisation of the skin occurs and connective tissue proliferation follows; lesions tend to be more heavily keratinised in older pigs. This lesion is thought to have an immunological basis and occurs after a period of sensitisation. Bacterial infection may also occur.

Clinical signs

Affected pigs scratch frequently, especially at mid-day. The first lesions appear as small red papules or weals and general erythema about the eyes, around the snout, on the inner surface of the pinna of the ears, in the axillae and on the front of the hock and tarsus where the skin is thin. Scratching results in the excoriation of these affected areas and the formation of brownish scabs on the damaged skin. Subsequently, the skin becomes wrinkled, covered with crusty lesions and thickened. The flanks become bare of hair and in badly-affected animals aural haematomas may form as a result of excessive head shaking. Reductions in productivity occur in infected herds. Litters' weight may be depressed 10% at weaning, sow feed use per piglet and per kg piglet are both increased by 5-10% and growth rates in finishing pigs are reduced by 5% or more.
Humane slaughter is not indicated as treatment is now as effective.

Pathology

The hyperkeratotic lesions of mange have been described above. Lesions may be obvious in the ears at post-mortem when the waxy crusts and inflamed internal surface of the pina can be clearly seen. Localised lesions occur elsewhere on the carcase as small (1-2 mm) round, slightly thickened lesions on rump, flank and abdomen. These can be seen most easily in animals which have been scalded after slaughter. Histological lesions are superficial and processing means that mites are rarely seen but an eosinophilic vasculitis is present in the dermis.

Epidemiology

Spread of infection is via pig to pig contact; infection of weaners usually occurs from the dam. Pigs may contact infection from infected pens after only 24 hours' contact. Mites may survive off the host for up to 3 weeks in the laboratory, but in piggeries, survival has only been demonstrated for 12 days at 7-18°C and 65-75% relative humidity. In warmer conditions, survival is shorter. Infections of man have been reported but disappear once contact with infected pigs stops.

Diagnosis

The clinical signs of scratching and rubbing, the presence of broken hairs on the flanks, crusts in the ears, crumpled ears and hyperkeratotic skin all suggest mange. The presence of red, pinpoint lesions on the skin after scalding are 92% specific for mange and have been used to score the severity of infection in a herd. Scores vary from 1 (mild lesions on the belly, head and buttocks, 82.5% specific) through 2 (lesions over flanks and back in low to moderate numbers, 98.6% specificity) to 3 (severe generalised lesions, specificity 99.5%).
Deep skin scrapings should be examined for the presence of mites, the finding of which is pathognomonic. The most likely sites in which to demonstrate the mite are the anterior portion of the inside of the ears and the face (80% of cases) and the skin of the tarsus (50% of cases). Mites may be found here and in the axillae in the carriers or in affected skin from clinical cases. Prior to scraping, the site should be smeared with 70% glycerine to bind the scraped material. Mites can be stimulated to leave crusts of skin or ear wax by subjecting small portions of

the latter to a combination of vibration and heat. Although recovery of mites is relatively easy in weaners, chronically affected sows often have few mites, the lesions being due to an immunological reaction. Where mites do not leave crusts they may be demonstrated by clearing scabs in 40% potassium hydroxide for 10 minutes. Eggs and mites may be demonstrated by dissolving ear wax in eosin - stained ethanol and filtering. Live mites and eggs are white.

Other similar conditions include swine pox which causes non-irritant lesions in the young pig, parakeratosis in which loose, dry, crumbly crusts occur with no irritation, exudative epidermitis mostly in young piglets with no irritation, and pityriasis rosea in which expanding ring lesions occur on the belly. Ringworm is rare, see fungi. Mites from old straw, mosquitoes and the Scottish midge may all produce lesions which may be confused with those of mange in SPF pigs. ELISAs using whole mite antigens can be used to detect antibody.

<u>Treatment</u>

Mange may be treated with ivermectin, amitraz or phosmet. Other substances such as doramectin have been shown to be effective but are not registered UK (1995). A single application of phosmet (Porect, SKB) poured on the back with part of the dose placed in the ears where obvious crusts are present, will treat the disease. Amitraz solution (Taktic, Hoechst) can be sprayed gently with a knapsack or pressure washer. The whole pig must be thoroughly treated. Treatment may have to be repeated within 7-10 days in order to kill eggs and larvae. It is particularly important to ensure treatment of ears. Ivermectin (e.g. Ivomec injection pigs MSD) can be given by subcutaneous injection at 300 µg/kg and kills mites in ears and on skin within 7-14 days, not instantly like the other products. Animals with severe crusty lesions in the ears should be treated again within 14 days as mites persist in the ear wax and such animals may represent a focus of infection.

<u>Control</u>

A typical control programme is shown below:

Boars	2-3 monthly intervals
Sows and gilts	at entry to farrowing house
Pigs	after weaning before moving/at moving
Purchased stock	isolate, treat.

With ivermectin and sows and boars may be treated by subcutaneous injection (Ivomec injection for pigs) and weaned pigs using the 2% premix for 7 days.

In all cases the efficacy of treatment is increased if animals are treated on entry into clean accommodation (rested 3 weeks or cleaned, disinfected and fumigated).

Treated and untreated pigs should not be mixed if best results are to be achieved. Regular treatments will reduce chronic infection and improve productivity. In studies in which ivermectin or phosmet have been used, an 8-10% improvement in daily liveweight gain and feed conversion efficiency has been gained under many different systems of husbandry.

Eradication

Phosmet and ivermectin can be used to eradicate mange from a farm, but only by treating all animals at appropriate intervals and by ensuring that treated animals enter cleaned accommodation. Although in theory a single treatment should be adequate, at least two treatments should be given, 14 days apart and accommodation should be sprayed with amitraz (1 g/20 m^2). Care should be taken when dosing neonates with organo phosphates as CNS signs such as head shaking can follow overdosing. When mange has been eradicated, purchased stock should be treated and isolated for 21 days in clean accommodation before being introduced or purchased from a mange-free herd.

References

Arends, J.J., Stanislaw, C.M., Gerdon, D. (1990). J.Anim.Sci. 68, 1495-1499. Effects of mange on lactating swine and growing pigs.

Courtney, C.H., Ingalls, W.L. and Stitzlein, S.L. (1983). Am.J.Vet.Res. 44, 1220-1223. Ivermectin for the control of swine scabies: relative values of pre-farrowing treatment of sows and weaning treatment of pigs.

Dalton, P.M. and Ryan, W.G. (1988). Vet.Rec. 122, 307-308. Productivity effects of pig mange and control with ivermectin.

Davis, D.P., Moon, D. (1990). J.Med.Entomology. 27, 391-398. Density, location and sampling of S.scabei (Ascaris, Sarcoptidae) on experimentally infected pigs.

Hewett, G.R. (1985) . Vet.Parasitol. 18, 265-268 . Phosmet for the systemic control of pig mange in growing pigs.

Lee, R.P., Dooge, D.J.D. and Preston, J.M. (1980). Vet.Rec., 107, 503. Efficacy of Ivermectin against S.scabei in pigs.

McMullin P.F., Jones, P.G.H., Hale C.J., Jones, M.A. Ryan, W.G. (1990). Proc.IPVS 11, 318. A survey of sarcoptic mange in cull sows in Great Britain.

McMullin, P.F., Guise, J., Cuthbertson, C., Jones, M.A. (1992). Proc.IPVS. 12, 373. A survey of the prevalence of S.scabei var suis in finishing pigs in Great Britain.

Morsy, G.H., Turck, J.J., Gaafar, S.M. (1989). Vet.Parasitol. 31, 281-288. Scanning electron microscopy of sarcoptic mange lesions in swine.

Sheahan, B.J. (1974). Vet.Rec. 94, 202-209. Experimental S.scabei infections in pigs: Clinical signs and significance of infection.

Sheahan, B.J., Kelly, G.P. (1974). Vet.Rec. 95, 169-170. Improved weight gains in pigs following treatment for sarcoptic mange.

Smith, H.J. (1986). Can.vet.J. 27, 252-254. Transmission of S.scabei in swine by fomites.

Demodectic Mange

Caused by Demodex phylloides, a long thin mite (0.25 mm in length). It is present in 10.3% cull sows (GB 1990) and is associated with small reddened or pustular lesions on the face and body. There is no treatment and severely affected animals should be killed.

Flies

A number of flies may be found in piggeries. The most important of these is probably Stomoxys calcitrans which sucks blood. This species and the non-parasitic Musca domestica may disturb piglets and sows and may lead to loss of condition. They breed in slurry and under uncleaned pen furniture and can spread disease within pens. Large powerful flies such as blue bottles (Lucilia sp. and Calliphora sp.) may spread disease from house to house or from farm to farm. They are normally controlled by baiting or sprays.

Ticks

These may occur on pigs from time to time. *Ornithodorus erraticus* occurs in Spain and is a reservoir of swine fever. *Ixodes ricinus* occurs on pigs in UK but only louping ill of the diseases it carries has yet been identified in pigs.

NUTRITIONAL CONDITIONS

Introduction

Nutritional deficiencies and excesses may both give rise to clinical disease in pigs and to reduction in productivity in both growing pigs and breeding animals. Overt clinical disease frequently results from:

1. Use of ingredients which have not been analysed so that accurate supplementation can take place. Examples include grains grown on selenium deficient soils and by-products such as bakery waste.

2. Spoilage of ingredients resulting from prolonged incorrect storage. This occurs when mould infections attack stored grains and when finished feeds and vitamin:mineral mixes are stored beyond their expiry dates.

3. The inclusion of high levels of normal nutrients as a result of errors in formulation or mixing. These occur most frequently following the addition of incorrect quantities of premix when mixing or the incorrect formulation of the premixes themselves. Occasionally the food itself may contain toxic levels of a nutrient such as salt or selenium.

    Overt clinical disease resulting from nutritional deficiency or toxicity is rare as the majority of pigs are fed on standard mixtures supplemented by carefully formulated premixes. Manufactured feeds are carefully supervised by qualified nutritionists and errors in formulation are rare. Most nutritional deficiencies or excesses require time to become apparent and fresh deliveries of feed (which may be normal) reduce the likelihood that nutritional disorders will develop. The following points should be borne in mind when considering a potential nutritional problem:

    i)   Nutritional disease giving rise to clinical or pathological signs can be recognised from the descriptions of the appropriate syndromes which follow.

    ii) Nutritional disease should be distinguished from infectious disease and poisonings. Feed refusal or depressed feed intake or growth rate may result from pneumonia or other infectious causes as may reduction in sow productivity.

    iii) Nutritional disease frequently occurs in groups of animals fed on the same ration (manufactured feed) or premix or raw ingredients fed on other farms.

    iv) Examination of the feed being given to the animals may reveal physical abnormalities. Samples may be taken for analysis.

    v)   There may be a history of prolonged storage of ingredients, of mechanical failure or incorrect incorporation of a particular nutrient or portion of the ration.

The examination of nutritional conditions is based upon the normal nutrient requirements of the pig. These are constantly changing as genetic advances and changes in husbandry develop. The guides to normal nutrient requirements given below are based upon historic requirements supplemented by recent publications and are a guide only.

Normal Nutrient Requirements

The figures given here form a basis for assessing the adequacy of a diet in terms of nutrients. For detailed consideration of pig feeding, books such as Practical Pig Nutrition and The Science and Practice of Pig Production should be consulted. The details of nutrient requirements have been reviewed in the A.R.C. technical review "The Nutrient Requirements of Pigs" 1981 and by the NRC in the US. Rapidly-growing pigs and those receiving porcine somatotrophin may have special requirements. Fat levels for lactating sows may be increased in lactation diets.

(a) Major Nutrients

Nutrient	Starter creep (4-28 days) Min.	Max.	Standard creep (4 wks - 40 kg) Min.	Max.	Grower (40-70 kg) Min.	Max.	Finisher (70 kg -) Min.	Max.	Pregnant sow Min.	Max.	Lactating sow Min.	Max.
DE (MJ/kg)	14.0	15.5	14.0	15.0	13.0	14.0	13.0	14.0	12.0	12.5	13.0	13.5
CP (%)	22.0	25.0	19.0	22.5	17.0	20.0	14.5	17.0	12.0	15.0	15.5	16.5
DCP (%)	18.5	20.0	15.0	16.0	13.5	14.0	11.0	12.0	9.0	9.5	12.5	13.5
Lysine (%)	1.2	1.5	1.0	1.3	0.8	1.5	0.8	0.85	0.60	0.70	0.7	0.8
Meth + cyst (%)	0.88	1.0	0.76	0.9	0.68	0.8	0.58	0.68	0.48	0.60	0.62	0.66
Calcium (%)	0.95	1.1	0.9	1.0	0.8	1.0	0.8	1.2	1.0	1.2	1.0	1.2
Phosphorus (%)	0.85	0.9	.78	0.82	0.6	0.8	0.6	0.8	0.6	0.8	0.8	0.8
Crude fibre (%)	1.0	3.0	2.0	4.0	2.0	5.0	2.0	6.0	2.0	7.0	2.0	6.0
Ether extract (%)	1.0	5.0	1.0	5.0	1.0	6.0	1.0	6.0	1.0	5.0	1.0	5.0

263

(b) Minerals: inclusion rates per tonne of air-dried mixed diet.

	Suggested in final mixed diet	Indicated as being provided in proprietary trace element
Calcium (kg)	8-12	
Phosphorus (kg)	7-11	4 - 9.2
Potassium (kg)		about 2.5
Salt (Sodium Chloride)(kg)	1.0-2.5	2 - 3.5
Magnesium (g)	400 - 800	10 - 75
Iron (g)	about 80	50 - 400
Zinc (g)	100-150	50-150
Manganese (g)	5 - 40	20 - 60
Copper (g)	3 - 10	5 - 175
Iodine (g)	0.16 - 0.5	1 - 4
Cobalt (g)	only in Vitamin B12	0.5 - 2
Selenium (g)	0.8 - 1.6	1.2

(c) Water requirements

Good quality water should be freely available by means of appropriate drinkers to all pigs even when it is provided in the diet. Water points or provision for watering should be available even pigs normally given wet feed in case of alteration in the dietary constituents or disease resulting in inappetence. Sucking piglets should also have access to water.

Sucking piglets		0.30 - 0.5 kg
Growing pigs:	15.0 kg body weight	1.5-2.0 kg
	90.0 kg body weight	6.0-12.0 kg
Sows: Non-pregnant		6-12.0 kg
Pregnant		10-20 kg
Lactating		25-40 kg

These requirements may be increased by a number of factors including the salt concentration of the diet, the ambient temperature and the use of leaky drinkers. Where water is freely available, flow rates should be 200 ml/minute in flat decks, 450 ml/minute in grower accommodation and 21/minute for sows .

The water requirements in the diet expressed as water: dry matter are usually:

Growing pigs	2.5 : 1	(restricted access)
	3.7 : 1	(ad lib)
Sows, non-pregnant	2.0 : 1	
pregnant	2.5 : 1	
lactating	3.0 : 1	

(d) Vitamins

	Liveweight and type of pig	Required per tonne of mixed dry diet	Normally provided as a supplement
Vitamin A	up to 20 kg	1.98 million i.u. (600 mg or 7.2g beta carotene)	yes
	20-50 kg	1.98 million i.u. (600 mg or 7.2g beta carotene)	yes
	50-90 kg	9.9 million i.u. (400 mg or 4.8g beta carotene)	yes
	sows	6.0 million i.u. (min.700 mg)	
Vitamin D3	up to 20 kg	3.5 mg	
	all other stock	0.2 million i.u. (3.0 mg)	yes
Vitamin E	all stock	10-20,000 i.u. (3.0-6.0 mg)	yes
Vitamin K	baby pigs	300 mg	sometimes
Thiamine	up to 90 kg	1.5 g	no
Riboflavine	up to 90 kg	2.5 g	sometimes
	sows	3.0 g	sometimes
Nicotinic acid	up to 20 kg	20 g	sometimes
	20 - 70 kg	14 g	
Pantothenic acid	up to 100 kg	10 g	yes
	sows	10 g	yes
Pyridoxine	up to 90 kg	2.5 g	no
	sows	1.8 g	no
Vitamin B12	up to 20 kg	18 mg	yes
	20 - 90 kg	10 mg	sometimes
	sows	15 mg	yes
Choline	up to 20 kg	800 g	no
	20-90 kg	850 g	
	sows	1000 - 1900 g	
Biotin	15-90 kg	1 g	
	sows	25 g	yes, usually
Folic acid	growing pigs	1 g	
	sows	5 g	no
Inositol) Vitamin C)	Dietary estimates not established		no
Essential fatty acids as linolenic acid	up to 30 kg	15 kg	not specifically
	30 - 90 kg	7 kg	not specifically
as arachidonic acid	up to 30 kg	10 kg	not specifically
	30-90 kg	5 kg	not specifically

Nutritional Deficiencies and Excesses

1.   Water

Water Deprivation and Salt Poisoning

Definition

a)   Effects on production

Limited water may cause depression of growth and production. Decreased water intake may result from inadequate supply, (water pressure, number of drinkers per pig, limited access or poorly maintained drinkers), the solids content of the water/sulphates) or disease. Water limitation is particularly important in the farrowing sow where it has been associated with lethargy and reluctance to rise and leads to increases in piglet mortality and depression of growth in the litter.

In other age groups it may reduce feed consumption and thus growth rate and in adult sows may lead to crystalluria and predispose to cystitis.

b)   Clinical disease (Salt poisoning)

Definition

Excess dietary salt or sudden water deprivation may lead to convulsions and abnormalities of gait and death or recovery within two days of exposure.

Incidence

Occurs sporadically, but may affect large numbers of pigs when water supply to a house is interrupted through cold weather, drought or burst pipes, when a high salt diet is fed or when an outbreak of diarrhoea such as T.G.E. increases water loss. It may also occur in individual pigs which are paralysed or otherwise unable to drink.

Aetiology and pathogenesis

The condition is most commonly associated with water deprivation on normal salt diets but high salt diets such as salted fish, buttermilk or pickling brines also predispose to the condition. The syndrome may follow the ingestion of large amounts of salt on limited water supplies or occur after sudden unrestricted access to water. It is thought that dehydration of tissues and an increase in the sodium content of the brain occur. High sodium levels in the brain inhibit anaerobic glycolysis and acetyl choline esterase levels and appear to be responsible. Sudden rehydration may exacerbate the condition.

Clinical signs

Peracute salt poisoning occurs after the ingestion of massive amounts of salt and results in prostration, running movements, coma and death. Acute salt poisoning following restricted water intake is most common. Pruritis, thirst and constipation are followed 1-5 days later by blindness, lack of interest in food or drink and failure to respond to external stimuli. Affected pigs may bump into obstacles and may circle, pivoting on one foot. Head pressing may occur. Convulsions occur regularly (every 7 minutes). Twitching of the snout is followed by contractions of the neck muscles, holding the head upright and by characteristic backing movements. Seizures last only a short time, but may end in rigidity and coma. Mortality may be high, but is usually 5% or less. Clinical signs may also develop after water is given following withdrawal.

Humane slaughter of affected paralysed pigs should not be carried out until after 24-36 hours as many recover.

Pathology

Gross changes are few. There may be congestion of the meninges and plasma sodium levels may be high. The microscopic changes are pathognomonic, and consist of meningoencephalitis with oedema and eosinophil accumulations around the vessels of the cerebral cortex and in the meninges. In later lesions, malacia occurs and cystic spaces are left.

Diagnosis

The history of water deprivation or salty diet is usually adequate, but organic arsenical poisoning and bowel oedema (absence of high pitched squeal) may resemble it. The histological findings are confirmatory and the presence of high plasma levels of creatinine phosphokinase and sodium (more than 160 m. eq/l.) may confirm. The absence of this level of sodium may only indicate that rehydration has occurred. Brain levels of sodium and chloride are not diagnostic. High salt levels in the stomach contents may also be suggestive. The condition may occur in any pig with chronic disease and inability to reach water.

Treatment

Spontaneous recovery may occur. The feed should be replaced and water intake controlled by giving small amounts at first to unaffected pigs and increasing gradually. Convulsing animals should be allowed to recover naturally, as dosing can lead to inhalation pneumonia. Water should be offered and animals may be sprayed with water. Betamethasone (2 mg/kg) may assist recovery and animals should remain in the dark and undisturbed for at least 24 hours.

Control

Ensure that pigs being placed in new pens can find the drinking water and check supplies, particularly in hot and cold weather. When salty rations such as whey and buttermilk are fed, water must be provided *ad lib*.

Reference

Marks, S.L., Carr, J. (1989). Vet.Rec. 125, 460. Water deprivation in weaned pigs.

2. Energy
Neonatal Hypoglycaemia

Definition

This condition arises from restriction of food intake in the neonatal pig and may result in death in convulsions. It may be exacerbated by factors such as low environmental temperature and infection.

Incidence

Common in poorly-heated farrowing houses and may be a predisposing factor in many infectious neonatal conditions. Responsible for 40% of all neonatal piglet mortality in the UK.

Aetiology

The prime cause of this condition is an inadequate intake of milk. This may be due to failure of the sow to provide sufficient milk for a number of reasons, including lack of sufficient functioning mammary glands, failure of secretion in case of agalactia, mastitis or systemic illness or for behavioural reasons. Death of the sow may also precipitate the syndrome in neonatal piglets. Failure of the piglet to suck may occur for a number of reasons, including congenital defects such as cleft palate or nervous signs such as splay leg and congenital tremor, infectious conditions such as colisepticaemia or arthritis and mechanical conditions such as foot damage. The presentation of the sow's udder may also be important as may be competition between piglets. Low environmental temperatures may exacerbate the condition and are very important contributory factors both in the UK and elsewhere.

Pathogenesis

The newborn piglet normally possesses carbohydrate reserves in the form of hepatic glycogen stores (10-14 mg/100 g) and blood glucose levels of 80-100 mg/100 ml (24 hours after birth). Fructose, the foetal blood sugar, is also present (50-60 mg/100 ml) but levels normally decline rapidly. Gluconeogenesis is not efficient until 7 days of age and glycogen reserves become depleted if the milk supply is inadequate. Blood sugar levels then depend upon dietary intake and are unstable. Feeding normally occurs every hour and provides adequate carbohydrate, but, if this pattern is interrupted, blood glucose levels may fall progressively until clinical signs of deficiency appear at a blood-glucose concentration of 50 mg/100 ml.

The original hepatic and muscular glycogen stores may be depleted by delay in parturition. Lower birth weight may cause increased heat loss and difficulty in competing with larger littermates for teats. There is no brown fat so the piglet cannot use fat to generate heat. Low environmental temperature (below 34°C for the single neonate or 25-30°C for the piglet able to huddle) lead to increased utilisation of glycogen reserves in liver and skeletal muscles and to the more rapid development of clinical signs. T.G.E. has also been shown to reduce effective glucose intake and precipitate clinical hypoglycaemia.

Clinical signs

Piglets aged less than 7 days are affected and, at blood glucose levels of 50 mg/100 ml, may show uncertain gait, and later support themselves by placing their noses on the ground and straddling their hind limbs. More severely affected pigs rest on their abdomens but eventually fall on their sides and develop convulsions. These consist of "galloping" of the forelegs, champing and frothing of the jaws in "air hunger" and are accompanied by bradycardia (to 80 beats/min), a decline in rectal temperature, shivering, dullness and, in the earlier stages, a weak squeal. Death normally occurs 24-36 hours after the commencement of the signs.

Animals which have entered a coma from which they cannot be revived by treatment should be killed humanely.

Pathology

Affected pigs have stomachs which are empty or contain a little curd. Blood glucose levels of affected pigs are usually less than 50 mg/100 ml and may be as low as 7 mg/100 ml. Hepatic glycogen is often absent in hypoglycaemic pigs.

Diagnosis

The clinical signs, including the finding of agalactia in the so should lead to consideration of hypoglycaemia.

Other diseases affecting baby pigs should be eliminated, e.g. neonatal septicaemia, neonatal diarrhoea, T.G.E., Aujeszky's disease and bacterial meningitis. Confirmation can be obtained from the response to treatment and from blood glucose and liver glycogen determinations and by response to treatment.

Treatment and prevention

Affected animals should be given i.p. injections of 15 ml of 5% glucose solution every 4-6 hours or oral glucose by stomach tube and kept at a minimum of 30-35°C (85-95°F). If the sow is unable to feed them, an artificial sow milk replacer should be given by stomach tube initially or they should be fostered onto another sow. Reduction in draughts and the provision of dry bedding for piglets may also improve survival.

References

English, P.R. and Morrison, V. (1984). Pig News and Information 5, 369-376. Causes and prevention of piglet mortality.
English, P.R. and Smith, W.J. (1975). Vet.Annual 15, 95-104. Some causes of death in neonatal piglets.

The Thin Sow Syndrome

Definition

A syndrome in which heavy weight loss occurs in sows in lactation and early pregnancy followed by failure to regain weight before farrowing again. This may become progressive and result in poor fertility and eventually emaciation and death.

Incidence

Not uncommon, particularly in stalled sows of lean breeds and in loose housed sows (including outdoor animals) where individual feeding is not practised.

Aetiology

The condition results classically from a combination of parasitism, low environmental temperatures and inadequate feed intake, particularly during lactation. Weight loss at this time may never be regained. Parasitism is less important in current UK systems where therapy is routinely carried out and feed supply to the group or to individuals is most important. Bullying may account for affected individuals but in the UK with its increasing outdoor pig population, low environmental temperatures are important Outdoor sows require at least 200 kg more feed per sow per year than indoor animals. Indoors the best environmental temperature is 22°C for thin sows in sow stalls and 21°C for sows in moderate condition. Any fall in temperature below this will require extra feed to maintain weight gain in gestation. Sow body condition should be condition score 3/4 or 6/10 (fat depth at P2 16-20 mm) at farrowing and may fall to condition score 2-2-5/4 or 4/10 (fat depth P2 12 mm) at the end of lactation. Unless these criteria are met, total weaning weight of the litter will be reduced, return to oestrus will be delayed and egg numbers will be reduced to give small subsequent litters.

Clinical signs

Emaciation in 30-90% of sows and boars in a herd, associated with hypothermia 36.5-38°C (97-100°F), depraved appetites, restlessness, apathy and later, difficulty in rising. The skin may be dirty and greasy and there may be surface abrasions. As the condition progresses, failure to return to oestrus and permanent infertility may occur.

Humane slaughter is only required in extreme cases of emaciation.

Treatment

Anthelminthic treatment should be considered and environmental temperatures restored to normal. Adequate feed intake during lactation and early pregnancy should be designed to maintain weight of the sow and to increase it by 10-15 kg between litters. This may be done by increasing the energy content of lactating rations with fat. It may be necessary to weigh sows after weaning in order to ensure that adequate weight gain has occurred between lactations, to assign them to groups for feeding at an appropriate level throughout pregnancy or to feed individually to condition.

Reference

Kirkwood, R.N., Nutaru, B.N., Gooneratne, A.D., Blair, R., Thacker, P.A. (1988). Canadian J. Animal Science 68, 283-290. The influence of dietary energy intake during successive lactations on sow prolificacy.

3. Protein and Amino Acids

The young weaned and actively-growing pig requires 26% crude protein, at 10 kg which should supply the following levels of essential amino acids: Lysine 1.45%, methionine + cystine 0.5-0.6%, L-isoleucine 0.6%, tryptophan 0.18-0.20%, threonine 0.65-0.7%. These figures do not apply to high performance transgenic pigs or to those receiving porcine somatotrophin in which protein levels of up to 30% may be required. Deficiency of protein or one of the amino acids listed above is first noted as a sub-optimal growth rate in growing pigs. Feed conversion is also less efficient, haemoglobin levels, haematocrit, albumin and serum transferrin levels are all depressed. In sows litter size may be reduced. Analysis of the diet or inclusion of the pure amino acid or a rich source may provide evidence for the causal role of the amino acid. Cystine and methionine deficiency may be a contributory factor in hepatosis dietetica.

4. Minerals

(a) Calcium and Phosphorus

Pig rations should contain at least 0.9% of calcium and 0.7% phosphorus (up to 1% in weaners). High levels of inclusion may be necessary if these minerals are not readily available in the diet. The maximum level of calcium should be 1.0% except for sows where it may reach 1.2%. Absolute or conditioned deficiency of calcium may occur and high phosphorus and low Vitamin D levels may contribute to the latter. Two syndromes are primarily associated with calcium deficiency, rickets in young pigs and osteomalacia in sows.

Rickets in Young Pigs

Definition

A syndrome in which rapidly growing pigs cease to grow, may be anorexic, develop lameness and skeletal changes which result in inability to stand and finally, in death.

Incidence

Rare, only likely to occur when home-mixed rations are grossly inadequate. An inherited form has been described.

Clinical signs

Affected pigs are usually 2-6 months of age, may become stunted, anorexic and lame over a period of weeks. In advanced rickets, animals may have obvious signs of skeletal abnormality, such as swollen joints, especially carpal and tarsal, elbow and stifle joints and bowing of the forelegs. Kyphosis may be obvious and affected pigs may be weak, unable to rise without knuckling and may scream weakly if forced to do so. Champing, frothing at the jaws and signs of depraved appetite may also be noted. Temperatures of 39.2-40°C (102.5-104°F)) are not uncommon. Many affected animals adopt a dog-sitting position.
Severely affected animals unable to walk should be destroyed humanely.

Pathology

The carcases of grossly affected animals are emaciated with changes in the skeletal system. Enlarged epiphyses are common in long bones and distortion or collapse of the soft cancellous bone may occur, particularly at the bearing surface of the joints. Pathological fractures of bones of the limbs or ribs may be present and a 'rachitic rosary' is usually present at the costochondral junctions. Histological lesions include enlargement of the epiphyseal plates and widespread deposition of osteoid and failure of even mineralisation. In less severe cases, microscopic lesions may be the only sign that disturbances in ossification are occurring.

Diagnosis

The clinical signs of rickets are distinctive and X-ray examination of bones or post-mortem examination will confirm poor mineralisation. History and the composition of the diet are of value. Plasma calcium levels may vary from 1.58 m mol/1-2.5 m mol/l (normal). Low calcium levels in feed and plasma may suggest primary calcium deficiency but Vitamin D levels in plasma are difficult to obtain in the UK. and a diagnosis of rickets due to Vitamin D deficiency may only be obtained by consideration of the amount entering the diet (minimum requirement 6-11 i.u./kg liveweight/day). Plasma phosphorus levels are low (less than 2.24 m mol/l) in Vitamin D and phosphorus deficiency. The condition must be differentiated from septic arthritis, by the absence of heat and pain in joints, from *M.hyosynoviae* infection (age affected and bony lesions) and osteochondrosis (reduced growth rate).

Treatment

Ensure that the calcium, phosphorus and Vitamin D levels of the finished ration are adequate. Injection of Vitamin D should not be considered until the composition of the ration has been restored to normal for some days. Animals with lesions which include pathological fractures are unlikely to recover or be economic to fatten and should be destroyed.

References

Pepper, T.A., Bennett, D., Taylor, D.J. (1978). Vet.Rec. 103, 4-8. Rickets in growing pigs and response to treatment.
Thompson, K.G., Robinson B.M. (1989). New Zealand Vet.J. 37, 155-157. An osteodystrophy apparently caused by vitamin D deficiency in growing pigs.

Growth depression

Growing pigs fed diets containing Ca:Pratios greater than 2.5:1.0 have reduced daily gain.

Hypocalcaemia and Osteomalacia in Sows

Definition

Hypocalcaemia may result in sudden death at farrowing, protracted farrowings, uterine prolapse and muscular weakness resulting in the adoption of the 'dog sitting' position. It may be accompanied by fever and respiratory distress at this time.

Incidence

May be common but rarely recognised because of lack of sampling of blood calcium levels in farrowing sows.

Aetiology and pathogenesis

Hypocalcaemia results primarily from low levels of calcium in the ration or its poor availability because of high phosphorus levels or some other reason. Commercial sow diets may contain low levels of calcium and some inclusion rates may be too low. Minimum figures of 0.6% have been considered adequate, but on low cost diets based on vegetable protein, this may be inadequate and a level of at least 0.9% and as much as 1.2% may be required. Low levels of dietary calcium lead to inadequate skeletal mineralisation and inadequate mobilisable calcium reserves at times of peak demand such as farrowing or late lactation. Lowered plasma calcium (normal is 2.5-2.7 m.mol/l in a normal modern hybrid sow) may lead to muscular weakness and problems with cardiac and myometrial function. In heavily lactating young sows or gilts with poor skeletal calcium reserves, this poor calcium status may be sufficient to allow pathological fractures of pelvic bones, femur or, more commonly, the vertebrae of the lumbosacral region. Osteodystrophia fibrosa may also occur and lead to changes in the alignment of the facial bones. Bone mineralisation may decline following restricted exercise.

Clinical signs

Sudden deaths in farrowing sows and the occurrence of a high incidence of prolapsed uteri or weakness and respiratory distress and fever may occur. Affected sows or gilts are usually unable to move their hind limbs and remain sitting or show degrees of posterior paralysis or lameness. Where broken bones are present, crepitus may be felt but the animals frequently guards the break with muscular rigidity or spasm and detection is difficult.

In some cases a large litter will be sucking. Occasionally newly-purchased gilts or boars mixed in yards or even finishing pigs will also be affected. Low blood calcium levels (2.0 m.mol/l) are present. Alkaline phosphatase levels are often raised.

Where broken bones are identified, or where animals are unable to rise within 1 hour of treatment, pigs should be humanely destroyed without moving them from the site.

Pathology

Few changes may be seen in animals which die suddenly but in those which have had osteomalacia, brittle bones, with thin cortices and pathological fractures especially of vertebral bodies may be seen. Bone ash levels in rib bones confirm hypocalcaemia.

Diagnosis

The clinical signs of spontaneous fractures, farrowing difficulties or of sows in a dog-sitting position with weakness of the hindlimbs are suggestive. Hypocalcaemia should also be considered in sudden death at this stage. Low plasma calcium levels, low calcium levels in bone ash from tibial bone biopsies, and a low calcium level in the feed will confirm. Post-mortem examination will allow differentiation of animals with pathological fractures from spinal abscess etc. In sudden death, bone ash will confirm a low calcium status and lesions of gastric torsion, *C.novyi* infection, endocarditis etc. should be obvious. Pigs may develop the dog-sitting position and pathological fractures following electrocution.

Treatment

Intravenous calcium borogluconate will restore affected sows to clinical normality and may need to be supplemented by subcutaneous injections. These should be given to all sows farrowing before the calcium level of the rations can be restored to 1-1.2%. Cull sows unable to rise as soon as practicable.

References

Ayliffe, T.R. and Noakes, D.E. (1985). J.Vet.Pharm. and Therapeutics 8, 212-214. The effect of oxytocin on the myometrium of the sow during experimentally induced hypocalcamia.
Combs, N.R., Kornegay, E.T., Lindemann, D.R., Welker, F.H. (1991). J.Anim.Sci. 69, 664-672. Evaluation of a bone biopsy technique for determining the calcium and phosphorus ratio of swine from weaning to market weight.
Jennings, D.S. (1985). Proc.Pig Vet.Soc. 14, 38-40. Hypocalcaemia in sows.

Maxson, P.F., Mahan, D.C. (1986). J.Animal Science 63, 1163-1172. Dietary calcium and phosphorus for lactating swine at high and average production levels.

b) Iron

Piglet Anaemia

Definition

A hypochromic microcytic anaemia of rapidly-growing piglets housed on concrete which results in poor performance and in the deaths of severely-affected animals. It is caused by a primary deficiency of iron in the diet.

Incidence

Rare under modern husbandry conditions but may occur in individual litters or where oral iron dosing is accompanied by diarrhoea. Subclinical disease may occur in outdoor pigs.

Aetiology and pathogenesis

The piglet is born with limited reserves of iron and copper and has a blood haemoglobin level of 12 g/100 ml at birth. Within the first 10 days of life, a physiological decline in blood haemoglobin levels to 8 g/100 ml occurs and the correct level is subsequently regained in normal healthy piglets with adequate available dietary iron.

During the first 4 weeks of life, the body weight of piglets may increase five-fold and active haemopoiesis is essential if the normal blood haemoglobin levels of 120-140 g/l are to be regained after the physiological fall. The dietary requirement for iron during this period of life is 15 mg/day, but only 1 mg/day can be supplied by the sow's milk in spite of supplementation of her diet with iron. The remaining requirement is supplied by iron present in the soil ingested by all piglets kept in extensive husbandry systems.

Where animals are farrowed and reared on concrete or outside on iron-free soil confined in soil-free creep areas, the requirement for iron outstrips the supply and a hypochromic microcytic anaemia develops as the blood haemoblobin levels continue to fall below the physiological low of 80 g/l. They may fall as low as 35 g/l by the age of 3-4 weeks. After this, the intake of creep feed becomes sufficient to supply the dietary requirement for iron and the blood haemoglobin levels normally begin to rise again in deficient pigs. Iron deficiency may reduce gastric and intestinal enzyme secretion and reduce neutrophil levels.

Clinical signs

The clinical signs appear most commonly in piglets of 3 weeks of age, by which time a severe anaemia may have developed, particularly in pigs in good condition.

Affected pigs may be plump, although their growth rate is up to 10% less than that of normal pigs. They appear pale, the ears, belly and the mucosae may be yellowish in colour. There may be oedema of the head and forequarters. Thin, pale, hairy pigs are more commonly seen. Diarrhoea is common, but the faeces are normal in colour. Affected pigs are lethargic and when disturbed, show dyspnoea and a prominent apex beat. Severely-affected piglets may die suddenly. Not all pigs in an iron-deficient litter may show clinical signs of the disease.

Humane slaughter is only indicated when animals are emaciated.

Post mortem findings

The carcases of affected pigs are pale, with thin watery blood and oedema of the muscles. Fluid exudates in the body cavities are common. The liver is enlarged in all cases and is a mottled greyish-yellow colour, due to fatty change. The heart is flabby and enlarged and there may be signs of enteritis.

Diagnosis

Diagnosis in piglets is based on the clinical signs outlined above and upon the history of no access to iron. Thrombocytopaenic purpura may also produce pallor and anaemia, but often produces jaundice. Navel bleeding and haemorrhage from castration, tail docking or internal injury may also occur. These are often individual rather than herd problems. Infections such as *C.perfringens* Type C and coccidiosis can cause anaemia as a result of blood loss. In older pigs pallor and anaemia can result from a number of conditions including bleeding from wounds, as a result of warfarin poisoning, gastric ulceration, proliferative intestinal adenopathy and a number of other conditions.

The diagnosis may be confirmed in piglets by the finding of low blood haemoglobin levels (below 70 g/l) in the third week of age and, in clinically affected animals, 40 g/l or less. A better indication is the red cell count which is less than 5 million per µl, and may be as low as 3 million per µl. The red cells are hypochromic and reduced in size. A rapid method of assay is to bleed from an ear vein into haematocrit tubes. Anaemic pigs may have a haematocrit of 10% or less compared with the normal 28-30%.

Treatment and control

Supplementation of the sow's diet cannot raise piglets' liver iron levels at birth or increase the amount of iron in the milk so piglets must be provided with 15 mg of iron per day to prevent the occurrence of anaemia. This may be provided in the following ways:

(i)   Intramuscular injection with iron dextran complex,
       or gleptoferron or other chelates

This is the most satisfactory method of prevention and treatment. For prevention, piglets should be injected in the neck rather than the hind limb at 1-3 days of age with at least, 200 mg of elemental iron. As the available preparations differ in their iron content, always follow the manufacturer's recommendations; 2 ml is the most common dose. Recently 200 mg in 1 ml have been given into the neck muscles where 3 week weaning is practised.

None of the preparations at present on the UK market appear to cause adverse reactions, but animals which have died may show yellowish staining of the hind limb muscles and brownish inguinal lymph nodes for some time after the injection in the hindlimb. This is normal. Fatal reaction to iron injections may indicate a low selenium or Vitamin E status in the piglets. Some preparations also contain cyanocobalamin (Vitamin B12) as an additional aid to haemopoiesis. Injection should be delayed during clinical infection ith PRRS.

(ii)   Oral iron supplements

Iron preparations are available in several forms, some of which are pastes containing various forms of reduced iron, usually as the citrate or fumarate given by individual oral dosing to piglets at birth and 14 days of age.

Granules containing iron dextran may also be given under lamps in the creep feed and pastes containing iron dextrans are also available for oral therapy. Recently soluble products for water medication have been used in piglet drinkers. In a few cases, farmers may wish to provide iron by including soil, peat or coal in the pen. The oral preparations suffer from the disadvantages that they may be missed out, that they are labour intensive, that, if given when diarrhoea is occurring, the iron may not be absorbed and that, if given in excess, they may cause diarrhoea. This is especially so with crude ferrous sulphate which may still be in use on some farms. Recent studies have suggested that supplementation of the sows' feed with iron allows the piglets to ingest sufficient iron from her faeces of which they eat approximately 10 g per day. This practice has recently been shown to produce uneven uptake and to be inferior to parenteral administration.

(iii)   Complex iron: copper deficiency

If iron therapy alone does not appear to cure the condition, copper supplementation may be necessary in addition. This is an unusual occurrence and is rarely necessary.

References

Caperna, T.J., Failla, M.L., Steele, N.C., Richards, M.P. (1987). J. Nutrition 117, 312-320. Accumulation and metabolism of iron dextran by hepatocytes, Kupffer cells and endothelial cells in the neonatal pig liver.
Daykin, M.M., Griffiths, A.J., Towlerton, R.G., (1982). Vet. Rec. 110. 535-537. Evaluation of the parenteral iron requirement of early weaned pigs.
Gleed, P.T., Sansom, B.F. (1982). Vet.Rec. 111, 136-139. Effects of feeding lactating sows on iron rich diet on piglet haematology and growth rates.
Larkin, H.A. and Hannan, J. (1983). Res. in Vet.Sci. 34, 11-15. Gastric structure and function in iron deficient piglets.
Larkin, H.A. and Hannan, J. (1984). Res. in Vet.Sci. 36, 199-204. Intestinal absorption and structure in iron deficienct piglets.

Excess iron

High levels of iron in the diet may reduce phosphorus absorption and result in rickets in growing piglets, so iron levels should not exceed 4 g/Kg.

c)   Copper

Few clinical signs other than anaemia, an increase in stillbirths, leg weakness, paresis/paralysis and ataxia have been directly related to copper deficiency, but experimental studies demonstrate cardiac enlargement, associated with failure to cross-link new collagen, increases in mitochondrial numbers and accumulations of glycogen.

Copper is commonly included (usually as copper sulphate) in growing pig rations at levels of 50-175 ppm. Copper, iron and zinc metabolism are linked and high levels of zinc may reduce liver copper as may iron. Copper toxicity may occur at 500 ppm or more and clinical signs include inappetence, depression of condition and weight gain, jaundice and the accumulation of copper in the hepatocytes of the liver which is yellow brown and fragile.

References

Pletcher, J.M. and Banting, L.F. (1983). J.South African Vet.Assn. 54, 43-46. Ataxia and posterior paresis in copper deficient weaners.

Pritchard, G.C., Lewis, G., Wells, G.A.H. and Stopforth, A. (1985). Vet.Rec. 117, 545-548. Zinc toxicity, copper deficiency and anaemia in swill fed pigs.

(d) Zinc

Parakeratosis of Swine

An absolute or conditioned deficiency of dietary zinc may result in depression of growth and the development of non-inflammatory proliferative lesions of the epidermis resulting in hyperkeratisation.

Incidence

May occur in subclinical forms in rapidly-growing pigs. The overt clinical form is rare.

Aetiology

Zinc may be deficient in the diet but in most cases absorption is inadequate due to interference from high levels of dietary phytic acid from soya, or wheat bran or from calcium. Rapid growth, low dietary concentrations of unsaturated fatty acids, dry feeding *ad libitum* and infections resulting in diarrhoea and malabsorption may all precipitate the condition.

Supplementation of the diet with linolenic acid appears to prevent the condition; zinc deficiency may produce its effect by reducing the biosynthesis of essential fatty acids and appears to produce its skin effects by damage to desmosomes linking cells and reducing keratohyalin synthesis.

Clinical signs

The condition occurs in pigs 2-4 months of age and is associated with depression of the rate of growth. Small erythematous areas develop on the ventral surface of the abdomen and inside the thigh. They become papules and then become elevated and scaly. The pastern, fetlock, knee and hock develop these crusty lesions which may spread to the shoulders and other areas of the body. Lesions are symmetrically distributed and are usually dry and crumbly. Cracking may occur, resulting in exudation of serum and secondary infection. Irritation is not a feature of this condition. Growth may be depressed and feed conversion efficiency reduced. Plasma levels down to 7.5 µg/ml may be found. Long-term feeding studies suggest that the effect of deficiency on reproduction is to increase problems at farrowing, more stillborn piglets and lower litter weights to 2 weeks of age.

Pathology

Changes are restricted to the skin. There is a subacute to chronic non-inflammatory change in all layers of the skin except for the stratum lucidum. Keratinization is incomplete and the stratum corneum is irregularly thickened and the cells within it retain their nuclei. The rete pegs penetrate more deeply into the dermis, there is an increase in the number of basal cells and dilation of the sweat glands and hypertrophy of sebaceous glands occurs. Parakeratosis of the oesophagus has been described in experimental situations and may occasionally be seen in natural cases.

Diagnosis

The age of the pigs affected and the distribution, texture and appearance of the lesions is suggestive of zinc deficiency. A skin biopsy may be of value in confirming diagnosis, serum zinc and alkaline phosphatase levels may be low. The lack of irritation and the absence of mites from skin scrapings differentiate the condition from sarcoptic mange. Exudative epidermitis usually occurs in younger pigs and is often associated with mortality.

Treatment

A dietary level of zinc of 100 ppm will restore health within 10-40 days. Supplementation of the rations with zinc carbonate, or sulphate should not exceed 200 ppm final zinc concentration. Toxicity due to excess zinc in the ration is difficult to produce as the diet is refused at high zinc levels but may be associated with copper deficiency. The pharmacological use of zinc oxide to 5,000 ppm does not appear to cause toxicity.

References

Hill, G.M., Miller, E.R. and Stowe, H.D. (1983). J.Anim.Sci. 57, 114-122. Effects of dietary zinc levels on sows' health and productivity of gilts and through two parities.
Hain, J.D., Baker, D.H. (1993). J.Anim.Sci. 71, 3020-3024. Growth and plasma zinc responses of young pigs fed pharmacologic levels of zinc.
Kalinowski, J. and Chavez, E.R. (1986). Canadian J.Animal Sci., 66, 201-216. Low dietary zinc intake during pregnancy and lactation in gilts.

(e)   Selenium

(i)   Deficiency

Cereals grown in selenium-deficient soils and some cereal varieties may contain less than the optimum level of selenium for animal growth. The addition of selenium to such diets to give a final concentration of 0.8-1.1 ppm increases growth rates in weaned pigs and reduces the incidence of hepatosis dietetica, diarrhoea, gastric ulceration and iron toxicity following iron injections. Selenium uptake is most efficient in the organic form (as methionine Se, cysteine Se) but inorganic selenium can also be absorbed.

Selenium levels in plasma are related to plasma glutathione peroxidase (GSH Px) activity and low levels of this enzyme indicate selenium deficiency. Serum levels of less than 0.025 ug/ml and liver levels of less than 0.10 mg/kg indicate selenium deficiency.

Studies of glutathione peroxidase levels suggest that selenium uptake may be inhibited by wheat bran and selenium excretion may be reduced by riboflavin in the ration. A genetic predisposition to low blood selenium has been detected and normal blood selenium levels fall at about 3 weeks of age in the absence of supplementation. Lesions of selenium deficiency are similar to those associated with Vitamin E deficiency and the complex is considered below under Vitamin E deficiency.

(ii)   Selenium toxicity

High levels of selenium in the diet may arise through the consumption of poisonous plants such as *Astragalus sp* and, more commonly, through the erroneous inclusion of high levels of selenium in mineral and vitamin premixes for pigs. Levels greter than 5-6 mg/kg (5 g/tonne) may induce toxicity and levels of 6.2, 8.1 and 17.2 mg/kg respectively were toxic when given to growing pigs. Earliest signs include reduction in feed intake followed by foelimb weakness, tremor, hyperaesthesis, recumbency, paresis and death. Hair loss and cracking of the hooves may be seen in chronic cases. Sows fed 2 mg/kg for the last part of gestation produced litters with high levels of stillbirths, and pre-weaning losses and piglets had haemorrhagic lesions of the anterior wall or sole of the feet. Animals which are recumbent should be destroyed humanely.

Affected animals have a polio encephalomalacia and lesions affecting the ventral grey matter. High levels of tissue selenium can be demonstrated (normal liver 0.7-1.8 mg/kg dry matter, kidney 5.0-11.5 mg/kg).

Withdrawal of toxic feed is the only appropriate treatment. Recovery from nervous signs in mobile pigs may taken 2 months.

Reference

Chavez, E.R. (1989). Pig News and Information 10, 167-171. Selenium nutrition of pigs; a review.

Mensink, C.G., Koeman, J.P., Veling, J., Gruys, E. (1990). Vet.Rec. 126, 620-622. Haemorrhagic claw lesions in newborn piglets due to selenium toxicosis during pregnancy.

Oldfield, J.E. (1985). Pig News and Information 6, 419-424. Some implications of selenium in pig nutrition.

Stave, H.D., Eavey, A.J. Granger, L., Halstead, S., Yamini, B. (1992). J.Am.Vet.Med.Assoc. 201, 292-295. Selenium toxicosis in feeder pigs.

5. Fats

A deficiency of essential fatty acids may result in the development of a scaly skin, particularly in adults. A weekly dose of cod-liver oil (10 ml per animal) is usually sufficient to correct this. The minimum levels of linolenic and arachidonic acids are given in Table C. These acids may also be essential for adequate prostaglandin formation. Indigestible fats in poor quality waste fat may result in diarrhoea when they are incorporated in feeds at high levels.

6. Vitamins

Vitamin A (Retinol) Deficiency

Definition

The absence of Vitamin A from the diet, its presence at low levels or poor absorption of the vitamin causes infertility and the birth of weak or non-viable piglets with congenital defects to sows with poor body reserves of the vitamin. Nervous signs, skin changes and reduction in the rate of bone growth may all occur in growing pigs.

Incidence

Rare now, but may occur in herds where home-mixed rations are given. Subclinical disease may be more common.

Aetiology and pathogenesis

Vitamin A is normally included in pig rations at levels of 3-9 million i.u. per tonne and can be produced in the liver from dietary carotene obtained from grass meal or fresh yellow maize. The presence of unsaturated fatty acids in the ration and the pelleting of feed may cause the destruction of Vitamin A incorporated in the ration and lead to the presence of low dietary levels of the vitamin. Vitamin A is necessary for the formation of visual purple, for normal bone growth, especially the remodelling of bones, for the normal development and function of secretory and epithelial cells and for normal embryological development. Uncontrolled bone growth in the spinal cord and cranium produces nervous signs associated with a rise in C.S.F. pressure. Clinical signs appear after 4-5 months on a deficient ration.

Clinical signs

Nervous signs such as incoordination, tilting of the head and eventual paralysis of the hind limbs with dog-sitting occur in growing pigs in which skin changes, especially splitting of the tips of the bristles, may occur. Sows, and, in particular, gilts, may produce stillborn or moribund piglets at full term in the most severe form of the disease. Stillborn piglets may have ascites and moribund animals are listless, weak and lie on their sides around the sow, making weak, paddling movements and squawking plaintively. Stronger animals may burrow in the bedding. Eye changes may be seen ranging from microphthalmia in all moribund piglets to minor iris or sclera defects in mildly affected animals.
Animals unable to walk should be destroyed humanely.

Pathology

In young growing pigs with posterior paralysis, demyelination of the spinal cord may be found. Signs that increased intracranial pressure may have occurred may also be present. In congenitally-affected piglets, oedema of the subcutaneous tissues is prominent and the body cavities are filled with sero-fibrinous fluid. Kidney abnormalities are common and the livers are yellowish grey (stillborn) or congested (moribund). Cerebellar hypoplasia and cardiac defects have been recorded. Plasma Vitamin A levels should exceed 7-8 ug (15-20 i.u.) per 100 ml. Normal sera contain about 23 ug (50-60 i.u.) per 100 ml. Liver should contain 60 ug (120-130 i.u.) per g, but clinical signs may not develop until levels of 2-5 ug (4-10 i.u.) per g are reached. C.S.F. pressures, normally 80-125 mm water rise to 200 mm or above.

Diagnosis

Based on history of home-mixed rations with no added Vitamin A, clinical and post-mortem findings and confirmed by analysis of liver biopsies or samples for Vitamin A.

Treatment and control

Commercial rations normally contain adequate Vitamin A, but home-mixed feed should be examined for Vitamin A content. If the condition is diagnosed, affected animals or those at risk can be treated parenterally with fat-soluble vitamins. Parenteral multivitamin and oral supplements also exist. Dose according to data sheet.

References

Brief, S., Chew, B.P. (1985). J.Anim.Sci. 60, 998-1004. Effects of Vitamin A and B carotene reproductive performance in gilts.
Goodwin, R.F.W. and Jennings, A.R. (1958). J.Comp.Path. 68, 82-95. Mortality of newborn pigs associated with a maternal deficiency of Vitamin A.

Vitamin A toxicity

If Vitamin A levels in the ration are high for long periods of time, lameness, decreased bone weight and depression of performance may occur. Diarrhoea has been described with short limbs, reduced long bone length flattening and caudal rotation of the humeral head and distal femoral condyles with narrow metaphyseal growth plates in the vertebrae. Liver Vitamin A levels are high.

Reference

Doige, C.E., Schoonderwoerd, M. (1988). J.Am.Vet.Med.Ass. 193, 691-693. Dwarfism in a swine herd : suspected Vitamin A toxicosis.

Vitamin D

Rickets

Rickets has been discussed under hypocalcaemia, but, if dietary calcium and phosphorus levels are adequate, treatment with parenteral ADE preparations such as those listed above, may be used as an aid to recovery. When high levels are fed, metastatic calcification may occur in kidneys, lung and heart, and it may be lethal or lead to depression of growth. A hereditary form of rickets has been described (see Congenital and Hereditary Conditions).

References

Pepper, T.A., Bennett, D., Taylor, D.J. (1989). Vet.Rec. 103, 4-8. Rickets in growing pigs and response to treatment.
Thompson, K.G., Robinson, B.M. (1988). New Zealand Vet.J. 37, 155-157. An osteodystrophy apparently caused by Vitamin D deficiency in growing pigs.

Vitamin E

Vitamin E Deficiency

Definition

Low dietary levels of Vitamin E (alpha tocopherol) are associated with a number of syndromes including hepatosis dietetica, nutritional muscular dystrophy (white muscle disease), mulberry heart disease, hertztod, yellow fat disease and infertility.

Aetiology

Caused by a deficiency of Vitamin E in the ration and exacerbated by low selenium, methionine and cystine levels and high fat levels in the diet. Oxidised fat, copper and the wet storage of cereals may all reduce the Vitamin E levels of diets. Only alpha tocopherol can be used by the pig and the descriptions which follow relate to this form of Vitamin E.

Pathogenesis

Alpha tocopherol acts both as an antioxidant and as a stabiliser of membrane lipids. It becomes bound to the membranes of mitochondria and microsomes. A specific loss of membrane bound arachidonic and linolenic acids occurs in Vitamin E deficiency and this is associated with low dietary levels of these acids. Selenium is related to this process in that it forms part of glutathione peroxidase, an enzyme which acts on oxidised polyunsaturated fatty acid radicals. Selenium therefore has a sparing effect on Vitamin E, the action of which in turn is related to methionine and cystine levels. Vitamin A is also spared by Vitamin E and is more rapidly destroyed in its absence. The major clinical signs of this complex deficiency appear to result from the effects on energy metabolism. The cells most severely affected in the pig are hepatocytes and muscle cells in the heart and skeletal muscles.

Vitamin E is normally present in cereal grains but can be destroyed if polyunsaturated fats, e.g. from fish oils, linseed oil or, mouldy or spoiled grain are included in the ration. Propionic acid treatment of barley may be important in the aetiology of the condition in the UK. The presence of low levels of selenium in grain grown on selenium deficient soils may exacerbate the condition and the now common practice of adding high levels of fat to rations may also be important.

Clinical signs

Sudden death is most commonly seen. Piglets affected by muscular dystrophy may be dyspnoeic with normal body temperature and no signs of enteritis. Clinical signs may appear in a few piglets in a litter at about 2 weeks of age. In older pigs, sudden deaths may occur after handling and affected animals within a group may show some signs of circulatory embarrassment such as lethargy, cyanosis and dejection. Muscle tremor may occur, especially at the shoulders. There may be stiffness, a limp or recumbency. In conditions such as dietosis hepatica and herztod, there may be evidence of poor growth rate. Anaemia may develop. Low levels of dietary Vitamin E may also depress fertility, increasing weaning to service intervals and reducing the percentage of returns to oestrus.

Affected pigs are rarely observed in life so humane slaughter is not usually required.

Pathology

Affected piglets with muscular dystrophy are in good condition and there may be some oedema of the subcutaneous tissues and pericardial fluid is commonly found. There is pulmonary oedema and the heart is enlarged. Pale, yellowish streaks are usually present on the ventricular walls. Fresh haemorrhagic streaks may be seen beneath the endocardium. The liver may be pale and there may be excess peritoneal fluid.

In older pigs, post-mortem features include heart lesions resembling those in piglets, necrosis of the liver which is pale and mottled or haemorrhagic. In long-standing cases where methionine and cystine deficiency may also occur, regeneration of liver lobules may be seen on the surface as reddish spots or tags in a yellowish liver. Rupture of the liver may occur, there may be an obvious fissure with an attached blood clot and the abdomen may be filled with blood. Gastric ulceration may be prominent. Oedema of the mesentery of the colon may be present. Muscles, especially the adductor muscle group in the hind limb, may be white or pale in colour. Lesions are often symmetrical.

Adipose tissue may be yellow (steatitis or yellow fat disease). The liver changes are often described as "hepatosis dietetica".

Histological findings include hyaline degeneration of individual muscle fibres both in the myocardium and in the longissimus dorsi, leg muscles, diaphragm and intercostal muscles. Where lesions precede degeneration of the arterioles and the presence of microthrombi may be seen, particularly in the cardiac muscle and in the liver.

Diagnosis

The clinical signs and post-mortem findings may suggest a diagnosis of one of the entities associated with Vitamin E deficiency (see hepatosis dietetica and mulberry heart). Confirmation depends on the demonstration of low dietary levels of alpha tocopherol. A level of 10 i.u. (60 mg)/kg dry matter [10,000 i.u. (60 g) per tonne] is considered adequate in sow feed and a minimum of 15 i.u. (5 mg)/kg dry matter (1,500 i.u. (5g) per tonne) in rations for pigs up to 90 kg. Histories of storage of grain in propionic acid, etc. are suggestive.

Levels of serum enzymes such as S.G.O.T., creatinine phosphokinase, ornithine carbamyl transferase and lactic dehydrogenase may all be raised in affected animals. Response to alpha tocopherol treatment is confirmatory although selenium may also have some effect.

Treatment

Parenteral treatment with alpha tocopherol or alpha tocopherol-selenium preparations is of value in affected groups of animals. Vitamin E is also available as a component of the fat soluble vitamin mixtures. Pregnant sows may be injected in order to reduce mortality in their litters, but for a period of 3-4 weeks, newborn piglets should be treated at birth until increased feed levels of the vitamin have raised maternal and foetal alpha tocopherol levels.

Control depends upon ensuring that adequate levels of dietary Vitamin E are present in the final ration. The suggestion that Vitamin E should be included at five times the fat percentage of the ration measured in mg/kg feed is usually adequate, but actively oxidising fats may need up to 20 times the fat percentage.

Vitamin E/Selenium Deficiency Related Syndromes

1. Steatitis (Yellow Fat Disease).

Yellow-brown discolouration of the fat may be seen in pigs at post-mortem examination or slaughter. This is due to the inclusion of high levels of unsaturated fatty acids in the feed (often swill) with a low level of Vitamin E. Vitamin E supplementation prevents the problem.

2. Hepatosis dietetica

This may occur in young growing pigs usually 3-4 months of age. Affected pigs may be depressed, vomit or stagger but are usually found dead. At post-mortem examination the livers are enlarged, mottled and may have bled into the peritoneal cavity. The lesions appear to be lobular in section with pale, haemorrhagic and apparently normal lobules. Microangiopathy underlies the changes and there may be evidence of muscular dystrophy.

The condition is associated with selenium deficiency more closely than with Vitamin E but both substances may be deficient and rations should be examined for both. A vegetable protein source such as soya and the use of high percentages of wheat offals with associated selenium-retaining bran and high fat may all predispose. Treatment by injection and then by correct ration formulation should be carried out.

3.   Mulberry Heart Disease

Definition

A syndrome in which acute heart failure and sudden death occur sporadically, usually in large fattening pigs with no history of stress. It can, however, occur in pigs from birth to adulthood.

Incidence

Common in Britain at present, occurs in some herds as sporadic deaths, particularly when least cost rations are used.

Aetiology and pathogenesis

Feeding propionic-acid-treated barley appears to predispose to the condition and Vitamin E deficiency appears to be involved. Toxic products of bacteria may contribute to the syndrome. Heredity may play a part as Landrace pigs have been said to be susceptible. In most cases selenium levels appear to be normal but tissue Vitamin E levels are low even when dietary levels are apparently adequate. The syndrome develops as a result of congestive heart failure, coupled with hydropericardium.

Clinical signs

Pigs of any age may be affected, but the condition occurs commonly in 20-50 kg animals. Affected pigs are anorexic and depressed with muscle weakness and lowered body temperature. They may become cyanotic before death which occurs within 24 hours of the onset of the clinical signs. Recovery has been recorded, but mortality is usually 100%. Humane slaughter is rarely possible.

Pathology

The carcase is usually in good condition with fluid and shreds of fibrin in all body cavities. The liver is enlarged and mottled. The pericardial cavity is full of gelatinous fluid and fibrin and the surface of the heart is streaked with haemorrhages running from base to apex. Similar haemorrhages occur in the endocardium. They lie immediately below the membrane and appear histologically as areas of free red cells with no obvious myonecrosis. Microangiopathy may be present and in most cases degeneration of the muscles may also be present (see Vitamin E).

Diagnosis

The heart lesions are characteristic. Bowel oedema, *Actinobacillus pleuropneumoniae* and *Streptococcus suis* Type II infection may also cause sudden death with fluid or fibrin in body cavities. Death from the porcine stress syndrome usually follows exertion. The histopathology and liver Vitamin E analysis usually confirm.

Treatment and control

The use of high levels of Vitamin E (2-3 times the recommended levels) prevents the development of the condition and implies a Vitamin E deficiency. Parenteral Vitamin E alone or with selenium may be used to treat animals in affected groups. Vitamin E may be restored to normal within a few hours by injection but may take 2 weeks by feed supplementation.

References

Kirby, P.S. (1981). Vet.Rec. 109, 385. Steatitis in fattening pigs.
Mortimer, D.T. (1983). Vet.Rec. 112, 278-279. Vitamin E/selenium deficiency syndrome in pigs.
Putnam, M.E. (1982). Proc.Pig Vet.Soc. 9, 178-183. Vitamin E for pigs.
Vleet, J.F. van. (1982). Am.J.Vet.Res. 43, 1180-1189. Comparative efficacy of five supplementation procedures to control Vitamin E selenium deficiency in swine.

Vitamin K.

Clinical disease associated with deficiency of this vitamin has been recorded in 5-6 week old pigs 1-2 weeks after weaning. Pigs were fed on rations without added Vitamin K and in one case housed in a flat-deck. Antimicrobials, including sulphadimidine, were being fed at therapeutic levels. Sulphadimidine is a Vitamin K antagonist and flat-deck housing prevents the consumption of faeces containing Vitamin K2 synthesised by intestinal microflora. Affected pigs fail to grow and develop subcutaneous haematomas, prolonged bleeding times, lameness and swelling of joints. Some became pale and some died (to 20% mortality).

The condition can be reproduced experimentally by feeding weaned piglets a low Vitamin K diet containing sulphadimidine (with or without other antibiotics) and housing them on wire. Defects in coagulation appeared after 35 days and the condition after 64 days. Conditioned deficiencies may also occur in coumarol/warfarin poisoning, and calcium excess and the condition must also be distinguished from mycotoxicosis.

Treatment with oral and injectable Vitamin K (l0 g menadione bisulphite per tonne or one i/m injection of 20 mg Vitamin K1 per piglet) provide treatment or prophylaxis.

Reference:

Newsholme, S.J., Cullen, J.S.C., Nel, P.W., Peyers, F. (1985). J.South African Vet.Ass. 56, 101-102. A haemorrhagic syndrome in recently weaned pigs ascribed to hypovitaminosis K.

Water soluble vitamins

Thiamine (Vitamin B1) Deficiency

Not likely to occur under natural conditions as a single entity unless pigs are fed rations containing large amounts of heat-treated carbohydrate, e.g. bakery waste in swill to which no balancer has been added. Up to 47% of thiamine requirements are met by bacterial synthesis in the gut. Requirements may be increased by high ambient temperatures and reduced by high fat concentrations in the diet. Thiaminases from bracken fern fronds or rhizomes

(*Pteridium aquilinum*) can cause death after sows have grazed infested pastures for 10 weeks but other thiaminases in food can cause disease.

Clinical signs include inappetence, poor growth rate, emaciation, a fall in temperature and respiratory rate resulting in death within 5 weeks from congestive cardiac failure in experimental conditions. There is cyanosis of the skin and mucous membranes. Sudden death, vomiting and depression have been reported in bracken poisoning. The post-mortem findings include enlargement of the heart, myocardial degeneration and fibrosis, pulmonary oedema, pleural effusion, pleurisy and pleural fibrosis. The thiamine status of pigs can be monitored by the levels of erythrocyte transketolase present. In deficiency they are low. Affected pigs may be treated with thiamine by injection.

References

Edwards, B.L. (1983). Vet.Rec. 112, 459-460. Poisoning .by *Pteridium aquilinum* in pregnant sows.
Lund, L.J. (1985). Proc.Pig Vet.Soc. 13, 96-97. Bracken poisoning in sows.
Gibson, D.M., Kenelly, J.J., Aherne, F.X. (1987). Canadian J.Anim.Sci. 67, 841-854. The thiamine status of pigs fed sulphur dioxide treated high moisture barley.

Riboflavin (Vitamin B2 Deficiency)

Clinical signs

Slow growth, some lameness, frequent diarrhoea, conjunctivitis, skin changes such as alopecia and matting of the hair with sebaceous secretions may be seen in growing pigs. Irregular oestrus, delayed oestrus and, eventually, anoestrus have been reported in deficiency in sows. Erythrocyte glutathione reductase levels appear to reflect riboflavine status and a 50% decline in active enzyme occurs before other deficiency signs appear. The birth of piglets with oedema of the forelegs has been recorded where sows have received deficient diets. Inclusion of 2.5g of riboflavine per tonne of feed prevent deficiency in fatteners but 3.2-3.3g/tonne may be required for pregnant sow rations.

Affected piglets should be killed humanely.

Niacin or Nicotinic Acid Deficiency

May occur when diets are fed in which maize, low in tryphophan (a nicotinamide precursor) and niacin itself, is the major ingredient.

In some cases the syndrome has been reported to result from the ingestion of antimetabolites such as 6 amino nicotinamide.

Clinical signs

These include inappetence, persistent diarrhoea and a dirty yellow skin with dermatitis, alopecia or coat abnormalities. Posterior paralysis in which swaying of the hindquarters, knuckling and even flaccid paralysis may occur has been described. Paralysed animals should be humanely destroyed.

Pathology

Haemorrhages in the walls of the stomach and duodenum may be seen, the mucosa of the small and large intestine may be swollen and friable and there may be ulceration of the large intestinal mucosa. Necrotic enteritis, resembling that seen in salmonellosis or intestinal adenomatosis, may be present. Histological lesions include a mucinous degeneration of the large intestinal mucosa differing from lesions of intestinal adenomatosis and focal lesions, especially destruction of glial cells may occur in the intermediate grey matter of the lumbar and cervical enlargements of the spinal cord. There may be widespread vacuolation of the white matter.

Treatment

Tryptophan supplementation of .ration should be carried out to give 2.7 kg/tonne or nicotinic acid should be added to give 14-20 g/tonne.

Reference

O'Sullivan, B.M., Blakemore, W.F. (1980) Vet. Pathology 7, 748-758. Acute nicotinamide deficiency in pig induced by 6-aminonicotinamide.

Pyridoxine (Vitamin B6)

Deficiency of this vitamin rarely occurs naturally. There is some suggestion that high fat diets may require supplementation and that supplementation may improve litter size in sows on maize and soya bean oilmeal. l.0 g/tonne additional pyridoxine is sufficient although 1.8 g/tonne has recently been suggested.

Reference

Easter, R.A., Anderson, P.A., Michel, E.J. and Corley, J.R. (1983). Nutrition Reports International. 28, 945-954. Response of gestating gilts and starter, grower and finisher swine to biotin, pyridoxine, folacin and thiamine additions to corn-soya bean meal diets.

Pantothenic acid deficiency

Definition

Deficiency of pantothenic acid occurs in pigs fed bakery wastes and results in nervous signs including the characteristic goose-stepping.

Aetiology and pathogenesis

Pantothenic acid is a coenzyme in the metabolism and synthesis of fats, carbohydrates and proteins. It is present at low levels in flour products such as bakery waste and levels are particularly low in cooked swill made from such waste. Levels may be barely adequate in some other types of ration especially where high oil levels and added copper are present. Its absence leads to demyelination of nerves.

Clinical signs

In weaned pigs a faulty action of the hind legs results in a mincing gait and progresses to posterior paralysis and collapse. Another type of disturbance begins as a snatching movement of the hind limb and progresses to a "goose-stepping" action in which the hind limb is snatched up to the belly and returns with the hock near the ground to cause a waddling or duck-like progression. There may be alopecia and a diarrhoea which is rarely watery. At least one of an affected group may be seen goose-stepping. In sows and young litters, diarrhoea may occur in the sow and loss of hair in the piglets.

Animals which are paralysed and recumbent do not recover readily and should be killed humanely.

Pathology

Oedema of the intestine, especially of the colon and degeneration of the peripheral nerves, posterior root ganglia and demyelination of the spinal cord are seen. The peroneal nerve is commonly affected.

Diagnosis

The goose-stepping is characteristic and further confirmation comes from the dietary history. Pathological findings are useful in confirmation and plasma pantothenate and dietary pantothenate levels can be determined by microbial assays. Dietary levels in deficiency are usually 4-10 mg/kg.

Treatment

Injection of individuals with multivitamins may be of value and the diet should be supplemented with 10-12 g/tonne of calcium pantothenate. In swill fed units a specially formulated mineral and vitamin mixture (low in salt as swill contains high levels) should be added after boiling and cooling. 10-12g calcium pantothenate per tonne will prevent the condition.

Biotin deficiency

Definition

A syndrome in which skin changes, hair loss and, in particular, hoof defects occurs in breeding herds. Reproductive performance is reduced.

Aetiology and Pathogenesis

Dietary biotin is normally present in adequate amounts in pig rations, although in feeds containing wheat or barley, the vitamin may be less readily available to pigs than in maize-based diets. Biotin is a cofactor in a number of enzymes especially carboxylation or transcarboxylation reactions. In growing pigs lipogenesis is affected through Acetyl CoA carboxylase. Deficiency in biotin on wheat and barley-based rations occurs quite commonly and at least 180 mg/tonne should be present for health.

Clinical signs

In field cases in the UK., the foot and skin lesions have been identified in sows. The foot lesions appear on the underside of the hoof and are only seen when the claw is cleaned. Others appear as longitudinal cracks on the wall originating in the coronary band. Heel and sole erosions and cracks also occur. High cull rates because of lameness, low numbers born, especially born alive and reared and long weaning to service intervals may also be seen. There may be alopecia and a dry scaly skin which may progress to give dermatitis with brownish crusts and petechial haemorrhages.

In the experimental syndrome, progressive hair loss occurs, the skin becomes dry and scaly and a white film and transverse grooves occur on the tongue. After 5-7 weeks on a deficient diet, claw defects occur. Erosion of the heel occurs first and is followed by cracking of the sole. Cracks appear in the now rubbery horn of the sole and the claw wall and result in lameness. Secondary infection may occur. Growth may be reduced in piglets receiving biotin deficient diets although this is not described in maize diets and skin and hoof defects have been recorded. Reproductive effects measured over 4 parities indicate that l-1.4 pigs per sow per year are lost, that weaning to service intervals may be increased by up to 4 days and that conception to first service may be reduced by 9%.

Pathology

In addition to the gross changes described above, the skin and claw lesions appear as areas of necrosis in the stratum corneum of the epithelium of the skin, oral and oesophageal mucosa and in the claws.

Diagnosis

The foot lesions resemble those of swine vesicular disease and this condition must be discounted before a diagnosis of biotin deficiency can be reached. Diagnosis can be confirmed by analysing the biotin content of the ration (100-220 ug/kg is the normal range), and noting the response to biotin supplementation of the diet. The reproductive effects can be confirmed only by supplementation of the diet in controlled studies. Populations with plasma levels of 60 ng/100 ml benefit from supplementation. An ELISA has recently been developed for plasma biotin.

Treatment

Supplement the diet with 400 mg-1250 mg/tonne of d biotin in all sow rations. Biotin is available as Rovimix H (1% d biotin, Roche) 40g premix/tonne is necessary for most purposes, for growing gilts, and pregnant and lactating sows to prevent foot lesions and improve litter size. Levels up to 3,000 mg/tonne may be necessary to reverse hoof lesions.

References.

Brooks, P.H. (1982). Pig News and Information 3, 29. Biotin in pig nutrition.

Brooks, P.H., Smith, D.A., Irwin, V.C.R. (1977). Vet. Rec. 101, 46-50. Biotin supplementation of diets, the incidence of foot lesions and the reproductive performance of sows.

Bryant, K.L., Kornegay, E.T., Knight, J.W., Webb, K.E., Notter, D.R. (1985). J.Anim.Sci. 60, 136-144. Supplemental biotin for swine: 1. Influence on feed lot performance, plasma biotin and toe lesions in young gilts.

Bryant, K.L., Kornegay, E.T., Knight, J.W., Webb, K.E., Notter, D.R. (1985). J.Anim.Sci. 60, 145-153. Supplemental biotin for swine: 2. Influences of supplementation to corn and wheat-based diets on reproductive performance and various biochemical criteria of sows during four parities.

Bryant, K.L., Kornegay, E.T., Knight, J.W., Veit, H.P., Notter, D.R. (1985). J.Anim.Sci. 60, 154-162. Supplemental biotin for swine. 3. Influence of supplementation to corn and wheat-based diets on the incidence and severity of toe lesions, hair and skin characteristics and structural soundness of sows housed in confinement during four parities.

Penny, R.H.C., Cameron, R.D.A., Johnson, S., Kenyon, P.J., Smith, H.A., Bell, A.W.P., Cole, J.P.L., Taylor, J. (1981). Vet. Rec. 109, 80-81. Influence of biotin supplementation on sow reproductive efficiency.
Penny, R.H.C. and others as above (1980) Vet. Rec. 107, 350-351. Foot rot of pigs ; the influence of biotin supplementation on foot lesions in sows.
Simmins, P.H. and Brooks, P.H. (1983). Vet.Rec. 112, 425-429. Supplementary biotin for sows : effect on reproductive characteristics.
Simmins, P.H., Brooks, P.H. (1988). Vet.Rec. 122, 431-435. Supplementary biotin for sows, effects on claw integrity.
Webb, N.G., Penny, R.H.C. and Johnston, A.M. (1984). Vet.Rec. 114, 185-189. Effect of a dietary supplement of biotin on pig hoof horn strength and hardness.

Cyanocobalamine (Vitamin B12)

Supplementation with this vitamin improves the rate of growth of pigs on diets composed largely of vegetable proteins but no specific deficiency syndromes have been identified. It is included in some piglet iron preparations, and such B12-supplemented products may improve growth rates of piglets. A suggestion that it may improve sow reproductive performance has been made.

Ascorbic acid (Vitamin C)

There is some evidence that Vitamin C supplementation of the diet may improve weight gain in young piglets and improve iron utilisation. It has also been shown to improve navel bleeding in piglets in some cases when fed to sows and may improve the numbers born alive and numbers weaned when given at I g./kg feed from day 105 of gestation. Vitamin C deficiency may arise as a recessive hereditary condition when foetuses may develop multiple haemorrhages and numbers born be decreased.

References

Kristensen, B., Thomsen, P.D., Palludan, B., Weger, I. (1986). Acta Vet.Scand. 27, 486-496. Mitogen stimulation of lymphocytes in pigs with hereditary Vitamin C deficiency.
Weger, I., Palludan, B. (1994). Vitamin C deficiency causes haematological and skeletal abnormalities during foetal development in swine.

Non-nutritive feed additives

These may be present in prepared diets and consist of:

(a) Therapeutic antimicrobials or other medicines.
(b) Growth promoters or "growth permitters".
(c) Probiotics.
(d) Substrates for microorganisms.
(e) Enzymes.
(f) Acidifying agents.
(g) Flavourings.
(h) Preservatives.
(i) Oral vaccines
(j) Inert carriers to improve the handling and dispersal of ingredients.

Labels of bags or specifications of bulk diets include additives (a) to (i) in EC countries.

(a) Veterinary medicines are only included upon prescription (a Veterinary Written Directive, UK) and can only be incorporated by someone registered under the Medicated Feedstuffs Regulations (UK). The medicines which may be incorporated have been mentioned in the text. A recent and unusual additive is zinc oxide which is included as an antidiarrhoeal agent for recently weaned pigs at levels of up to 3,000 g/tonne.

(b) Growth promoters are antimicrobials or minerals (Copper to 175 ppm) included to improve daily liveweight gain and feed conversion efficiency by 5-10% or more. Their effect in S.P.F. pigs and in herds with a high health status is minimal. It appears, therefore, that they suppress subclinical disease. Hormonal growth promoters are no longer used in the UK, their place having been taken by the use of uncastrated boars. Growth promoters include inorganic compounds such as copper, and organic compounds such as antibiotics and synthetic antimicrobials. Some disadvantages of antimicrobial growth permitters have been:

1. The development of resistance to the same antimicrobial used for therapy, e.g. tylosin. There is, however, some doubt now whether low levels of antimicrobials do induce resistance to therapeutic levels of the drug.

2. Interference with other antimicrobials, e.g. the interaction between salinomycin and tiamulin.

3. The reduction in natural B vitamin synthesis in the gut.

4. Overgrowth of elements of the 'normal' gut flora may occur following withdrawal of a growth promoter and subclinical or clinical disease may result from this recolonisation of a non-immune gut. This type of disease is as yet poorly documented.

5. Resistance to antimicrobials such as chloramphenicol may develop amongst some gut bacteria and cause concern in Public Health.

6. Residues of medicines or additives may persist in carcase meat and in this case an age range is normally specified for their use and withdrawal times are given. Withdrawal times should be strictly observed and the widespread introduction of tests for residues in meat now ensures that this is done. Many growth promoters are not absorbed. Some, such as copper may be limited on environmental grounds.

(c) Probiotics are dried but still viable cultures of microorganisms such as lactobacilli, streptococci and yeasts which are said to colonise the intestine and prevent colonisation by disease causing agents. The main points in the pig's life where they are of theoretical value are in the neonate, after weaning and after antimicrobial treatment. Their value has not been demonstrated unequivocally by controlled scientific studies of the type which have proven the efficacy of antimicrobial growth promoters. Probiotics may be killed by antimicrobial use.

(d)   Substrates for microorganisms such as fibre have been included in some rations for reasons mentioned above and with similar results.

(e)   Enzymes such as proteases and amylases are sometimes included to aid digestion.

(f)   Acidifying agents such as fumaric and citric acids or proprietary agents such as (SmithKline Beecham) lower gastric pH and inhibit microorganisms such as E.coli and salmonella in feed. There is experimental evidence to support an effect on performance.

(g)   Flavourings may give a feed an unexpected smell or colour but the feed may be perfectly wholesome.

(h)   Preservatives such as salt or formalin may be present in whey or skim and antioxidants such as ethoxyquin when used to preserve wet stored barley are often present in many feeds. Propionic acid may be associated with low levels of Vitamin E and rapid destruction of fat soluble vitamins. Some labile constituents such as antimicrobials may be enteric coated.

(i)   Bacterial antigens. Intagen (Hoffman LaRoche) is an example. For use see E.coli.

(j)   Inert carriers such as bentonite may be included to enable the successful mixing and dispersal of ingredients.

Processing

Heating destroys B Vitamins such as thiamine, drugs such as penicillin G and bacteria such as salmonellae. Heat is generated during pelleting and this should be taken into account when considering heat labile feed ingredients. The boiling of swill also affects heat-labile vitamins but this heat treatment may also increase the digestibility of some waste foods.

Storage

Feed should not be used after the expiry date printed on the label and should be protected from heat and moisture. Mould growth may occur in bins (see mycotoxins) and rodent and bird contamination may give rise to infections. Fodder mites may infest feed and make it unpalatable and they and their eggs may appear in faeces. Storage of premixes beyond their expiry date commonly leads to problems.

Introduction

A number of abnormalities may be seen in the newborn piglet or may appear shortly after birth. Such congenital conditions may be produced by one of the factors outlined below. Others are of genetic origin but do not become apparent until much later.

1. Spontaneous developmental abnormality
2. Heritable abnormalities
3. Infectious agents
4. Nutritional deficiency or poisoning
5. Unknown cause.

In investigating a problem involving congenital conditions, it is important to recognise those under genetic control, and those caused by infection, nutritional deficiency or poisoning as the methods of control used in each case are so different. Those which are expressed later like lymphosarcoma and the porcine stress syndrome must be differentiated from other conditions in older pigs.

1. Spontaneous developmental abnormality

This may occur sporadically in any pig herd but may be more common where late matings have occurred (old egg or sperm), or where old breeding stock are used. Hermaphroditism, some hernias, cardiovascular abnormalities, cleft palates, monsters, Siamese twins etc. may be spontaneous and not controlled by heritable genetic abnormalities, but in general, developmental abnormalities are relatively uncommon. Should they become so within a herd, a genetic, infectious or nutritional origin should be considered.

2. Heritable conditions

A number of congenital conditions in pigs are heritable or are predisposed to by genetic factors. These include a number of breed characteristics. Some of these conditions are described below. Where genetic factors are influenced in their expression by nutrition or other environmental factors such as infection this will be indicated.

Hernias "Ruptures"

These are one of the commonest congenital defects of pigs (up to 1.5%, currently 0.3% UK) and may be inguinal or umbilical. Their production is, in some cases of inguinal hernia governed by a double recessive gene or is polygenic. The heritability of inguinal hernia has been shown to be 0.29-0.35 depending on breed. Inguinal hernias are usually unilateral and are only expressed in the male. Hernias cause problems in a number of ways:

a) by enlarging to such an extent that they touch the ground and ulcerate

b) by being damaged during fighting

c) at castration

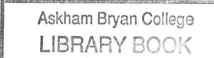

d) strangulation may occur when intestines or omentum become trapped following peritonitis, Glasser's Disease, fighting and enteritis. Once intestines become trapped, animals show signs of abdominal pain and distension and the hernia becomes tense. The intestines present cannot be manipulated back into the peritoneal cavity and the skin over it becomes discoloured and necrotic.

When hernias reach the ground, ulcerate severely or become strangulated, the animal should be destroyed humanely unless surgical relief is to be carried out.

Treatment

Surgical reduction of inguinal hernias is commonly practised at castration but as castration becomes less common for economic and welfare reasons, it is likely that surgical correction will become less common. The procedure must be of economic benefit to be carried out.

Control

Suggest the culling of sows giving rise to affected litters or boars whose progeny have a high incidence of the condition if the incidence is sufficiently high to make this an economic proposition. Animals with large hernias may require self-certification as casualties and be penned separately on transport for slaughter.

Hermaphrodites

True hermaphrodites have both testicular and ovarian tissue sometimes as an ovotestis. Hereditary, less common than male pseudohermaphroditism in which male gonads are present but the reproductive tract has a number of female features such as fallopian tubes and uterus or reduced penis size. The external genitalia are generally female in form. Overall incidences of 0.09% have been recorded UK. Pregnancy has been recorded in hermaphrodites, also mosaicism.

References

Pond, W.G. (1961). Cornell Vet. 51, 394.
Hunter, R.H.F. (1988).   Proc.Pig Vet.Soc. 21, 135-139. Intersexuality in domestic pigs.

Cystic kidneys

Inherited cysts of tubular origin in both Landrace and Large White pigs occur congenitally. Their production is governed by an autosomal dominant mode of inheritance but the actual numbers produced may be under polygenic control. Recruitment to the cyst population appears to occur throughout life. There appear to be no clinical consequences during normal adult life but kidney condemnations may reach 47.5% at slaughter.

Piglets in affected herds may remain stunted after weaning and become pot-bellied. They should be killed humanely. At post-mortem examination polycystic kidneys with or without hydronephrosis may be found.

295

References

Wells, G.A.H., Hebert, C.N., Robins, B.C. (1980). Vet. Rec. 106, 532-535. Renal cysts in pigs : prevalence and pathology in slaughtered pigs from a single herd.
Wijeratne, W.V.S. and Wells, G.A.H. (1980). Vet. Rec. 107, 484-488. Inherited renal cysts in pigs : results of breeding experiments.

Hypoplastic kidney and renal agenesis

A condition in which small kidneys or no kidneys are found in piglets of up to 8 weeks of age. Governed by an autosomal recessive gene and often results in death. Ureters may be capped with undifferentiated mesenchyme.

Reference

Mason, R.W., Cooper, R. (1985). Aust.Vet.J. 62, 413-414. Congenital bilateral renal hypoplasia in Large White pigs.

Polycystic disease

An inherited polycystic disease with cysts in kidneys, bile ducts, epididymus, uterus and pancreas. Affected piglets die within 1-3 days.

Cystic lymph nodes

Cysts in ileal mesenteric lymph nodes, caecocolic lymph nodes and colonic lymph nodes up to 2 cm in diameter may be found in otherwise normal pigs.

Inverted nipples

More than one nipple may be affected in this simple recessive system. The mechanism of inversion appears to be due to proliferation of fibrous tissue at the base of the teat resulting from a lack of oestrogen receptors. It has been suggested that boars producing 4% or more affected female progeny in 40 litters should not be used for breeding. Environmental damage may also cause inverted nipples.

Reference

Done, J. T. (1980). Vet. Annual. 20, 246-254. Teat deficiencies in pigs.

Cryptorchidism

A sex-linked autosomal recessive character governed by 2 loci with a heredity of 0.057. The testicles may be at the inguinal ring or further into the peritoneal cavity. Not important unless boars intended for breeding are concerned in which case they should be rejected. May be associated with boar taint in countries where castration is routine, but both aromatase and oestrogen secretion by cryphorchid testes is lower than from scrotal testes. If slaughter is delayed boar taint may be a problem. An overall incidence of 0.24% has been recorded UK, but 2.26% in Germany and up to 8% by experimental breeding. The left testis is three times as likely to be affected as the right.

Reference

Rothschild, M.F., Christian, L.L., Blanchard, W. (1988). J.Hered. 79, 313-314. Evidence for multigene control of cryphorchidism in swine.

Atresia ani

A common condition in which the rectum fails to open to the exterior. A thin membrane or a considerable band of fibrous tissue may be present. Male pigs usually have swollen abdomens and die within 3 weeks of birth, but in females the rectum may open into the vagina and the animal survives in 50% of cases. The condition may be governed by a recessive gene, probably with incomplete (50%) penetrance and may not occur in more than 50% of an affected litter. It may also arise as a result of environmental or developmental abnormality. It may be present in 0.3% pigs in the UK. A heritability of 0.009% has been suggested.

Treatment

Mild cases may be treated surgically, badly affected piglets should be killed humanely.

Control

If a genetic mechanism is clearly involved in the outbreak in question do not breed from affected gilts or from the sibs of affected animals. Cull breeding stock if cost effective and do not use the same boar on the same sow.

Congenital meningoencephalocoele

Recorded in Landrace and Large Whites and inherited. Affected pigs have exposed meninges protruding through incomplete fusion of parietal or frontal bones and the mortality rate is high. An autosomal recessive condition. If it becomes a problem, a cost benefit analysis will decide whether culling is worthwhile.

Reference

Wijeratne, W.V.S., Beaton, D., Cuthbertson, J.C. (1974). Vet. Rec. 95, 81-84.

Hereditary dwarfism

A simple autosomal recessive causing dwarfism and chondrodysplasia has been reported from Denmark. Another type affecting the limbs only has been described from Czechoslovakia. Affected pigs required humane slaughter.

Reference

Jensen, P.T., Nielsen, D.H., Jensen, P. and Bille, N. (1984). Nord.Vet.Med. 36, 32-37. Hereditary dwarfism in pigs.

Kaman, J., Drabek, J., Zert, Z. (1991). Acta.vet.Brno. 60, 237-251. Congenital dysproportional chondrodysplasia.

Inherited Thick Forelegs

The forelegs are markedly enlarged below the elbows and the skin is tense and may be discoloured. Mortality due to crushing and starvation is common. A simple autosomal recessive character governs the condition which appears to operate by causing a periosteal detachment distal to the elbow with subsequent new bone formation.

References

Doize, B. and Martineau, G.P. (1984). Canadian J.Comp.Med. 48, 414-419. Congenital hyperostosis in piglets : a consequence of a disorganisation of the perichondrial ossification groove of Ranvier.
Kay, M.M. (1962). Canad.J.Comp.Med. 26, 218.

Crooked Tails or Kinky Tail

Absence or malformation of the tail occurs commonly in the Landrace and Large White breeds and is thought to be inherited. May be dominant but with low penetrance. Incidence UK is 1.7%.

Legless Pigs

An autosomal recessive lethal factor leading to absence of leg bones.

Reference

Johnson, L.G. (1940). J. Hered. 31, 239.

Cleft Palate

Affected piglets die of starvation after a few days as they cannot create sufficient vacuum in their mouths to suck milk. Affected piglets should be killed humanely. Governed by an autosomal recessive gene in most cases but can also result from chromosomal trisomy and poisoning by hemlock (*Conium maculatum*).

References

Koch-Weimar, P. and Neumuller-Jena, O. (1932). Dt. Tierarzte.Wschr. 40, 353. Genetic.
Painter, K.E., Keeler, R.F., Buck, W.B. (1985). Am.J.Vet.Res. 46, 1368-1371. Congenital skeletal malformations induced by maternal ingestion of *Conium maculatum* (poison hemlock) in newborn pigs.

Syndactyly (mule-foot)

Dominant to normal cloven foot.

Reference

Detlefsen, J.A., Carmichael, W.J. (1921). J.Agric.Res. 20, 595.

Polydactyly (Supernumerary digits)

Inherited and appears to be an autosomal dominant which is lethal in the homozygote and expresses polydactyly in the heterozygote.

Reference

Malynicz, G.L. (1982). Annals de Genetique et de selection Animale 14, 415-420. Complete polydactylism in Papua New Guinea village pigs with otocephalic homozygous monsters.

Arthrogryposis

In this condition joints, usually of the limbs are fused. Affected piglets die but can also delay farrowing. This may result from a simple autosomal recessive gene, from neural or muscular defects and has been attributed to poisoning with thorn apple, hemlock (*Conium maculatum*) or *Nicotiana* (tobacco). Affected pigs should be destroyed humanely.

Reference

Lomo, O.D. (1985). Acta Vet.Scand. 26 419-422. Arthrogryposis and associated defects in pigs: indication of simple recessive inheritance.

Hereditary Rickets

Identified in German Landrace as an autosomal recessive vitamin D dependent rickets type 1. Also in other breeds. Homozygotes grew slowly and developed hypocalcaemia with severe secondary hyperparathroidism and hypophosphataemia by 8 weeks of age. Cholecalciferol injections reverse the syndrome and it appears to be due to low 1, 25 dehydroxy Vitamin D3 levels in plasma.

Reference

Fox, J., Maunder, E.M.W., Randall, V.A., Care, A.D. (1985). Clinical Science 69, 541-548. Vitamin D dependent rickets type 1 in pigs.

Skin conditions

Dermatosis vegetans

A relatively rare hereditary disease of young pigs characterised by lesions of the skin and hoof and a giant cell pneumonitis which is usually fatal. It is governed by a semi-lethal factor with recessive autosomal inheritance and has been seen in Landrace pigs in Britain which are descendants of an original carrier Swedish Landrace import.

Skin lesions. These may be present at birth or develop at 2-3 weeks of age from raised pink swellings on the abdomen or inside the thighs, spreading and passing through a pityriasis rosea-like stage, and, after 5-8 weeks become thickened and covered with greyish-brown or black crusts.

Foot lesions. "Clubfoot" are less common but are always present at birth with swelling and erythema in the coronary area of the hoof and the production of defective horn on the walls, sole and bulb of the foot.

Giant cell pneumonitis. This is the characteristic finding and essential to the diagnosis in older pigs. In pigs of more than 1 week of age, the giant cells may be demonstrated and nodules of them appear as firm red-brown bodies 13 mm in diameter throughout the lung. These may regress to leave alveolar fibrosis in pigs which survive until 1 year of age.

Course of the disease. A decline in growth appears after 5-6 weeks and most affected pigs are dead within 6 months. Affected pigs should be humanely destroyed.

Control

Breed affected sows with Large White boars.

References

Done, J.T., Loosmore, R.M. and Saunders, C.N. (1967). Vet. Rec. 80, 292-297. Dermatosis vegetans in pigs.
Evensen, O., Bratberg, B. (1990). Res.Vet.Sci. 49, 50-55. A sequential light microscopic study of the pulmonary lesions in porcine dermatosis vegetans.

Pityriasis rosea

A common condition of unknown aetiology, possibly governed by an autosomal dominant gene with incomplete penetrance and seen in young pigs. The condition may be more common in Landrace and has recently been given the name porcine juvenile pustular psoriaform dermatitis.

Clinical signs

The condition may be seen in individual animals or whole litters, but usually only occurs in 2-3 pigs per litter. The lesions appear at 2-4 weeks of age as a few 2-3 cm hyperaemic patches on the flanks, groin or thighs and expand rapidly to form reddish rings with a normal centre. The normal area gradually expands as the condition continues. The condition is self-limiting with a course of about 2 months and resolves completely. Pruritis is not seen even at the height of the disease when the lesions may cover a large amount of the surface area. Weaners may be disfigured at sale time and may not command their true price.

Control

Change the boar if a large number of cases occur in a herd.

Reference

Corcoran, C.J. (1964). Vet. Rec. 76, 1407-1409. Pityriasis rosea in pigs.

Epitheliogenesis imperfecta (Congenital ectodermal defect)

This appears as raw patches with raised edges on the skin and may be mistaken for wounds. In Britain they have been recorded in Saddleback and Large White Pigs and are thought to be hereditary, possibly due to a single autosomal recessive character. Healing may occur or infection may result in death. Animals with large lesions should be humanely destroyed.

Reference

Parish, W.E. and Done, J.T., (1962). J. Comp. Path. 72, 286. Seven apparently congenital non-infectious conditions of the skin resembling congenital defects in man.

Hairless Pigs

Hairlessness is dominant to normal coat with incomplete penetrance and so heterozygotes can be picked out. Iodine deficiency may also cause it.

Reference

Roberts, E. and Carroll, W.E. (1931). J. Hered. 22, 125.

Congenital Porphyria

An uncommon condition in which excess porphyrins are produced and discolour the bones and teeth. Porphyruria is difficult to demonstrate and there appear to be few effects upon health although anaemia has been described. Photosensitsation does not occur. Autosomal dominant genes are involved. Has been identified in Duroc pigs in Japan where it may be recessive.

Reference

Jorgensen, S.K. (1959). Brit.Vet. J. 115, 160-175. Congenital porphyria in pigs.

Muscular Conditions

Congenital splay leg (Myofibrillar hypoplasia)

This important (up to 1.5 per cent) condition occurs as an additive polygenic trait with no clear evidence of dominance, especially in Pietrain, Landrace and Welsh pigs. It appears to occur twice as frequently in males and a maternal effect has been identified, apparently mediated through larger litters which have more affected piglets and a shorter (0.9 day) gestation period. There are too few Type I myofibrils in the fibres of muscles of the foreleg, lumbar group and, most important, the hindleg. The condition appears to represent a failure of muscle fibres to mature in sufficient numbers to provide adequate support at birth. The semitendinosus muscle is most severely affected in the hindlimb.

Affected piglets are unable to stand, and are often found with a hindlimb extended anteriorly along the axis of the body with the opposite member abducted. If not killed by crushing and if able to feed, affected piglets become normal within 10 days of birth. Affected piglets may develop sores on the perineum and erosion of the base of the tail. Up to 50% of affected piglets may die if not assisted. They are particularly prone to chilling.

The condition becomes apparent 2-3 hours after birth and 2-3 piglets may be affected in each litter. Affected piglets may be kept warm and reared artificially for 2-3 days and returned to the sow. Non-slip floors and the use of elastic bands on the hindlimbs may improve viability. Crossing Landrace or Welsh sows with Large White boars reduces the incidence. The use of physostigmine has been suggested as an aid to recovery in piglets 12 hours or more of age. Repeated massage of the hindlimbs improves survival dramatically.

Humane killing may be appropriate where severely affected animals, or those with extensive ulceration, lose condition and cannot be nursed.

The incidence of splayleg may increase when PRRS outbreaks occur and in zearalenone poisoning.

References

Blackburn, P.W. (1988). Proc.Pig.Vet.Soc. 21, 185-186. Splayleg piglets : treatment.
Bradley, R., Ward, P.S., Bailey, J. (1980). J.Comp.Path. 90, 433-466. The ultrastructural morphology of the skeletal muscles of normal pigs and pigs with splayleg from birth to one week of age.
Thurley, D.C., Gilbert, F.R. and Done, J.T. (1967). Vet. Rec. 80, 302-304. Congenital splayleg of piglets : myofibrillar hypoplasia.
Ward, P.S. (1978). Vet. Bull. 279-295. The splayleg syndrome in new-born pigs : a review I.
Ward, P.S. (1978). Vet.Bull. 48, 381-399. The splayleg syndrome in new-born pigs : a review II.

Pietrain creeper syndrome

A progressive, familial myopathy of Pietrain pigs has been described in one herd in Britain, features of it have been detected in another and also in Landrace pigs. the onset of the disease occurs in pigs of either sex at 2-3 weeks of age in up to 30% of an affected litter. Tremor of the hindquarters appears and within a few days occurs in the forequarters. The limbs become partly flexed and a "tip-toe" gait is adopted. Reluctance to stand becomes progressively more common and affected piglets walk on permanently flexed carpal joints and on the digits of the flexed hindlimbs. Creeping continues until around 65 days after the onset when permanent recumbency develops and the pigs must be destroyed. They remain alert and feed and grow normally.

Muscle cells in the proximal limb muscles vary greatly in size, may have internal nuclei and many are degenerating. The condition appears to be inherited as an autosomal recessive.

References

Wells, G.A.H., Pinsent, P.J.N. and Todd, J.N. (1980). Vet Rec. 106, 556-558. A progressive familial myopathy of the Pietrain pig : the clinical syndrome..
Bradley, R., and Wells, G.A.H. The Pietrain 'creeper' pig: a primary myopathy. In Animal models of neurological disease, eds. Rose, F.C. and Behan, P.O. Pitman Medical (1980) 34.

The Porcine Stress Syndrome (P.S.S.)
Pale Soft Exudative (P.S.E.) Muscle and Malignant Hyperthermia

Definition

A complex of conditions associated with an autosomal recessive gene of variable penetrance. Animals of well muscled strains may die suddenly during transport (P.S.S.), give rise to pale, watery pork at slaughter (P.S.E.) and develop malignant hyperthermia when exposed to halothane anaesthesia. Back muscle necrosis may also develop.

Incidence

The incidence of this condition may be based on the number of clinical cases, usually deaths in transport, the number of animals which have tested positive for the nomozygous or heterozygous forms by phenotypic assessment (principally the halothane test) and most recently and accurately, figures produced since 1991 for the distribution of homozygous and heterozygous carriers of the gene in the pig populations in a breed or an area. Examples of the incidence of clinical disease include figures from the Netherlands, where deaths in pigs transported to slaughter reached 0.7% in 1980 and P.S.E. occurred in up to 30% of carcases. In Britain, deaths during transport were fewer, 0.08% in 1974. Phenotype testing suggests that the condition occurred in the Dutch, West German (68%) and Belgian (86%), Landrace, the prevalence of the condition was about 11% (1980).

Figures obtained for the presence of the gene give a definitive picture of prevalence. This tests in US, Canada and UK (1993) showed that 97% Pietrain, 35% Landrace, 15% Duroc, 19% Large White, 14% Hampshire, 19% Yorkshire and 16% Crossbred pigs carried the gene with gene frequencies of from 0.72 (Pietrain) to 0.07 (Hampshire). 1% of pigs were homozygous and 20% pigs tested were carriers. In a French study the French Landrace animals tested were completely free from the gene.

Aetiology

The cause of the condition is the substitution of cytosine (C) for thymidine (T) at position 1843 on the ryr 1 gene on chromosome 6 P11 921. The gene codes for ryanodine, responsible for gating (controlling) the calcium (Ca^{++}) channel in the sarcoplasmic reticulum of skeletal muscle. The point mutation of C for T results in the replacement of the aminoacid arginine at position 615 in the ryanodine peptide with cysteine, thus altering its function. The altered protein facilitates the opening of the calcium channel and inhibits its closure. The flow of calcium ions stimulates contracture of the muscle and sets in train all the other consequences described below. The altered channel can be stimulated by lower concentrations of Ca^{++}, ATP and caffeine in muscle of genotype MHnn (Malignant Hypothermia homozygote) than in normal animals (MHNN). Inhibition of gating by Ca^{++} and Mg^{++} is also damped down, so responses continue longer. Anaesthetics such as halothane and stress raise Ca^{++} and ATP levels so that further Ca^{++} release occurs and the muscle becomes unresponsive to inhibition. The heterozygote MHNn is intermediate between the two homozygotes in terms of Ca^{++} flows.

The mutation appears to have arisen once and to have spread to all affected breeds. The ryr 1 gene was previously designated for halothane sensitivity n for sensitive i.e., affected pigs were Hal nn, normals Hal NN and is transmitted as an autosomal recessive with high or complete penetrance.

The homozygote Hal NN and the heterozygote Hal Nn are both resistant to the effects of simple halothane anaesthesia. The Hal (MH) gene is linked to a series of other characters, some of which have been used to identify stress susceptibility. They are as follows in apparent order of linkage: S (the suppressor gene of the AO blood group), Phi (phospho-hexoisomerase), Hal MH (the halothane susceptibility gene), H (a blood group) Po2 (serum post albumin protein 2) and Pgd (6 phosphogluconate dehydrogenase. The linkage can be expressed S(AO)-Phi-Hal-Po2-Pgd. Possession of the gene is associated with heavily muscled or lean breeds and the selection of pigs for meatiness and carcase conformation has aided spread by selection and by the use of breeds with a high prevalence of the gene such as Pietrains as sires for slaughter pigs.

Pathogenesis

The condition occurs as a result of a switch of energy utilisation in the muscles of susceptible pigs from aerobic to anaerobic metabolism resulting from the increased Ca^{++} flux in the calcium channel of the sarcoplasmic reticulum and the prolonged activity which follows. An enormous increase in lactate production, an increase in body heat production and poor production of A.T.P. result. Body temperature rises partly due to a peripheral vasoconstriction and accumulation of lactate. Muscle damage leads to increases in plasma creatine phosphokinase and, in some cases, potassium ions. Calcium uptake and release from the sarcoplasmic reticulum appears to be critical in the pathogenesis of the condition. Noradrenaline levels are high and it appears to be metabolised less quickly than in normal pigs. High cortisone levels and an increased rate of thyroxine and triiodothyronine utilisation also occur in affected pigs. Triggering of the mechanism can result from stress of movement, some anaesthetic agents and slaughter when anaerobic glycolysis also develops.

The possession of the halothane susceptible gene leads to an increase of carcase lean, a slower growth rate and, in sows, 1.16 fewer births and 1.76 fewer weaned pigs per litter than in resistant litters. Heterozygotes are economically superior to either homozygote.

Clinical signs

Pigs of 9 weeks of age and especially heavy hogs or adults, are affected. Early signs of stress include muscle and tail tremor which progress to dyspnoea, blotched red and pale skin, an increase in body temperature to more than 41.5°C. followed by collapse, muscle rigidity and death. Some of these changes may be induced by anaesthesia. The condition is more common when the environmental temperature rises above 22°C. The changes are so rapid that humane slaughter is rarely an option.

Pathology

Few changes are seen, but there is some oedema and collapse of the lung. Rapid development of rigor mortis occurs. Pale, soft exudative muscle develops in 60-70% of stress-susceptible pigs within 15 minutes of death and can be seen as pale areas contrasting with the deeper red unaffected muscle bundles when the longissimus dorsi or ham muscles are cut in section. Muscle pH falls to pH 6.0 or less within 45 minutes of death. There may be some necrosis and change in cardiac muscle. Histological lesions include the presence of degenerating and regenerating muscle fibres, but these may represent previous episodes of the condition.

Diagnosis

The clinical signs of blanching of the skin and rigidity following stimulus are suggestive if seen. The rigid carcase and the presence of pale soft exudative lumbar or ham muscles with a low pH may also suggest the condition. The body conformation, breed, a history of stress or high ambient temperatures are often helpful. Other causes of sudden death in large pigs such as anthrax, twisted bowel, bloody gut, gastric torsion, electrocution, vegetative endocarditis etc. should be ruled out. Susceptible pigs can be identified in life by the polymerase chain reaction for the normal and altered genes in blood or tissue. This test is available commercially and animals which have been screened and found to be negative may bear a tag N 1843. Heterozygotes and homozygotes for the MHn gene are also identified.

Where this test is not available, the phenotype can be determined by older tests such as the halothane test, using halothane 3 or 5% for 3-5 minutes in young pigs 9 weeks of age. Affected pigs become rigid and sometimes develop raised rectal temperatures. Anaesthesia should be discontinued or death will result. This test reliably detects susceptible homozygotes but a repeat test for 3 minutes coupled with succinylcholine at 0.75 mg/kg may reveal heterozygotes amongst apparently negative animals. Intravenous halothane and the use of halothane anaesthesia on adult pigs induced using barbiturate may also be used. Raised plasma levels of creatinine phosphokinase or pyruvate kinase may also be helpful, also the detection of Phi B,, Pgd B, the absence of the AO blood groups and the presence of the Ha/Ha blood groups may also be helpful. The use of caffeine solutions on the contractibility of isolated biopsied muscle specimens has also been used. The use of carcase meat conductivity and pH measurements may also be useful at slaughter. 45 minutes after slaughter reactors may have a meat pH of 5.9 or less. New DNA hybridisation tests are being developed and one for Phi has been described.

Control

Clinically affected animals or those prone to stress should be given adequate ventilation, cooled with water drips or sprayed in hot weather, starved for 12 hours before transport and not transported at environmental temperatures exceeding 22°C (72°F). Tail lifts help reduce transport stress. Any mixing likely to result in fighting should be avoided. Access to sugar solutions in the lairage may prevent P.S.E. Pentobarbitone anaesthesia should be used in stress-susceptible pigs. Stress can be reduced by the use of azaperone or carazalol prior to movement.

As selection programmes for lean carcases and large hams tend to increase the prevalence of stress in susceptible pigs, some countries and companies have adopted a policy of testing for and eliminating stress susceptible animals. Others have used homozygous stress susceptible sire lines on resistant dam lines to combine the economic advantages, carcase quality and prolificacy of the heterozygote. The success of companies and countries in reducing the incidence of the gene in individual lines has now been confirmed using PCR gene testing and a number of breeds and lines are now free from the gene. Both sow and boar lines which combine the meaty phenotype with the MHNN (stress free) genotype are now commercially available and the presence of stress susceptible animals (MHnn) in a herd is now unnecessary.

References

Allen, W.M. Harding, J.D.J. and Patterson, D.S.P. (1970). Vet. Rec. 87, 64-69. Experimentally induced acute stress syndrome in Pietrain pigs.

Evaluation and control of meat quality in pigs. A seminar in the EEC Agricultural Research Programme held in Dublin, Ireland 21-22 Nov. 1985. (1987) Proceedings of Conference, Martinus Nyhoff.

Fujii, J., Otsu, K., Zorzato, F., DeLeon, S., Khanna, V.K., Weiler J.E., O'Brien, P.J., MacLennan, D.H. (1991). Science 253, 448-451. Identification of a mutation in porcine ryanodine receptor associated with malignant hyperthermia.

Gregory, N.G. and Wilkins, L.J. (1984) J.of Science of Food and Agriculture 35, 147-153. The intravenous halothane test as an experimental model for quantifying stress sensitivity in pigs.
Mabry, J.W., Christian, L.L., Kuhlers, D.L. and Rasmussen, B.A. (1983). J.Heredity 74, 23-26. Prediction of susceptibility to the porcine stress syndrome.
MacLennan, D.H., Duff, C., Zorzato, F., Fujii, J., Phillips, M., Korneluk, R.G., Frodis, W., Britt, B., Worton, R.G. (1990). Nature 343, 559-560. Ryanodine gene is a candidate for predisposition to malignant hyperthermia.
O'Brien, P.J., Shen, H., Cory, C.R., Zhang, X. (1993). J.Am.Vet.Med.Ass. 203, 842-851. Use of a DNA-based test for the mutation associated with porcine stress syndrome (malignant hyperthermia) in 10,000 breeding swine.

Associated conditions

a) Back Muscle Necrosis

Necrosis of the longissimus dorsi is a sporadic condition of sudden onset in pigs of more than 50 kg in bodyweight. Pain and difficulty in movement, pyrexia and unilateral or bilateral swelling of the back occur. A proportion of pigs die in the acute stage from lactic acidosis and cardiac insufficiency. The condition appears in herds in which the porcine stress syndrome occurs.

Lesions include discolouration of the skin over the affected area, generalised congestion and some petechiation. Ruptures, areas of pallor and haemorrhage are present in the back muscles. The pH of affected muscle is lower than that of adjacent unaffected muscle. Local haemorrhage, loss of myofibrillar material and calcified muscle cells and other degenerative changes were seen in histological sections.

Diagnosis is based on the clinical signs, and should be supported by measurements of plasma creatinine phosphokinase levels which are raised. Post-mortem findings are confirmatory but both longitudinal and transverse sections of the affected muscle mass should be carried out.

Reference

Bradley, R., Wells, G.A.H. and Gray, L.J. (1979). Vet.Rec. 104, 183-188. Back muscle necrosis of pigs.

b) Malignant hyperthermia

This occurs during halothane anaesthesia of stress-susceptible pigs or when the ambient temperature rises above 28°C. Beyond this temperature heat loss cannot occur in the absence of water and body temperatures climb to 41.5°C or beyond and death results. Water cooling and tranquillisers may reduce mortality.

c) Pale soft exudative muscle (P.S.E.)

This results from excessive glycolysis in stress-susceptible pig muscle at slaughter and causes low pH (less than 6) and high temperature (41°C or more) 45 minutes after slaughter. m ere is excessive drip and taste is impaired.

Asymmetric hindquarter syndrome

A disparity of the size of one hindleg in which fat and muscle cell distribution in the muscles of the posterior thigh are abnormal. Careful examination and dissection are required for diagnosis. Appears at 2-3 months of age, may be of genetic origin.

Reference

Done, J.T., Allen, W.M., Bailey, J., De Gruchy, P.H., Curran, M.K. (1975). Vet. Rec. 96, 482-485. Asymmetric hindquarter syndrome (AHQS) in the pig.

Nervous Conditions

Congenital Tremor

Three of the types of tremor present in piglets are known to be heritable. They are:

Congenital Tremor AIII
(Congenital cerebrospinal hypomyelinogenesis)

A severe, coarse tremor of the head and forequarters with side to side undulation of the hindquarters sometimes accompanied by squealing may be seen in male Landrace piglets at birth. The clinical signs disappear when the animal is asleep, and are accentuated by stress such as cold or the ingestion of cold liquids, or being made to walk backwards.

The condition is governed by a sex-linked recessive gene carried by the sow and is due to a deficiency in the number of oligodendrocytes and a resulting inability to myelinate CNS nerve fibres. A low proportion of litters are affected, and in these, 25% of piglets show signs. The condition recurs in successive litters of the same parents.

Affected piglets are prone to starvation and crushing and a high proportion of affected piglets die. The condition may be seen as a faint shimmer of movement of the head and shoulders in adult Landrace boars, especially when they are forced to walk backwards.

Control

Mate Landrace sows with Large White boars of unaffected Landrace boars.

Reference

Harding, J.D.J., Done, J.T., Harbourne, J.F., Randall, C.T., Gilbert, F.R. (1973). Vet. Rec. 92, 527-529. Congenital tremor type A III in pigs: an hereditary sex-linked cerebrospinal hypomyelinogenesis.

Congenital Tremor AIV

A hereditary tremor seen in a low proportion of litters in British Saddleback pigs and occurring in 25% of the litter. The condition is recessive but not sex-linked and is due to a defect in the lipid metabolism of the CNS which results in demyelination and remyelination. Not common. The condition causes high mortality in affected piglets and recurs in subsequent litters of the same parents.

Saddleback X Large White Tremor

A monogenic autosomal recessive tremor has been recorded in Large White X Saddleback mating and is distinct from AIV. There is ataxia, dysmetria, perverse movement and a loss of righting reflex. It is a progressive cerebellar disorder.

Reference

Kidd, A.R.M., Done, J.T., Wrathall, A.E., Pampligione, G., Sweesey, D. (1986) Br.Vet.J. 142, 275-285. A new genetically-determined congenital nervous disorder in pigs.

Circulatory disorders

Willebrand's disease

A haemophilia-like condition has been described and occurs in both sexes. Factor VIII is reduced and platelets are more stable than normal. Clotting times are 15 minutes or more. Autosomal recessive. Other conditions may also occur.

Reference
Thiele, G.L., Rempel, W.E., Fass, D.N., Bowie, E.J.W., Stewart, M., Zoecklein, L. (1986). J.Heredity 777, 179-182. Inheritance of a new bleeding disease in a herd of swine with Willebrand's disease.

Thrombocytopaenic purpura and Haemolytic Disease of the Newborn.

Definition

Thrombocytopaenic purpura is a disease of young piglets characterised by multiple haemorrhages and death of the whole or part of a litter 3 or 14-30 days of age after they have ingested colostrum containing antibodies to their platelets.

Incidence

Low, less than 1%.

Aetiology

Thrombocytopaenic purpura is caused by the formation of antibodies to foetal thrombocyte antigens in the sow by isoimmunisation. the ingestion of these antibodies in the colostrum and their absorption by the piglets results in a fall in the circulating levels of thrombocytes to about $200 \times 10^9/l$ at 2 days of age (normally higher, 250-300). Recovery takes place to $400 \times 10^9/l$ at 5 days and from the 9th day onwards declines to a level of $50 \times 10^9/l$ when purpura appears. Megakaryocytes and other cells in the bone marrow are affected and replacement of circulating thrombocytes does not occur. Pigs which die from purpura frequently have no circulating thrombocytes.

The uneven effect of the condition in a litter appears to be related to growth and the ingestion of colostrum, well-grown piglets which have sucked most colostrum being most severely affected. In order for the disease to occur, the thrombocyte type of the boar must differ from that of the sow and she must have had at least one previous litter to a boar of that thrombocyte type.

Clinical signs

The disease appears in piglets of 14-30 days of age with a lesser peak at 3 days of age. In most cases only a quarter of the litter is affected. Most affected piglets die. Death may occur without clinical signs but affected piglets are often pale and listless with an increased respiratory rate. A blotchy, purple skin, haemorrhages, mainly on the belly, and vivid scratch marks may be seen. m e mucous membranes are usually pale and the faeces may be blood stained. There is no fever.

Pathology

Affected pigs are in good bodily condition. Haemorrhages of varying sizes are seen in the epicardium, myocardium, pleura, joints and skeletal muscles. All lymph nodes are engorged with blood.

No megakaryocytes are present in the bone marrow. Platelets are low in numbers (50xl0/l or less) or absent from the blood of affected pigs.

Epidemiology

The condition is not uncommon and affects the second and subsequent litters of sensitised sows bred to the same boar. It has been recorded most frequently in Large White and Landrace pigs and is particularly common when a Large White boar is used on a Landrace sow.

Diagnosis

The characteristic clinical and post-mortem picture may be confirmed by platelet counts. Septicaemic conditions should be ruled out.

Treatment and prevention

Affected piglets should be kept warm and offered fluid replacer, given multivitamins and antimicrobials for 3 or 4 days as supportive treatment. The use of Vitamin K has not been reported. When a sow has been bred to the same boar after having a litter of affected piglets, they too will be affected. The condition can be prevented by transferring the litter to another sow for 24 hours or until the colostrum containing the antibody is used up. Artificial feeding can also be practised. The same boar should not be used on sows which have had affected litters and, if the problem is widespread in a herd it may be economic to change the boar to one of a different breed.

References

Saunders, C.N.,Kinch, D.A. (1968). J. Comp. Path. 78, 513-523. Thrombocytopaenic purpura of pigs.
Saunders, C.N., Kinch, D.A., and Imlah, P. (1966). Vet.Rec. 79, 549.

Haemolytic disease of the newborn

A condition in which isoantibodies produced by the sow to foetal red cells are absorbed by the piglets in the colostrum, causing intravascular haemolysis which results in jaundice and, sometimes, death in piglets aged 2-3 days. This condition resembles thrombocytopaenic purpura in its aetiology and pathogenesis and frequently occurs with it. It may be differentiated from thrombocytopaenic purpura by the early deaths (2-3 days of age), the presence of jaundice and by the demonstration of low red cell counts in the blood of the affected piglets.

Control in the same way as thrombocytopaenic purpura.

Reference

Hall, S.A., Rest, J.R., Linklater, K.A. and McTaggart, H.S. (1972). Vet. Rec. 91, 677. Concurrent haemolytic disease of the newborn and thrombocytopaenic purpura in piglets without artificial immunisation of the dam.

Hereditary scurvy, Vitamin C or ascorbic acid deficiency

Described as an autosomal recessive in Denmark, affected pigs lack the ability to synthesise ascorbic possibly because of the absence of gluconolactone oxidase in the acid liver. Piglets are born normal but, after weaning, plasma hydroxyproline and alkaline phosphatase levels fall. These plasma changes are followed by inappetence and reluctance to move. Subperiosteal haemorrhages and lesions of the metaphyses of the bones are seen When sows are deprived of Vitamin C the changes noted above occur *in utero* and piglets may be born with them.

Reference

Thode Jensen, P. *et al.*, (1983). Acta Vet.Scand. 24, 392-402
Wegger, I., Palludan, B. (1994). J.Nutrition. 124, 241-248. Vitamin C deficiency causes haematological and skeletal abnormalities during foetal abnormalities in swine.

Hereditary Lymphosarcoma

Hereditary lymphosarcoma has occurred at least once in a Large White herd in which it appears to be produced as an autosomal recessive gene. The condition occurs in 25% of the progeny of carriers. Affected piglets become stunted and pot-bellied with enlarged peripheral lymph nodes. They become affected by 6 months of age and do not survive beyond 15 months of age, never reaching sexual maturity. Circulating lymphocyte levels may be raised and blast cells may occur in the circulating blood.

The pathological findings are of a multicentric lymphosarcoma with enlargement of all lymph nodes, especially those of the alimentary tract and bronchus. 5 mm foci of tumour may be seen in peripheral nodes. The liver may be enlarged with white focal lesions as is the spleen. The thymus is involuted. diagnosis of a lymphosarcoma can be reached on pathological grounds, but the involvement of a genetic component requires breeding studies or studies of the incidence of the condition.

Reference

Head, K.W., Campbell J.G., Imlah, P., Laing, A.H., Linklater, K.A., MacTaggart, H.S. (1974). Vet. Rec. 95, 523-526. Hereditary lymphosarcoma in a herd of pigs.

Barking Piglets

A syndrome in which piglets are born with features of immaturity, including domed heads, sparse erect hair, failure to develop normal respiration (a barking grunt occurs) and soon die. Inadequate lung expansion is present with an absence of surfactant and the thyroid is small and functions poorly. An autosomal recessive.

References

Gibson, E.A., Blackmore, R.J.J., Wijeratne, W.V.S., Wrathall, A.E. (1976). Vet. Rec. 98, 476-479. The 'barker' (neonatal respiratory distress) syndrome in the pig. Its occurrence in the field.

3. Congenital defects resulting from infectious conditions

Congenital Tremor AI. (Myoclonia congenita)

This results from infection of the sow by swine fever (hog cholera) virus either of high virulence, low virulence or sometimes, vaccine strains at 10-50 days' gestation and was responsible for 12% of all outbreaks of trembling in piglets seen between 1963 and 1965 in the U.K. A high proportion of the litters are affected, more than 40% of pigs within a litter are affected and mortality may be medium or high. Piglets of both sexes and dams from any breed are affected. It does not recur in successive litters from the same parents. Affected piglets show various degrees of muscular tremor, ataxia and inability to stand and suck. When placed on their feet, they may collapse. The tremor is still noticeable after 2-3 weeks. Outbreaks may last up to 4 months.

At post-mortem examination, the cerebellum is abnormally small with almost complete absence of the vermis. This cerebellar hypoplasia may only be obvious in mildly affected animals after comparing the cerebellum:brain weight ratios (0.04-0.08 if affected). Spinal cord changes are most repeatably seen at the level of the third cervical vertebra. There are fewer myelinated axons than in unaffected piglets, apparently because of subnormal or delayed myelination. Maternal antibodies to swine fever can be detected and in some animals (see swine fever) virus may be isolated.

Diagnosis

It is important to differentiate this type of congenital tremor from other causes. The high proportion of litters affected, the high mortality and the presence of the condition in piglets of both sexes born to sows of any breed are useful characters. The presence of cerebellar hypoplasia at post-mortem examination distinguishes it from all but AII and AV. In the latter there is usually a history of organophosphorus treatment and the outbreak lasts for only a month, in AII mortality is low. Virus isolation or demonstration or antibody studies will confirm Swine Fever.

Control

Notifiable and controlled as Swine Fever.

References

Bradley, R., Done, J.T., Hebert, C.N., Overby, E., Askaa, J., Basse, A. and Bloch, B. (1985). J.Comp.Path 93, 43-59.
Harding, J.D.J., Done, J.T. and Derbyshire, J.B. (1966). Vet. Rec. 79, 388-390. Congenital tremors in pigs and their relation to swine fever.

Congenital Tremor AII (Myoclonia congenita)

Other infections or unknown conditions in the dam may give rise to congenital tremor. A fairly clearly-defined infectious condition occurs in most pigkeeping areas of the world. Infection in adults is asymptomatic except for the production of affected litters. A high proportion of litters are affected and more than 80% of the piglets within these litters are born with tremor but little mortality occurs (a difference from AI). Piglets of both sexes may be affected, and affected litters may be born to dams of any breed. The condition does not recur in successive litters from the same parents and the outbreak lasts about 4 months. Affected piglets which suck usually survive and have only slight tremor by 6-8 weeks of age. The disease can be reproduced by infecting pregnant sows with brain suspension from affected piglets at day 30. A virus is suspected, possibly a retrovirus.

Cerebellar hypoplasia may occur and varying degrees of hypomyelinogenesis are found. Viruses have been demonstrated in infectious brain tissue but have not yet been characterised. Antibody to Swine Fever and Bovine Viral Diarrhoea is absent. The condition may otherwise be difficult to distinguish from AI. Control may involve the exposure of non-pregnant sows and gilts to infected piglets in an attempt to reduce the length of an outbreak. Trembling in neonatal piglets may be associated with Aujeszky's disease and may not necessarily be congenital.

Reference

Done, J.T., Wooley, J., Upcott, D.H. and Hebert, C.N. (1986). Br.vet.J. 142, 145-150. Porcine congenital tremor Type AII: spinal cord morphometry.
Vanderkerckhove, P., Maenhout, D., Curvers, P., Hoorens, J., Ducatelle R. (1989). J.Vet.Med. (A). 36, 763-771. Type A2 congenital tremors in pigs.

Weak piglets

A number of infectious conditions can lead to the birth of weak piglets. These include leptospirosis, Brucella (not UK), enterovirus and PRRS infections and possibly, parvovirus infections. Premature farrowing or late abortion due to a number of infectious agents may also lead to the birth of weak piglets. These may be born early as a result of direct infection of the foetus (toxoplasmosis) or due to fever e.g. erysipelas. In utero infections may also cause stunting, reduce birthweight and thus liveability.

Stillborn animals often accompany litters of weak pigs.

4. Congenital conditions attributable to nutritional deficiencies or poisoning

Congenital Tremor AV

Exposure of the dam to Trichlorfon or Neguvon between days 45 and 79 (especially 75-79) of gestation can result in the birth of a high proportion of litters containing trembling piglets. 90-100% of piglets of both sexes within affected litters may be born with rhythmic tremor, may stumble and fall and have difficulty in sucking. The mortality rate is high. Outbreaks may last about a month, but where the chemical is applied routinely (in some mange treatments), it may occur for longer periods. Severity of the tremor is dose-related.

The most consistent pathological features are cerebellar hypoplasia (cerebellum:whole brain ratio often 4%), reduced spinal cord size and hypomyelinogenesis. History will separate AV from AI and AII.

Reference

Wells, G.A.H. (1977). Pig Farming 25,73-76. Haloxon neurotoxicity.
Pope, A.M. et al. (1986). J.Am.Vet.Med.Assn. 189, 781-783.
Trichlorfon-induced cerebellar hypoplasia in neonatal pigs.

Mulberry Heart Disease

Mulberry heart disease may be found in young piglets and has been seen in piglets in utero. It has been described in more detail under Vitamin E deficiency.

Cleft palate

Cleft palate may result from Hemlock poisoning (Conium maculatum). See also arthrogryposis.

Splayleg

Splayleg may result from Fusarium intoxication in the sow as a result of eating mouldy rations.

Weak piglets

These may result from a deficiency of vitamins such as Vitamin A (accompanied by microphthalmia and generalised oedema with herniation of the cerebellum through the foramen magnum and abnormalities such as cleft palate). Vitamin E (weak with some splayleg) and pantothenic acid deficiency. There may also be weak piglets in litters affected by zearelenone and ergot posoning. The use of prostaglandins in herds with improperly recorded service dates may lead to the birth of premature, weak piglets.

Hairless pigs may result from iodine deficiency.

5.   Conditions present at birth but of unknown cause

Congenital Tremor Type B

Congenital tremors of unknown cause with no consistent gross or microscopic lesions are assigned to Group B. At least three types appear to exist. One may have cerebellar hypoplasia and lowered levels of cerebroside and lipid in the spinal cord, another has none of these features and yet others have few if any distinctive changes at all. It seems likely that more aetiological agents and conditions will be distinguished in this area. At least one of these types may be due to a virus as it appears to be transmissible.

The bleeding navel syndrome

This has occurred in a few pig herds. Affected piglets bleed to death as a result of failure of closure of the umbilicus or relaxation of previously closed vessels 2-6 hours after birth. Large, pale piglets, often covered with blood are found. There may be an underlying immaturity of collagen. Attendance at farrowings and ligation of the umbilicus with Holliston baby navel clamps can reduce mortality but recent studies have shown the condition may be prevented in some cases by feeding ascorbic acid (1-5 g per sow per day) to sows for at least six days prior to farrowing. Vitamin K injections given to sows have also been reported to have some effect.

Reference

Sandholm, M., Honkanen-Buzalski, T. and Rasi, V. (1979). Vet. Rec. 104, 337-338. Prevention of navel bleeding in piglets by preparturient administration of ascorbic acid.

THE INVESTIGATION AND CONTROL OF CONGENITAL DISORDERS.

Congenital abnormalities occur in about 1-5% of all pigs born. Obvious abnormalities or those which cause death e.g. atresia ani tend not to be passed on as such animals are not selected for breeding. m ere is thus a tendency for abnormal pigs to be eliminated and for any inherited component of the condition to be eliminated as well.

Dominant genetic traits are rapidly seen and eliminated as they are expressed in all animals carrying them (AA).

Recessive genetic traits will only be expressed by homozygotes (aa) but not by heterozygotes (Aa). An incidence of 1% of recessive trait indicates that 18% of the population are heterozygotes.

Sex linked conditions are only expressed in males but if mated with a carrier, females homozygous for the trait may express it.
Recessive genetic traits may be identified by the familial pattern recorded in an existing closed herd but are less easily identified where breeding stock of unknown carrier status is regularly introduced. A repeatable incidence of 25% of the progeny in successive matings of the same boar and sow would indicate a recessive genetic trait. In a few conditions such as PSS or pityriasis rosea this may happen, but in other conditions such as atresia ani the results are less clear-cut and a genetic influence can only be determined because of a high incidence of the trait following carrier matings or mating carriers with recessives.

Chromosomal or developmental abnormalities appear spontaneously and, unless associated with genetic transmission or a particular environmental cause will be sporadic.

Environmental factors such as nutrition, infection and poisoning may be distinguished by history of disease in sows at the relevant stage of gestation e.g. swine fever.
They may also occur in sows of different breeds on the same farm and the abnormality may fail to reappear in any sow mated with the same boar on a subsequent occasion. Some congenital abnormalities of infectious origin may only occur in the litters of recently-introduced gilts. In some cases the condition responsible can be identified and in others transmission can be proved

experimentally. Nutritional deficiencies such as Vitamin A deficiency or excesses such as selenium toxicity can be identified by analysis of the ration if they continue. Toxins and poisonings are usually associated with exposure of sows to a toxin such as trichlorphos at the appropriate stage of gestation and either fail to recur in subsequent litters or occur in animals on other farms receiving the same treatment or food.

Control

This should rely on the correction of environmental factors such as nutrition, toxin exposure and infection whenever possible.

Where a genetic component is suspected, it is

(1)   Common practice not to retain affected individuals for breeding unless, as in P.S.S., there is an economic advantage.

(2)   Culling of the affected individual, its sibs and, possibly, its parents may also be commonly practiced if the incidence of the trait is less than 3% particularly if this will have no effect on genetic progress.

(3)   When the incidence of the trait is more than 3%, full sib culling may be carried out, but only if advantageous.

(4)   Test mating of possible carriers with homozygous recessives can be carried out with subsequent elimination but to reduce the frequency of a recessive gene from 0.5% to 0.25% would require 6 generations of selection solely against that gene.

(5)   The identification of carriers by means other than test mating (as in PSS) leaves decisions as to control to be based solely on economics and the genetic advantages to be gained by retaining or eliminating the gene e.g. the use of PSS-resistant sire lines and PSS-sensitive dam lines.

References

Bampton, P.R. (1994). Pig J. 32, 68-82. The investigation of genetic and hereditary disorders of pigs.
Huston, R., Saperstein, G., Schoneweis, D. and Leipold, H.W. (1978). Vet.Bull. 48, 645-675. Congenital defects in pigs.
Steane, D.E. (1985). Proc.Pig Vet.Soc. 12, 38-49. Congenital abnormalities.
Wrathall, A.E. (1988). Proc.Pig Vet.Soc. 21, 116-134. The boar and congenital problems.

Definition

Mastitis in sows may be localised to a single gland or may involve more than one to cause fever, depression and death. Losses due to piglet mortality may be considerable. Coliform mastitis and the sporadic chronic mastitis affecting single glands are described separately as is agalactia.

a) Coliform mastitis

Definition

Coliform mastitis may be caused by any enterobacterial organism. Infection may be localised to a single gland or may involve more than one to cause fever, depression and death. Agalactia is common and piglet mortality and growth depression may be considerable.

Incidence

May be a major cause of loss in affected herds.

Aetiology

The acute and severe forms of this condition are often associated with *Klebsiella spp.* and may occur in outbreaks of fatal disease often associated with the trauma of a particular type of sawdust bedding. A wide variety of *E.coli* serotypes may be isolated, often differing from gland to gland. Other coliform organisms may be identified. Recent studies suggest that the *E.coli* types all possess fimbriae and can adhere to epithelial surfaces.

Pathogenesis

In many cases, traumatic injury resulting from unclipped piglet teeth, sawdust bedding (particularly important in Klebsiella mastitis), or poor quality flooring is a contributory factor in initiating infection. One, or both glands supplying a single teat may be infected. Infection usually enters via the teat canal and bacteria multiply in the gland. In some cases, infection may be transient, producing an endotoxin-mediated cellular response and a shift to the left in blood white cell counts and in others, colonisation, multiplication and acute mastitis with systemic signs and agalactia apparently caused by the effect of *E.coli* endotoxin on prolactin production. Introduction of either endotoxin or interleukin I to the mammary gland will cause mastitis and agalactia and endotoxin can be detected in the blood in mastitis.

Clinical signs

Acutely affected sows are usually depressed, inappetent and pyrexic (temperatures of 40.5-42°C (105-107°F) are not uncommon). The udder is usually swollen and oedematous, often with massive congestion. Any secretion that may be obtained after oxytocin injection is purulent. Pain in the udder may lead to restlessness in the sow when piglets attempt to suck. The litter rapidly loses condition. The condition occurs within 1-3 days of parturition in most cases and death frequently results. Coliform mastitis appears to regress within 3-4 days although in severe cases the lactation may cease entirely if death does not occur. Subacute infection or infection in one or more glands occurs much more commonly and may be recognised by the increased hardness of the gland and, in its early stages, by a square area of reddening of the skin over the affected gland. The litter loses condition. The litter loses condition and in subclinical *E.coli* mastitis this loss of condition may draw attention to its presence. Secretion may appear grossly normal in subacute or subclinical infection but cytology demonstrates raised cell counts ($>10^6$/ml).

Euthanasia is only indicated in acute disease when the body temperature falls below normal, the animal can no longer rise and respiratory distress develops.

Pathology

At post-mortem examination, the carcase muscle and the liver may be pale and the subcutaneous tissue over the affected mammae is oedematous. The cut surface of affected mammae is diffusely or focally reddened. An acute inflammatory reaction and necrosis of the alveolar epithelium is present. *E.coli, Klebsiella* spp. or other coliform organisms may be isolated from the affected glands, although in many cases the organisms have already been eliminated. Sows with subacute or subclinical mastitis rarely die. Lesions are restricted to the few glands affected. Often only one of the two glands supplying 1 teat is reddened and engorged with milk.

Epidemiology

Outbreaks occur on individual farms and are frequently associated with faecal contamination or wetness of bedding. In the case of Klebsiella mastitis, infected sawdust may be associated with the outbreak. There appears to have been a reduction in the acute form of the disease causing death in recent years.

Diagnosis

Acute mastitis is easily recognisable. Subclinical mastitis may only be detected after cell counts on expressed milk. Cell counts in infected glands may reach 2.0×10^8/ml with 75% polymorphs but levels of 4.0×10^7/ml may be found in involuting unsucked normal glands. Normal milk contains 1×10^6 cells/ml. Chronic mastitis is easily palpable upon inspection during lactation and easily seen in dry sows. The isolation of the bacteria from milk may also be of value.

Treatment and control

Acutely ill sows may be saved by parenteral treatment with antibiotics such as neomycin, tetracyclines, ampicillin, amoxycillin, streptomycin or by the use of trimethoprim: sulphonamide injections for 2-4 days. Oxytocin should also be given. In some cases treatment is effective. The litter should be fostered or reared artificially. After recovery it may be necessary to cull the sow. In severely affected cases the prognosis is poor but rehydration with saline given intravenously by flutter valve may cause a dramatic improvement in moribund animals. Other supportive treatment should be given and recent studies suggest that some anti-inflammatory drugs such as flunixin meglumine (Finadyne, Schering Plough, not registered for pigs UK) may have some value. In subacute cases, rehydration is not necessary.

Control depends upon the use of hygiene, use of soft bedding other than sawdust, clipping piglets' teeth, early treatment and, possibly, the use of commercial *E.coli* vaccines may reduce the incidence if the condition is due to *E.coli*. Prophylactic treatment with trimethoprim:sulphonamide at 15 mg/kg given in the feed from day 112 of gestation to day 1 post-partum may prevent the condition as may feed medication with other agents. Animals which have had severe or repeated bouts of mastitis should be culled.

References

Backstrom, L., Morkoc, A.C., Connor, J., Larson, R. and Bryce, W. (1984). J.Am.Vet.Med.Assn. 185, 70-73. Clinical study of mastitis metritis agalactia in sows in Illinois.
Jones, J.E.T. (1979). Vet. Annual, 19, 97. Acute coliform mastitis in the sow.
Martineau, G.P., Smith, B.B., Douze, B. (1992). Veterinary Clinics of North America: Food Animal Practice : Swine Reproduction 8, 661-684. Pathogenesis, prevention and treatment of lactational insufficiency in sows.
Smith, B.B. and Wagner, W.C. (1985). Am.J.Vet.Res. 46, 175-180. Effect of *E.coli* endotoxin and thyrotropin-releasing hormone on prolactin in lactating sows.
Wegmann, P. and Bertschinger, H.U. (1984). Proc.Int.Pig Vet.Soc. 8, 287. Sequential cytological and bacteriological examination of the secretions from sucked and unsucked mammary glands in and without mastitis.

b) Sporadic or chronic mastitis

Definition

Mastitis may affect single glands particularly in older sows to result in abscess formation and loss of the individual gland often with few systemic clinical signs.

Incidence

In one UK survey 18.8% of culled sows were affected. Only one gland was infected in 60% of affected sows.

Aetiology and Pathogenesis

A(C).pyogenes, streptococci, staphylococci, *Bacteroides* spp. fusobacteria and clostridia may all be isolated. The organisms enter the gland as does *E.coli* but do not usually cause the systemic reaction seen in coliform mastitis.

Clinical signs

Often noted only when an affected gland fails to return to normal after weaning. It may be noted as local inflammation and pain over that portion of the udder during lactation and pus may be expressed. As oedema may spread over more than one gland, the exact location of the affected gland may not be identifiable. There is often teat injury. Culling should be carried out when multiple abscesses or ulceration are present but humane slaughter is rarely indicated.

Pathology

Abscessation and fibrosis, often coupled with physical damage to the teat or its end may be found. The bacteria listed above may be isolated.

Epidemiology

Bedding and unclipped teeth, flooring such as perforated metal which predispose to teat damage may all allow organisms to colonise the udder and cause the condition.

Diagnosis

Clinical signs as above, confirmed by expression of pus and isolation of organisms.

Treatment and control

Parenteral antimicrobials including penicillin if staphylococci or streptococci are involved. Oxytocin administration may be of value Control can be established by improving husbandry. Affected sows should only be retained if they have sufficient functioning teats.

Reference

Delgado, J.A. and Jones, J.E.T. (1981). Br. Vet. J. 137, 639-643. An abattoir survey of mammary gland lesions in sows with special reference to the bacterial flora of mammary abscesses

The Mastitis, Metritis, Agalactia Complex (M.M.A.), the Periparturient Hypogalactia Syndrome (P.H.S.)

Definition

A complex syndrome in which hypogalactia or agalactia occur within 12-72 hours of parturition. Fever, anorexia, vulval discharge and mastitis may all accompany the basic change and the growth rate and survival of the litter are usually affected.

Incidence

Recent surveys suggest that the most severe forms are becoming less common.

Aetiology

Unknown. It has been considered to be due to bacterial invasion of the mammae and subsequent production of endotoxins which are absorbed to give the systemic signs. A similar syndrome can be reproduced experimentally in some cases, by the intravenous injection of endotoxin into sows. Endotoxin cannot, however, always be demonstrated in the plasma of affected animals, neither can bacteria or mastitis be identified in the mammary glands. Bacteria in the gut or in endometritis may be the source of endotoxin but the available evidence suggests that endometritis is not the source of endotoxin. ß-haemolytic streptococci and coliforms have been associated with the condition and in many cases mastitis may be present in one or more glands.

Hormonal causes have been suggested as levels of a number of hormones may be depressed following parturition. It may be that these represent the effector mechanism, but the initiating factors have not been identified. Hormones involved in lactation include insulin, cortisone and prolactin, oxytocin, oestrogen and progesterone and changes in the levels of all these have been demonstrated in pigs with agalactia. Levels of oxytocin are often half those in normal sows. Prolactin levels may be dramatically reduced by small volumes of endotoxin and recent studies suggest that the inhibition of prostaglandin F2 alpha production in the uterus (possibly by infection) may remove an important stimulus to prolactin secretion. Management and nutrition appear to be important in the aetiology and low exercise, high nutrient density rations, overfeeding and poor hygiene all appear to predispose to the condition. The importance of water intake and stress or disturbance during parturition is not yet clear.

Clinical signs

The syndrome usually occurs within 12 hours - 3 days of parturition. Inappetence is commonly the first sign to be noted, followed by depression, restlessness when being suckled and loss of condition in the litter. Affected sows may have a slight fever, 39.5-41°C, unless mastitis is present. Vulvar discharge and constipation are frequently with associated with this condition but neither may be present. The disease lasts for a minimum of 3 days and then resolves spontaneously. By this time the litter may have been lost. The condition may be preceded by delays in parturition (>5 hours) and may vary in its intensity. In mild cases of hypogalactia unaccompanied by mastitis or other elements of the complex, depressed daily liveweight gain in piglets (<105 g/day, normal 125 g/day) may be the only indication of the problem.

Affected sows recover but hypoglycaemic piglets which do not respond to treatment, may require euthanasia in extremis.

Pathology

Neither mastitis nor metritis is a constant finding. Where mastitis occurs, it appears to be patchy within a gland and of an acute catarrhal nature. Oedema of the subcutaneous tissue and inflammatory changes in the draining lymph nodes occur where mastitis is present. Histologically the glands of affected pigs often resemble those of sows at 110 days' gestation.

Epidemiology

The condition sometimes occurs in batches It is particularly common where hygiene is poor and where sows are fat.

Diagnosis

Clinical signs are the main method of diagnosis. Confirmation of bacterial mastitis may be made by the examination of milk samples. Disease in the litter, such as diarrhoea, septicaemia or hypothermia, may lead to decreased intake of milk and overstocking of the udder. When fever is present, other disease (e.g.

erysipelas) may be the cause. A history of difficulty in farrowing, or small litters or incomplete cleansing, may indicate retention of a foetus or placentae. Examination per vagina, if within 24 hours of parturition, will establish this. In some cases mycotoxins such as trichoethecenes may be involved.

Treatment

Affected sows should be given frequent doses of oxytocin. Parenteral broad spectrum antimicrobial may be given and is advisable when mastitis, metritis or fever are present. Ampicillin, tetracyclines, trimethoprim sulphonamide or enrofloxcin may be given. Anti-inflammatory drugs such as flunixin meglumine have been reported to improve recovery. The value of corticosteroids is equivocal.

Control

Hygiene, and exercise of the sows prior to farrowing and during the early stages of lactation may help. Restriction of the feed for the last two or three days before farrowing and replacing part of it with bran, may help reduce the incidence. Reduction of feed intake to 1 kg/day from 100 days, gestation and use of vegetable protein reduced the incidence of hypogalactia.

The use by farmers of oxytocin in early cases of agalactia may be helpful and reduce the need for veterinary involvement. Treatment should begin when sow body temperature is 39.4°C 12-18 hours post farrowing. Routine injections of antibiotic and oxytocin post farrowing have been shown not to be helpful. Recent studies have indicated that treatment with trimethoprim: sulphonamide in the feed at 15 mg/kg bodyweight from day 112 of gestation to day 1 *post partum*, reduces the incidence of the disease markedly as may in-feed medication with other sulphonamides or tetracyclines. The use of long acting tetracycline (Terramycin LA, Pfizer) injections given 1 day before farrowing has been shown to be beneficial in some herds. Recently some studies have shown significant decreases in agalactia in sows which have farrowed early as a result of prostaglandin use. Other studies have found no difference.

References

Goransson, L. (1989). J.Vet.Med. Series A 36, 505-513. The effect of feed allowance in late pregnancy on the occurrence of agalactia *post partum* in the sow.
Kensinger, R.S., Collier R.J., Bazer, F.W. (1986). J.Anatomy 145, 49-59. Ultrastructural changes in porcine mammary tissue during lactogenesis.
Liptrap, R.M. (1987). Veterinary Annual (1987). 27, 134-138. Lactational failure in the sow.
Martineau, G.P., Smith, B.B., Douze, B. (1992). Veterinary Clinics of North America : Food Animal Practice : Swine Reproduction 8, 661-684. Pathogenesis, prevention and treatment of lactational insufficency in sows.
Peter, A.T., Huether, P., Doble, E., Liptrap, R.M. (1985). Res.vet.Sci. 39, 221-229. Prostaglandin F2 alpha and prolactin in experimental hypogalactia in sows.

"Actinomycosis" of the Udder

Chronic mastitis may sometimes involve more than one teat and spread along the udder to cause a large swelling which is hard to the touch and may touch the ground. It is frequently ulcerated. It normally results from the retention of animals with chronic mastitis. *Actinomyces sp.* may be isolated from fewer than 50% of cases but a variety of other organisms are present. Amyloidosis may occur in the kidneys of affected animals. Affected animals should be culled, but severely affected animals with lesions too large for transport should be destroyed humanely.

Vulval Discharges

Discharges from the vulva may be physiological when they occur immediately post-partum and as semen leakage post service but may also be pathological. They may originate from the uterus in endometritis, from the vagina in vaginitis, from the vulva itself or from the urinary tract in cystitis and pyelonephritis. Vulval discharge is not always apparent in these three underlying syndromes and apparently unaffected animals may prove to be affected upon further investigation. Cystitis and pyelonephritis have been dealt with under bacterial disease, post-partum and post-service vulval discharges and endometritis are considered below.

Post-partum Vulval and Vaginal Discharges
(Post-farrowing vulval discharges, PFD)

Definition

Discharges from the vulva occur in sows after farrowing. They are often copious and may then be linked with depression of production parameters such as performance of the litter and subsequent productivity. They may indicate the presence of metritis.

Incidence

Extremely common worldwide (92% farms Australia). Also present in a high proportion of some farms (to 60%).

Aetiology

A number of bacterial species including ß-haemolytic streptococci of Groups G and L, *A.pyogenes, Actinobacillus suis, Bacteroides spp. Clostridia* and *Haemophilus spp* may be isolated. Coliforms may also be present as may be staphylococci. The bacteria appear to colonise the physiologically-disturbed uterus and vagina. The exact predisposing factors are not yet clear, but the incidence may be reduced by antimicrobial cover from before farrowing and by hygiene.

Pathogenesis

Some of these bacteria are present or identifiable prior to farrowing but with the normal post-parturient flow of materials from the involuting uterus, they increase in numbers and give rise to histological evidence of inflammation in the walls of the vagina and/or give rise to endometritis. The discharge eventually resolves but may be accompanied by mild cystitis or by metritis. The mechanism of infection is not yet clear but infection is probably ascending and often follows interference at farrowing.

Clinical signs

Post parturient vulval discharge occurs initially (12-36 hours) as a clear mucoid, serous or bloody discharge and may in normal circumstances dry up. In some cases (up to 60-70% of sows in a herd) it may persist for 5-7 days. For some days after this pus may be seen during urination or may be found on the floor behind the sow. When post-parturient vulval discharge is prolonged, extended weaning to service intervals may be recorded although recovery is apparently complete before weaning. Subsequent fertility may be reduced by 10% in animals recovered from discharge.

Direct inspection by vaginoscope can distinguish between endometritis, vaginitis and vulvitis. In endometritis, the onset may be early (1.6 days), discharge volume high (100 ml) and the discharge may be white-yellow in colour. Systemic signs of metritis include rectal temperature >40°C, (104°F), inappetance and agalactia in severe cases. Death (5%) may occur and the farrowing rate may be half that of unaffected sows.

Vaginitis is twice as common as metritis, has a later onset (day 4) and produces less discharge (11-30 ml) less inappetance, no deaths and little effect on subsequent fertility. Vulvitis represents only 10-72% of all discharges, appears on day 3, produces the least volume (scant-6 ml) lasting for 2 days and is least likely to affect appetite and has little effect on fertility.

Humane slaughter is only indicated in recumbent animals with metritis which have not responded to treatment or are unable to rise.

Pathology

Pus may be found in the vagina and may originate from the uterus in metritis or from vaginitis alone. Larger than normal numbers of neutrophils may be seen migrating through the vaginal wall in histological sections. Endometritis may be found and appreciable volumes of pus may be present in the uterine lumen.

Epidemiology

The condition appears to be present in individual herds and to occur in cycles.

Diagnosis

Easily seen in the early stages, a speculum may be required to see pus or inflammation later in the disease and relatively easily distinguished from cystitis. In early cases incomplete parturition should be considered. Late cases or those with a closed endometritis may only be suspected following the systemic signs. Swabs for bacteriological examination should be guarded or a speculum used to reduce vulval contamination.

Treatment and control

Antimicrobial therapy may be given parenterally, locally by irrigation of the vagina or placement of pessaries or by the inclusion of antimicrobial at therapeutic level in the feed over the period of farrowing and for 7 days afterwards. Control of the problem has been achieved by routine antimicrobial injection at farrowing. Antimicrobials used include tetracyclines, ampicillin and trimethoprim sulphonamide.

Hygiene is important in prevention. Faecal accumulations behind sows should be removed before and after farrowing, all interference at farrowing should

323

be carried out using clean hands and antimicrobial treatment should be considered immediatey interference has been carried out. Sows with endometritis should be culled after confirmation.

References

Bara, M.R., Cameron, R.D.A. (1994). Proc.IPVS. 13, 400. A study of the incidence, characterisation, effect on reproductive performance and predisposing factors associated with post-farrowing vulval discharges.
Madec, F., Miquet, J.M., Leon, E. (1993). Rec.Vet.Med. 168, 341-349. La pathologie de la parturition chez la triue. Etude epidemiologique dans cinq elevages.
Taylor, D.J. (1984). Proc.Int.Pig Vet.Soc. 8, 151. Clinical and bacteriological effects of antimicrobial therapy on naturally-occurring post-partum vulval discharge in sows following service.

Post Weaning Vulval Discharge (Post-weaning Discharge, PMD)

Definition

Vulval discharges of vaginal or uterine origin occur from 7 days post-service onwards and may be copious. They are associated with a high rate of return to service.

Incidence

Worldwide, 24% of herds affected in a UK survey 1980-85 with individual cases possible in almost any herd. 28% Australia 1994.

Aetiology and pathogenesis

Apparently associated with ascending infections with bacteria such as *E.coli*, *Proteus* spp., *streptococci*, *S.hyicus* and *A.pyogenes*, although the actual organisms initiating the syndrome are not yet identified. The source of infection may be faecal or slurry contamination of the vulva or service by individual boars kept under poor hygienic conditions. Vaginitis may result or infection may progress to endometritis. Uterine infection may result in death of the eggs or developing embryos and delayed return to service. *A.pyogenes* has been shown to be capable of this.

Clinical signs

Vulval discharge appears first as tacky mucus on the vulval lips 15-20 days post-service. A creamy discharge then develops and may persist until at least 80 days post-service. Returns to service usually follow. Discharge is more common in older sows and rare in gilts or first parity animals. Endometritis, vaginitis and cystitis may all occur and may be distinguished by endoscopy. Volumes of discharge are usually highest (90 ml) in endometritis and fertility is lowest (farrowing rate 14%) and depression of appetite is most severe. Vaginitis occurs in fewer cases of PMD than endometritis, has a later onset (12-30 days) produced lower volumes of discharge (14-26 ml) has a 70% farrowing rate and is not fatal.

Pathology

Vaginitis and endometritis alone or together may be present in culled sow Necrotic embryos may be present.

Epidemiology

Frequently associated with poor hygiene and poor crate design. Individual boars, boars kept in dirty conditions or purchased from several sources may be strongly associated with the condition.

Diagnosis

Based on inspection. The presence of blood or mucus in the discharge indicates cystitis or pyelonephritis. Frequently found during investigation of high rates of return. Discharge may be visible only on the underside of the tail, on faeces or on the backplate of the crate. It is difficult to detect in loose-housed sows. Discharge may pool in the anterior vagina and be visible only through a speculum or endoscope. Bacteria may be identified in culture.

Treatment and control

Sows can be treated parenterally with antimicrobial such as long-acting oxytetracycline at the first signs of discharge but this may not save the pregnancy or cure the problem. Prevention involves injection at weaning followed by feed medication with oxytetracycline at therapeutic level for 21 days. Boars should be treated also by washing the preputial sac and instilling an oxytetracycline intramammary preparation daily for 5 days. Treatment should be accompanied by rigorous cleaning and disinfection of sow and boar accommodation and consideration should be given to lowering slurry levels in dry sow houses and to altering the back plates of stalls. The poor farrowing rate of endometritis affected sows makes culling advisable.

References

Bara, M.R., Cameron, R.D.A. (1994). Proc. IPVS. 13, 399. A study of the incidence, characterisation, effect on reproductive performance and predisposing factors associated with post-mating vulval discharge (PMD).
MacLachlan, N.J. and Dial, G.D. (1987). Veterinary Pathology 24, 92-94. An epizootic of endometritis in gilts.
Muirhead, M.R. (1986). Vet.Rec. 119, 233-235. Epidemiology and control of vaginal discharges in the sow.

Endometritis in Sows with no vulval discharge

A large number of organisms may be found in metritis. They include *E.coli*, *Bacteroides spp*, Clostridia, streptococci especially *S.equisimilis*, *C.pyogenes*, aerotolerant campylobacters, sporolactobacilli and staphylococci. In many cases the organisms enter at farrowing or service, reach high levels and are then eliminated but some remain, particularly after difficult farrowings. Where vulval discharges are absent, returns to service may indicate endometritis or pyometra. The latter may be detected by ultrasound. Metritis is present in approximately 30%

of sows culled for infertility and its prevention may only be feasible if a programme such as that described above is adopted or if strategic antibiotic injections are given over farrowing and service. The economics of this practice have to be considered for each individual herd.

References

Berner, H. (1984). Proc.Int.Pig Vet.Soc. 8, 284. Pathogenesis, clinical signs and bacteriology.
Muirhead, M.R. (1984). Vet.Annual 24, 118-126. The investigation and control of a production problem in pigs: low litter size, vaginitis and endometritis.

Preputial Ulceration and Disease in Boars

Ulcers and inflammation of the preputial diverticulum may occur and lead to pain and swelling. there may be enlargement of the superficial lymph nodes and it may be possible to detect the inflamed organ. Eversion of the sac under anaesthetic will confirm. It may be excised surgically or the animal may be treated.

Rotting Prepuce Syndrome

Has occurred in uncastrated boars of 50-75 kg The ventral prepuce becomes abraded, erythematous, oedematios and exudative and may heal or progress within 48-72 hours to necrosis of prepuce and adjacent abdominal wall. Lesions may reach 30 cm in length. Affected pigs may die and should be sent for slaughter or killed humanely.
The syndrome may be a form of transit erythema occurring on wheat straw.

Reference

Marriott, D.W. (1993). Pig.Vet.J. 31, 152-159. The rotting prepuce syndrome.

Stomach ulcers

Ulceration occurs in the pars oesophagea of the stomach to give a clearly-defined syndrome of major importance in the pig industry and also in the glandular part of the stomach where its significance is not yet clear.

1.   Gastric ulceration (Ulceration of the pars oesophagea)

Definition

Gastric ulcers of the pars oesophagea are common in pigs kept under modern husbandry conditions and may cause clinical disease or death when haemorrhage or perforation occurs. In the majority of cases, they are an incidental finding at slaughter.

<u>Incidence</u>

Gastric ulceration has been identified in most pig-rearing countries. The incidence found at slaughter may vary between 2% and 50% although it may be higher in individual herds. Figures for incidence are complicated by the influence of pre-slaughter handling where increased holding time increases lesions and recording of changes as true ulceration (5.9%) erosions (11.4%) hyperkeratosis (36.7% Minnesota 1994 figures). Healed ulcers indicate a higher incidence if recorded. The mortality from the condition may reach 10% in outbreaks in fattening pigs and farrowing sows.

<u>Aetiology</u>

The aetiology of gastric ulceration in pigs is unknown. A number of factors have been suggested as the cause, but the condition may be one of multiple aetiology in which more than one of these factors is involved. The aetiology does not appear to be connected with age as pigs of all ages are affected. No evidence of breed incidence or hereditary transmission has been found.

a) Infection

Gastric ulceration has been observed in a number of infectious conditions, e.g. swine fever, T.G.E. and *S.choleraesuis* infection but this is usually in the fundic area. Studies of the organisms associated with the bases of ulcers have shown that staphylococci and streptococci are often present. In some cases, pure cultures of streptococci have been isolated. Although *Candida albicans* is present in many cases, experimental evidence is lacking for its causal relationship to gastric ulceration.
Pneumonia is strongly associated with gastric ulceration.
Ulceration of the glandular portion of the stomach has also been associated with infection by <u>Hyostrongylus rubidus</u> and may occur following achlorhydria in chronic enteric disease.

b) Toxicity

Copper toxicity has been suggested as a contributory factor in losses from gastric ulceration. In one study, the addition of copper to the ration at 50 ppm raised the death rate from the condition from 1% to 3%.

c) Nutrition

A number of attempts have been made to protect pigs from gastric ulceration by the addition of vitamins, etc., to the feed. Some success has been claimed when selenium, alpha tocopherol, cystine or methionine supplements are given or when the proportion of unsaturated fatty acids in the diet is lowered. High levels of oxidised unsaturated fatty acids may play some part in the aetiology of the condition. It has been suggested that zinc supplementation may reduce the incidence.

d) Feed processing

Studies of the effects of the particle size of feeds and their fibre content have shown that finely-ground pelleted feeds may predispose to gastric ulceration. It has been suggested that the increased moisture content of the stomach contents of pigs fed on finely-ground feed may allow better mixing of the enzymes and closer contact of ingesta and the epithelium of the oesophageal area. Pepsin levels are higher in the stomachs of pigs fed on finely-ground and pelleted feeds.

e) Season

Seasonal changes in incidence have been observed, but probably produce their effects through stress.

f) Stress

Gastric function has long been known to be affected by stress and stresses such as transport, starvation, mixing, overcrowding, increase the incidence of gastric ulceration in pigs. The exact mechanism whereby stress produces or enhances gastric ulceration is not clear, but may be concerned with the increased secretion of hydrochloric acid and digestive enzymes during stress. Ulceration appears more common in pigs of middle social rank.

Pathogenesis

Hyperkeratosis of the pars oesophagea proceeds to erosion and then to ulceration. Ulcers may remain open and blood vessels may rupture. Healing may occur at any stage but is accompanied by scarring if ulceration has occurred.

Clinical signs

The disease may vary from peracute to subclinical. Peracute cases are often found dead in good condition. Animals of any age may be affected, but sows before and after parturition and rapidly growing pigs between 20 and 40 kg are most commonly affected. Animals which survive the acute intragastric haemorrhage become recumbent, breathe rapidly and may grind their teeth in pain. They refuse to eat or drink, the body temperature is low and all visible mucous membranes are cold and pale. Affected pigs may vomit and stand with a rigid back. Pain can be elicited by pressure at the xiphisternum. Subacute cases may show intermittent melaena, passing dark, dry faeces, with anorexia and a reduced growth rate. The subclinical form is most commonly seen at slaughter. Affected pigs grow significantly more slowly than unaffected animals especially when cicatrisation of the oesophagus has occurred.

Pathological findings

Stomach ulcers occur most commonly in the oesophageal area surrounding the cardia which is covered with stratified squamous epithelium. There may also be ulcers or gastritis in mucus and acid-secreting regions. There may be linear, raised parakeratotic lesions of the eosophageal epithelium.

Changes ranging from thickened, rough yellow-brown epithelium through slight, light brown superficial erosions to ulcerations reaching the deeper layers may all be seen. The bases of the ulcers may be covered with necrotic material and clotted blood may be seen adhering to exposed blood vessels. Chronic ulcers may appear as craters floored by the smooth muscle. Scarring may reduce the size of the cardiac sphincter.

Pigs which have died as a result of haemorrhage from an ulcer are pale, the stomach is often distended with clotted blood and the intestines are filled with blood which may be altered. The haemorrhage may be traced to the edge or floor of an acute ulcer or to the sides of a chronic one. Perforation may also occur.

Ulcers may also heal with scarring. Histological sections of early lesions show inflammation of the lamina propria, swelling of the cells of the epithelium and extension of the rete pegs into the lamina propria. The bases of ulcers are usually infiltrated with eosinophils, mononuclear cells and neutrophils. In chronic ulcers, fibrosis of the base may occur. Fibrinonecrotic membranes containing bacteria may be present. Healing ulcers become covered with epithelium and are fibrotic.

Diagnosis

Gastric ulceration is difficult to diagnose in the live pig. The presence of tarry blood in the faeces for 3-8 days without the presence of fever or other signs and pallor of the mucous membranes or white parts of the animal, and raised plasma pepsinogens (5.15 affected 1.5 normal), are suggestive of gastric ulceration. In younger pigs, proliferative haemorrhagic enteropathy produces similar signs. Gastric ulceration must be differentiated from swine dysentery which normally affects all the pigs in a group. The faeces of pigs affected with swine dysentery normally contain mucus and fresh blood and when the blood-stained intestine is rinsed, the mucosa appears congested and inflamed. In gastric ulceration, clotted blood washes off. Salmonellosis is usually associated with fever and a putrid diarrhoea.

Treatment and control

Treatment by blood transfusion or i.v. fluid therapy can relieve the clinical signs and ranitidine syrup may be given orally at 300 mg/sow/day. Antimicrobial cover may also assist the recovery of valuable individual animals. Gastric ulceration may be reduced by removing stress, relieving overcrowding, using proper ventilation and also by reducing the growth rate of young stock by omitting growth promoters from the rations and by increasing fibre levels in the diet, particularly by the use of oats or sugar beet pulp. Zinc, selenium and Vitamin E levels should be supplemented if inadequate. The most important preventive measure is to increase the particle size of the ration to that passing a screen of 3.55 mm (4.68 mm may be optimum) and ensuring that it is fed as meal rather than pellet. Particle size in pellets may also be increased. The pH of whey should be checked and very acid whey should not be fed.

References

Davies, P.R., Grass, J.J., Marsh, W.E., Bahnson, P.B., Dial, G.D. (1994). Proc.IPVS 13, 471. Time of slaughter affects prevalence of lesions of the pars oesophagea of pigs.
Kavanagh, N. (1994). In Practice 16, 209-213. Gastric ulcers in pigs.

2.   Ulceration of the glandular parts

Ulceration of the fundes, pylonis and cardia occurs in a number of specific infectious diseases such as T.G.E. *S.cholerae suis* infection and swine fever. Gastritis occurs as a result of *H.rubidus* infection in the stomachs of adults and gastritis of varying degrees of severity follows the achlorhydria associated with diarrhoeic disease. Recent studies suggest that there may be an association between the *Helicobacter pylori*-like or *Gastrospirillum suis* spiral organisms long known from the crypts and ulceration of this part of the stomach. Clinical signs, pathogenesis and economic importance (if any) of this widespread condition have not yet been evaluated.

Gastric Torsion in Sows

A condition in which sudden death from gastric torsion follows feeding. The condition occurs most commonly following once-daily feeding and can be prevented by feeding twice daily, preferably rapidly, using automatic feeders. In one recent survey in the UK it was responsible for up to 12% of sow deaths with intestinal torsions.

Affected pigs are found to have stomachs grossly distended with food and twisted about the mesenteric axis. Splenic torsion and, sometimes, associated splenic rupture, may also be present. It is thought that rapid ingestion of feed, possibly coupled with fermentation of the food mass, leads to dilatation and, in conditions of excitement, to torsion. If pigs are seen at the dilated stage, exercise may prove beneficial.

Retroversion of the Bladder (in Sows)

Detected at farrowing when exhausted sows may be found to have a mass occluding the anterior vagina. This is the bladder which has been reflected. If the sow is made to stand, the bladder can be manipulated out of the way. Death may otherwise occur.

The Intestinal Haemorrhage Syndrome
"Bloody Gut"/Whey Bloat

Definition

A syndrome in which large pigs 35 kg - adult become pale, have distended abdomens and die suddenly. At post-mortem examination, the small intestine is distended with blood-stained fluid and there may be gaseous distension of the colon. Volvulus may be present and there is usually blood-stained fluid in the abdomen. The carcase is pale.

Aetiology

a) Whey. In whey-fed pigs, an anticlockwise torsion of the whole intestinal mass allows the caecum to point cranially. The large and small intestines are involved and the twist occurs at the root of the mesentery and does not involve the duodenum. Affected pigs may be seen live. Some appear bloated and recover, others die. Excessive gas production from whey reaching the colon has been suggested as a cause of this condition (Whey bloat or Colonic bloat).

b) Manipulation. Animals turned when anaesthetised have developed the condition.

c)   Allergy. Allergy to milk protein or some other component of the diet has been suggested as a cause. The evidence for this view is the presence of large numbers of eosinophils in the lesions.

d)   Non whey fed pigs. A similar syndrome may be seen in pigs fed on skim milk, or wet or dry meal. Volvulus may or may not be present and in some cases there is no gas in the caecum. The aetiology is unknown.

e)   Infection. Ileal symbiont *intracellularis* has been suggested as a contributory cause in cases in which no volvulus occurs and enteropathogenic *E.coli*, *C.perfringens* type C and enterotoxigenic *Clostridium perfringens* Type A may be involved in some A enterotoxin may be involved in some.

Clinical signs

Found dead or seen with abdominal colic and mild rise in body temperature and, sometimes, pallor of the body.

Pathology

The gross pathological changes are described above. The small intestine is almost always autolytic but in animals seen to die there is massive inflammatory change with shedding of the small intestinal villous epithelium, loss of villi and migration of inflammatory cells into both the lamina propria and the lumen which is filled with cells, red cells and bacteria.

A wide variety of clostridia can be isolated from these lesions including both sporulating and vegetative *C.perfringens* Type A and *C.perfringens* enterotoxin has also been demonstrated.

Epidemiology

In whey fed units, deaths occur more commonly as the whey concentration rises. Elsewhere deaths occur sporadically, usually with one or two pigs dying in any one pen.

Diagnosis

Based on characteristic post-mortem findings.

Treatment

As deaths occur suddenly, treatment can rarely be given. A spasmolytic may be of value and may be accompanied by injection of an antibiotic. Trimethoprim:sulphonamide was used successfully on one farm where the problem occurred frequently. Change of diet may be preventative. Reduction in the whey concentration can reduce mortality but also reduces growth rate.

References

Todd *et al.* (1977). Vet. Rec. 100, 11.
Noyes, E., Pijoan C., Ruth, G., Raffe, M. 1988). Vet.Rec. 122, 47-48. Intestinal torsions in swine under anaesthesia.

Colitis

Definition

A diarrhoea of weaned pigs of any age from weaning to slaughter the cause of which is not immediately apparent and which may result in loss of performance.

Incidence

Present in 5% of herds in the UK (1986) but possibly more common at present. Identified in France, Belgium, Denmark, The Netherlands, Canada, the U.S. and Eire.

Aetiology and pathogenesis

The syndrome is currently poorly defined and the aetiology and pathogenesis is unknown at present. In many cases described in the literature agents known to cause disease in this age group have not been sought. Two main areas have been considered important, nutrition and infection.

Nutrition has been considered relevant because field observations suggest that the syndrome occurs on a particular feed and that when that feed is changed the disease disappears. In many cases the use of this 'suspect' feed on other farms is not associated with the syndrome. Firmer evidence comes from studies in which the same diet was fed as pellets, meal and as ground pellets. Disease occurred on the pelletised ration and not on the meal. Pigs fed ground pellets were intermediate between the groups. Pelleting may caramelise carbohydrates, alter particle size, destroy micronutrients or growth promoters and involve the use of pelleting agents or binders.

Nutritional factors known to affect digestion include the presence of trypsin inhibitors in peas, beans and raw soya and the effects of poor quality fat. Infection may also be important. The pig is now weaned at 3 weeks of age when lactogenic immunity is withdrawn. Serum antibody to pathogens does not decline until 6-10 weeks of age. Exposure of pigs to colonisation or infection with a wide range of agents occurs from that time onward at a rate which depends upon exposure to the agent and the immune status of the individual pig. Enteric pathogens may be suppressed by antimicrobial growth promoters and the mixing and change in growth promoter which occur when housing is changed enhance the spread of agents to which immunity is lacking.

Infection of the growing pig with rotaviruses, epidemic diarrhoea and enteroviruses is common. T.G.E. may also occur in immune herds at this period. Torovirus may also infect the colon at this stage. Bacterial diseases which occur in this age group include E.coli enteritis associated both with classic enterotoxigenic strains but also with attaching and effacing E.coli and with those of haemorrhagic colitis type PE, salmonellosis, swine dysentery, spirochaetal diarrhoea, Yersinia enterocolitica and the campylobacter infections all affect this age group and affect the colon. Recent studies with C.perfringens type A have shown that this organism can initiate a syndrome resembling some forms of "colitis" and Bacteroides fragilis strains have also been shown to be capable of causing diarrhoea.

Parasites such as Oesophagostomum and Trichuris suis may also damage the large intestinal mucosa. In younger pigs coccidia such as I.suis may still be present and the Eimeria species may also affect the large intestine. Cryptosporidia are often present in the intestines of affected pigs and both Balantidium coli and Trichomonas spp. may colonise lesions caused by other agents.

These infectious agents must be considered when studying the aetiology and pathogenesis of the syndrome. They may interact with nutrition by lowering the absorptive capacity of the large intestine.

Clinical signs

Softening of the faeces and the occasional passage of mucus. Diarrhoea can also develop. Individual pigs may be affected for 3-20 days and appear hollow-flanked, dirty and restless. Growth rates may be depressed and feed conversion may be affected. The syndrome is most common in the 8-10 week age group but can occur later. The faeces of affected pigs may froth and bubble immediately after taking from the rectum.

Pathology

In classic 'colitis' only the large intestine is affected. The contents are fluid, contain bubbles and sometimes have an oily sheen. In early cases the mucosa appears to be normal even histologically, and on scanning electron microscopy. Local loss of microvilli from colonic epithelial cells may occur. In some cases there may be more obvious colonic lesions.

Epidemiology

Present within individual farms, transfer from farm to farm may occur with breeding stock. The condition may be present more commonly under unhygienic conditions.

Diagnosis

Diagnosis is based on the clinical signs and the absence of the comprehensive list of agents listed above. The small intestine should be examined post-mortem and the respiratory tract should be examined where poor growth rate is a problem, to confirm that pneumonic conditions are not contributing to the poor productivity.

Treatment and control

In the short term, changing the feed for meal or for that produced to another specification may improve the situation. Accommodation should be cleaned and all-in, all-out housing adopted.

Other diseases such as pleuropneumonia, which contribute to growth depression in this age group should be eliminated and other enteric diseases identified should be treated and controlled. In cases where spirochaetal diarrhoea has been identified, tiamulin or dimetridazole have been used successfully. Where C.perfringens type A is important avoparcin inclusion as the growth promoter has dramatic effects. Where Y.enterocolitica is present, tetracyclines may be of value.

Rectal Stricture Syndrome

Definition

A syndrome in which the rectum of fattening pigs becomes fibrosed and the animal dies with megacolon.

Incidence

The condition occurs in outbreaks affecting up to 10% of finishing pigs but is sporadic.

Aetiology and pathogenesis

The aetiology is unknown, but it often follows untreated rectal prolapse in which sloughing has occurred and may follow any enteritis in which excoriation of the rectal mucosa and associated mucocutaneous junction is a feature. This area has a blood supply from the posterior haemorrhoidal artery and from the perineal arteries but a poorly-vascularised zone exists at the junction of the two blood supplies. Any mucosal ulceration or arteriolar thrombosis may cause damage to the mucosa and results in scarring. In male pigs the presence of the retractor penis muscle lying across the rectum at this point may exacerbate changes. The circulatory and inflammatory changes have been considered to be due to salmonella infections but in the UK this is not always the case. In some cases the syndrome follows the use of an antimicrobial such as tylosin and it has been said to result from overgrowth by *Candida spp.* and other yeasts which may be isolated from affected colons. Another site at the brim of the pubis may be inflamed in the chronic stage of enteric disease. Bacteria such as selenomonas appear to be associated with the lesions and chlamydia and *IS.intracellulare* may be present.

The condition often develops within 10 days of a dietary change and is often preceded by stickiness and erythema at the mucocutaneous junction accompanied by a marked reluctance to defaecate.

Clinical signs

Affected pigs become dull, depressed, anorexic and cease to grow. The abdomen becomes grossly distended and the outline of the swollen colon may be seen. In some cases the partially occluded rectum allows the passage of soft ribbon-like motions.

Humane slaughter should be carried out when complete rectal stricture is present and when two successive weighings one week apart show no growth.

Pathology

A grossly distended large intestine is seen. A band of fibrous tissue, sometimes with abscessation on its dorsal side, may be found at the anus, 3-4 cm proximal to it or at the brim of the pubis up to 10 cm cranial to the anus.

Diagnosis

The presence of a pig aged 5 weeks or more with a distended abdomen depressed and standing in the corner of a pen is suggestive and the diagnosis can be confirmed by the insertion of a thermometer or gloved finger into the rectum when an obstruction will be met 2-4 cm into the rectum. Post-mortem examination will confirm.

Treatment and control

It is technically possible to exteriorise the constricted rectum dorsal to the anus while the pig is anaesthetised. The rectum can be cut proximal to the obstruction and sewn in to the perineum to form a new anus. A rubber ring can be used to exteriorise the caecum or mid-colon in a colostomy. Surgically treated pigs may grow rapidly to gain market weight or may develop fresh strictures. Animals which fail to gain weight for the first three weeks post-operation should be destroyed. The syndrome may be reduced in incidence by the prompt repair of rectal prolapses (see below) and the treatment of outbreaks of chronic diarrhoea in animals at risk. A mixture of penicillin, chlortetracycline and sulphadimidine has been found to eliminate the early inflammatory lesions of the rectal wall and to prevent the disease.

Rectal Prolapse

Rectal prolapse may occur in pigs of any age but is more common in males aged 14-16 weeks. In male piglets it may follow straining resulting from the impaction of phosphate crystals in the urethra. In weaned pigs it may follow medication with tylosin and to a lesser extent other antimicrobials and is often accompanied by soft faeces and by coughing. The rectal mucosa protrudes visibly and can be damaged when pigs are mixed and fight due to the raised abdominal pressure of the alarm calls. The hyperoestrogenism associated with zearelenone may predispose to the condition in sows but most commonly it is a consequence of tethering heavily gravid sows with the hindquarters lower than the body or hanging over a drop.

The consequences are similar in all cases. The prolapsed rectum may become reduced naturally, become strangulated, necrotic and drop off or be bitten off by the other pigs. Rectal stricture, death from loss of blood or peritonitis may all occur. Animals may recover if separated from their fellows, the prolapse may be reduced under anaesthetic and secured by a purse-string suture or amputated surgically. Animals may be treated in their groups by the insertion of an 18-20 cm helical corrugated plastic tube of 1.5 cm diameter for weaners and fatteners and 2-3 cm diameter for sows into the prolapse. Heavy duty rubber bands are placed over the prolapse near the anal ring. Tube and prolapse drop off after 5-7 days.

Affected animals of slaughter weight may be penned separately and transported for slaughter but extensively and irreparably-damaged animals should be slaughtered humanely.

References

Douglas, R.G.A. (1985). Vet.Rec. 117, 129. A simple method for correcting rectal prolapse in pigs.
Gardner, I.A., Hird, D.W., Franti, C.E., Glenn, J. (1988). Vet.Rec. 123, 222-225. Patterns and determinants of rectal prolapse in a herd of pigs.

Uterine and Vaginal Prolapse

Similar in the sow to rectal prolapse but may also follow parturition, damage at service or the intake of zearalenone. May be reduced and secured under anaesthetic or amputated if necrotic. Uterine prolapse reduction is so traumatic that humane slaughter should be considered.

Heat Stroke

As environmental temperatures increase from 22°C to 40-41°C, pigs seek shade, water, mud or slurry in order to wallow and cool themselves. Animals in transit, stressed and unable to cool themselves - in sow stalls, farrowing crates or in full sun become dyspnoeic, salivate, breathe with difficulty and become restless. They may later become frenzied, cyanotic and die. A body temperature of 41°C (106°F) - 43°C (110 F) may be recorded. Pathological findings include blood-stained foam in the nostrils and trachea, congestion and haemorrhage in the carcase and some oedema, particularly in the lungs. Productivity may be depressed as may be feed intake. Diagnosis is based on history of high temperature and absence of other causes of death.

Treatment involves tranquillising affected pigs, e.g. with azaperone, cooling the limbs and belly with water and injecting a corticosteroid. Prevention: increase ventilation or, in hot countries, provide cold running water or sprinklers in each pen. N.B. The porcine stress syndrome may develop in environmental temperatures of 22°C+.

References

McGlone, J.J., Stansbury, W.F., Tribble, L.F. (1987). J.Animal Science 65, 456-462. Effects of heat and social stressors on young pig performance. Also
McGlone, J.J., Stansbury, W.F., Tribble L.F. (1988). J.Anim. Sci. 66, 885-891. Management of lactating sows during heat stress.

Sunburn

A cause of dermatitis in White pigs outdoors. Reddening, oedema and then crusting and peeling occur. Affected pigs may be very hot to the touch. Shade or wallows are sufficient to prevent and cure. Vesicles may result from contact with celery or parsnip leaves and exposure to the sun.

Frostbite

Occurs following exclusion of sows from shelter by other sows of the group.

Electrocution

This occurs when electrical wiring is directly available to pigs or when faulty electrical connections result in current passing through metal cage fittings. Some affected pigs are found dead and may have burn marks at the point of contact. The carcases are congested, there may be froth on the lips.

Survivors may be found in a dog-sitting position with posterior paresis, lame, unwilling to feed. There is froth in the trachea and oedema of the lungs. Blood splashing of the heart and musculature is common. Examination of the skeleton frequently reveals fractures of vertebrae, particularly in the thoracic region, of the humerus and especially of the neck of the scapula, the pelvis and the neck of the femur. Decomposition often occurs rapidly following death by electrocution.

The skeletal damage, burn marks and proximity to electric wiring differentiate sudden death from this cause from many other causes of sudden death including cardiac failure, septicaemias such as anthrax and erysipelas. Bacteriology or classic gross lesions distinguish the condition from the bacterial septicaemias, gastric torsion, gastric ulceration, vegetative endocarditis, the porcine stress syndrome, heatstroke and *C.novyi* infection.

When electrocution is suspected ensure that all metalwork and dead pigs are no longer live before investigation. In view of the deep fractures, animals unable to walk home or rise should be killed humanely on site and not transported for slaughter.

Salt Poisoning

Salt poisoning is usually due to water deprivation and has been dealt with under that heading.

Carbon Monoxide Poisoning

Dramatic increases in the stillbirth rate may accompany the use of faulty gas heaters in poorly ventilated farrowing accommodation. Stillbirth rates up to 53% have been recorded. 50 ppm carbon monoxide is the acceptable upper limit and at levels of 120-150 ppm abortion and stillbirth occur. At 150-200 ppm, foetal blood reaches carboxy haemoglobin saturation point within 24-48 hours and the foetus dies. Affected piglets' tissues are cherry-red, there are serosanguineous pleural effusions, hypoxic leuco-encephalopathy and extramedullary haemopoiesis. Levels of 200-300 ppm impair the growth and activity of newborn piglets. No changes are seen in the sow. 200 ppm. does not appear to affect weaners but 200-300 ppm. may reduce performance.

Carbon monoxide can affect man and should be cleared before investigation of the accommodation is carried out.

References

Dominick, M.A. and Carson, T.L. (1983).Am.J.Vet.Res. 44, 35-40. Effects of carbon monoxide exposure on pregnant sows and their foetuses.

Morris, G.L. Curtis S.E., Simon, J. (1995). J.Anim.Sci.61, 1070-1079. Perinatal piglets under sublethal concentrations of atmospheric carbon monoxide.

Morris, G.L., Curtis, S.E., Widowski, T.M. (1985). J.Animal Science 61, 1080-1087. Perinatal piglets under sublethal concentrations of atmospheric carbon monoxide and perinatal pigs and 1080-1087 weaned pigs.

337

Ammonia

Reduction in growth rate and feed conversion rate of up to 24% can result when atmospheric ammonia levels reach 150 ppm.

Nitrate and Nitrite Poisoning

Definition

The ingestion of nitrate or nitrite results in gastroenteritis and dyspnoea, weakness, cyanosis and death.

Incidence

Occurs as outbreaks in fattening pigs on whey diets and where pigs have access to nitrates or more commonly, nitrites.

Aetiology and pathogenesis

Nitrate in straw and ammonia in slurry can be converted to nitrite by microbial action. Nitrite is available to the pig in drainage water and in water of condensation in badly-ventilated accommodation where concentrations may reach 8-10,000 ppm. Nitrites may also occur in whey as a result of cheese-making. The lethal dose of potassium nitrite appears to be 22 mg/kg and for sodium nitrite is 88 mg/kg. Nitrogen dioxide may also be produced by other farm processes such as silage making. Ingested nitrate may be turned to nitrite in the gut. Nitrite is absorbed and causes methaemoglobinaemia. When 75-90% of the haemoglobin is converted to methaemoglobin, deaths occur. The clinical signs and pathology are largely due to anoxia.

Affected pigs have a raised respiratory rate with a rapid, weak pulse. Salivation, passage of large amounts of urine, dilated pupils, convulsions and opisthotonus all occur. Weakness and then cyanosis develop shortly before death.

Methaemoglobin can be detected in the blood, but samples need to be analysed by spectrophotometry or using the diphenylamine blue test. Recumbent animals which cannot be treated should be slaughtered humanely.

Pathology

The carcase may be brownish in colour and a brownish discolouration of the blood may be noted. Petechiae may be present on serous surfaces and oedema and emphysema of the lungs may be seen. The gastric and intestinal mucosa may be haemorrhagic and if care is taken upon opening the stomach, brown nitrogen dioxide gas may be seen.

Diagnosis

The afebrile nature of the condition and a history of whey feeding or poor ventilation, coupled with the post-mortem findings, may suggest this condition. It must be distinguished from the intestinal haemorrhage syndrome which may occur under similar conditions. Samples of gut contents or urine for nitrite determinations should be mixed with chloroform to arrest microbial nitrite production. The Nitur-test (Boehringer, Mannheim) may be used on gut contents.

Treatment

Methylene blue i.v. 1-2 mg/kg bodyweight will improve affected animals. Good ventilation, removal of the source of nitrite and access to unlimited fresh water will all be beneficial.

Reference

McLoughlin, M.F., McMurray, C.H., Dodds, H.M., Evans, R.T. (1985). Vet.Rec. 116, 119-121. Nitrogen ioxide (silo gas) poisoning in pigs.

Phenol or Coaltar Poisoning

Skin lesions: Phenols (in disinfectants) may cause teat necrosis and coronary band ulceration in piglets and cause pimples and weals on the skin when pigs are put into pens still wet with concentrated disinfectant.

Poisoning: Ingestion of phenols, cresols and coaltar products such as tarred paper and clay pigeon fragments (outdoor pigs) can cause sudden death, sometimes preceded by weakness, depression, inappetence, abdominal tenderness and, occasionally, pallor and icterus of visible mucous membranes. Ictric or collapsed pigs should be slaughtered humanely.

Dead pigs have enlarged, friable red and yellow mottled livers. Excess fluid may be present in the body cavities, the kidneys may be enlarged and the lymph nodes haemorrhagic. Centrilobular necrosis and haemorrhage into the lobules are the most striking histological changes.

Treatment

Little or none; skin poisoning cases should be washed.

Warfarin Poisoning

This occurs occasionally in pigs and may present as lameness, weakness and anaemia with bleeding from all orifices, especially those of the head.
Low red cell counts and prolonged clotting times may be found in blood samples and haemorrhages into the carcase are found at post-mortem examination.Treat with Vitamin K preparations, e.g. Menadione (Bimeda Vitamin K injection V).

Monensin poisoning

Monensin levels of 20 mg/kg-50 mg/kg body weight given orally cause anorexia, diarrhoea, ataxia, lethargy, dyspnoea, myoglobinuria and death. Electrocardiographic abnormalities are observed. Serum aspartate aminotransferase and creatine kinase levels are raised at the time that muscle and myocardial damage occurs. Pigs which have died from monensin toxicity have bilaterally-symmetrical pale areas in the diaphragm, thigh muscles, triceps, intercostal and longissimus muscles. Left atrial damage is seen in the heart, there is necrosis followed by degeneration of muscle cells and subsequent lysis and phagocytosis of cells. In damaged skeletal muscle there is hyaline necrosis, macrophage infiltration and eventually regeneration of fibres and their function. The urine is reddish-brown.

Monensin poisoning occurs in pigs given excess monensin (maximum therapeutic level 100 ppm) or when other ionophores such as salinomycin are included at levels such as 166 ppm (8 mg/kg) and when tiamulin is included at therapeutic levels of 150-200 ppm in fed containing monensin. Similar toxicity may be seen with salinomycin, narasin and maduromycin.

Affected pigs may be killed humanely if recumbent and convulsing, but animals with posterior paresis normally recover within 10-20 days..

References

Kavanagh N.T., Sparrow, D.S.H. (1990). Vet.Rec. 127, 507. Salinomycin toxicity in pigs.
Vleet, J.F. van, Amstutz, H.E., Weirich, W.E., Rebar, A.H. and Ferrans, V.J. (1983). Am.J.Vet.Res. 44, 1460-1468. Acute monsensin toxicosis in swine: effects of graded doses of monensin and protection by pretreatment with selenium Vitamin E.
Vleet J.F. van, Amstutz H.E., Weirich, W.E., Rebar, R.H., Ferrans, V.J. (1983). Int.J.Vet.Res. 44, 1469-1475. Clinical, clinicopathologic and pathologic alterations of monensin toxicosis in swine.
Umemara, T., Kawaminami, A., Goryo, M., Itakura, C.(1985). Vet.Pathology 22, 409-414. Enhanced myotoxicity and involvement of both Type I and Type II fibres in tiamulin:monensin toxicosis in pigs.

Arsanilic acid poisoning

This may occur in pigs receiving organic arsenicals when water is not freely available e.g. cold, interrupted supplies etc. Signs of toxicity include tremor of the head and incoordination later progressing to paralysis. Blindness may occur and death may result. Withdrawal of the drug and provision of unlimited fresh water normally allows recovery. Humane slaughter is advised for pigs which remain recumbent 2-3 days after withdrawal of drug.

3-nitro 4-hydroxyphenylarsonic acid poisoning

The ingestion of 5 times the recommended dose of 3-nitro 4-hydroxyphenylarsonic acid (187.5 mg/kg) gives rise to muscle tremors and clonic convulsions after exercise. Eleven days after these signs appear paresis occurs and by 22 days after the first signs animals may be paraparetic with paraplegia occurring on day 33. Paralysed animals should be slaughtered humanely.

References

Kennedy, S., Rice, D.A. and Cush, P.F. (1986). Veterinary Pathology 23, 454-461. Neuropathology of experimental 3-nitro-4-hydroxyphenylarsonic acid toxicosis of pigs.

Rice, D.A., Kennedy, S., McMurray, C.H. and Blanchflower, W.J. (1985). Res.in Vet.Sci. 39, 47-51. Experimental 3-nitro-4-hydroxyphenylarsonic acid toxicosis in pigs.

Furazolidone toxicity

Furazolidone given at 70 mg/kg in the feed causes pigs to develop ataxia, paresis and signs of thrombocytopaenia. Higher levels cause vomiting, slight ataxia and feed refusal.

Carbadox toxicity

Three times the recommended levels (150 ppm) for 5 weeks results in dry faeces, reduced abdominal volume, reduced feed intake and loss of condition with altered hair coat. The colon is reduced in size with dry contents and there are adrenal and renal lesions.

Olaquindox toxicity

Ten times the recommended rate (500 ppm) resulted in inappetence, episodic paralysis and reduction in growth rate. Affected pigs were hairy. Lesions occur in the zona glomerulosa of the adrenal.

Reference

Newsholme, S.J., Walton, J.R., Elliot, G. (1986). Vet.Rec. 119, 554-555. Poor growth episode paralysis and adenocortical injury in swine after accidental olaquindox overdosage.

Reaction to Tiamulin

Reddening of the skin and, in severe cases, death may occur rarely when large pigs housed in deep manure or dirty conditions are treated for chronic swine dysentery with tiamulin at 150-200 ppm in feed. The reaction develops within 72 hours of first feeding and affects areas of faecal or manure contact. Dead pigs may have cardiac haemorrhages and the skin lesions consist of inflammation and necrosis of the epidermis. Removal of medicated feed, washing with water and provision of clean bedding cures the condition.

Reaction to Penicillin

Injections of procaine penicillin may cause an immediate reaction. Pigs may vomit, shiver and tremble and become depressed. Rarely they die.

Osteochondrosis and Epiphyseolysis

Definition

Osteochondrosis is a generalised skeletal disease with leg weakness occurring in animals less than 18 months of age. Changes are seen in the ossification process, particularly in the medial femoral condyle of the knee, the distal growth plate of the ulna and the 6th-8th costochondral junctions. Eventually the changes lead to erosion of the articular cartilage and to painful osteoarthrosis of the joint. When the changes occur in the proximal growth plate of the femur the femoral head may be lost in epiphyseolysis.

Incidence

Some degree of change may be present in up to 80% of some breeds, particularly in meaty animals such as Dutch Landrace or Swedish Landrace or Duroc.

Aetiology and pathogenesis

The aetiology is not known but histological lesions have been demonstrated in piglets 1 day of age and may therefore be congenital. They become more obvious with age although developing and healing lesions may occur at any one time. Areas of inadequately ossified cartilage remain in bone developing from the cartilaginous physis or growth plate separating epiphyseal and metaphyseal bone and at the epiphyseal-articular surface. These cartilaginous areas in bone lead to structural weakness and fracture or distortion of the bone, the separation of the cartilage from the underlying bone and to clefts in the epiphyseal plate. The underlying cause appears to be a defect in the chondrocytes which do not undergo normal hypertrophic maturation, but accumulate rough endoplasmic reticulum, lipid droplets and mitochondria. The surrounding matrix contains deposits of electron-dense material which may prevent normal vascularisation and thus ossification. Such lesions may eventually heal and ossify. Growth rate and heredity appear to affect their development but there appears to be no effect of diet or flooring type.

These changes lead to abnormal growth and change in the shape of bones and joints, including the vertebrae. One of the commonest sequelae identified in the UK is epiphyseolysis in which the head of the femur is shed in rapidly grown animals giving rise to leg weakness in animals approaching puberty.

Clinical signs

These include shortening of the step, knock and buck knees and swaying of the forelimbs. In the hindlimb the feet may be positioned too far forward, and pigs stand with their legs apart and show weakness at the pastern and swaying of the hindquarters. Changes increase with age. Epiphyseolysis may lead to sudden hindlimb lameness and pain at the hip but not necessarily at the stifle or hock. The affected leg is shorter than the unaffected but the thickness of the muscle mass makes palpation difficult. Animal may be unable to rise, adopt a dog-sitting position and resent movement. It occurs commonly in young gilts when first delivered or at service.

Osteochondrosis is a common cause of leg weakness and lameness in young breeding stock but may progress to arthrosis and deformation of affected bones. Kyphosis may also develop as animals attempt to spare affected limbs. Animals unable to rise should be humanely slaughtered on the spot.

Pathology

The thickening of the cartilage with separation from underlying bone is the most prominent feature and in joints, flakes of cartilage may become 'joint mice' and give rise to synovitis. Deformation may take place at affected points in long bones or even fracture (femoral head). The microscopic changes have been described above.

Epidemiology

Common in heavy rapidly growing meaty pigs on hard flooring, but still present even in animals reared on grass or deep litter. Forelimb weakness is obvious in some Duroc boars.
The clinical signs are suggestive. The condition can be confirmed by radiography 100 days + and identified at slaughter. Must be separated from inflammatory joint conditions such as erysipelas and mycoplasmal arthritis. Joint ill is usually confined to smaller pigs and foot lesions such as vesicular diseases and laminitis should be obvious. Epiphyseolysis may be confused with fracture of the femur especially pathological fracture in hypocalcaemic gilts.

Control

The growth rate of breeding stock can be reduced and it has been suggested that calcium and phosphorus levels of high nutrient density diets may need to be increased in order to supply adequate levels of these minerals in the rapidly-growing pig. Exercise may be beneficial and gilts intended for breeding may be kept in straw yards. There is evidence that the condition may be under genetic control. It is much less common in Large White than in Landrace pigs and genetic studies with Duroc boars suggest that it can be selected against.

References

Blowey, R.W. (1994). Vet.Rec. 134, 601-603. Trochanter fracture and patellar osteochondrosis as causes of lameness in pigs.
Farnum, C.E., Wilsman, N.J. and Hilley, H.D. (1984). Vet.Path. 21, 141-151. An ultrastructural analysis of osteochondritic growth plate cartilage in growing swine.
Hill, M.A., Ruth, G.R., Hilley, H.D. and Hansgen, D.C. (1984). Am.J.Vet.Res. 45, 903-916. Dyschondroplasias, including osteochondrosis in pigs between 29 and 150 days of age. Histological changes.
Hill, M.A., Hilley, H.D., Feeney, D.A., Ruth, G.R., Hunsgen, D.C. (1984). Am.J.Vet.Res. 45, 917-925. Dyschondroplasia, including osteochondrosis in boars between 25 and 169 day of age. Radiologic changes.
Hill, M.A., Ruth, G.R., Hilley, H.D., Torrison, J.L., Bagent, J.K. and Leman, A.D. (1985). Vet.Rec. 116, 40-47. Dyschondroplasias of growth cartilages (osteochondrosis) in cross-bred commercial pigs at 1 and 15 days of age.

Foot Lesions

Foot lesions are an important cause of debility in pigs and occur in a number of systemic and nutritional conditions. In addition, foot lesions of the baby pig occur in response to the quality of the flooring and, in the adult, poor quality slatted flooring causes a posture leading to compression of the spinal nerves and eventual paralysis.

Foot Lesions in Baby Pigs

Erosion of the sole, bruising on the heels and of the accessory digits and erosion of the knees can all occur in sucking piglets when expanded metal flooring of the wrong mesh size or eroded concrete are used as flooring. Once the skin has been eroded, infection enters and can give rise to septic arthritis of the pedal joints or to synovitis and permanent lameness. Such conditions have a marked effect on growth rate and may impair it permanently.

All the lesions with the exception of tenosynovitis, are transient. Bruising of the sole occurs within 24 hours of birth, reaches a peak at 6-8 days of age and disappears by 14 days of age. Erosion of the sole reaches a peak at 5-7 days. Bruising and erosion of the heels also disappear by 14 days of age as do accessory digit injuries which reach peak incidence at 7-8 days. Necrotic skin lesions are also transient.

Prevention depends on relaying concrete, painting it with resin or rubber paint and on the use of mats. Plastic coating can be put on floors or they should be replaced with a gap size of 10 mm or less.

Infected foot lesions do not respond completely to antimicrobial treatment in all cases. Where lesions do not resolve by weaning, the condition of the pig should be assessed and animals which are thin or unable to stand should be killed humanely.

Foot abscess (tenosynovitis) has been shown to be more common in the piglets of multiparous sows with disease. Prompt control of sow disease and routine antimicrobial injection of piglets with tetracycline 100 mg at birth may reduce incidence.

Reference

Gardner, I.A., Hird, D.W., Sullivan, N.M., Pierce, R.J. (1990). J.Am.Vet.Med.Ass. 196, 1791-1794. Clinical, pathologic and microbiologic findings of foot abscess in neonatal pigs.
Gardner, I.A., Hird, D.W. (1994). J.Am.Vet.Med.Ass. 204, 1062-1067. Risk factors for development of foot abscess in neonatal pigs.

Foot Lesions in Older Pigs

One third of all sows culled in the U.K. are culled because of lameness.

1. ## Foot-rot.

A term used to describe a variety of septic conditions affecting the claws of pigs of all ages. The primary lesion is some form of defect or penetration of wall or bearing surface of hoof which provides point of entry for secondary bacterial invasion. These include erosions of sole, heel and toe, fissures in the wall (Sandcrack) and separation of wall from sole at the white line. Infection spreads in the hoof in 3 possible ways - a deep necrotic ulcer may develop involving the laminae and coronary band, necrotic tracks may reach the coronary band and form ulcers, or infection may penetrate deeply and involve the deep digital flexor tendon, or phalangeal bones or joints. When abscesses burst at the coronet, the condition is known as "bush-foot". Abrasive and chemical effects of newly-laid concrete contribute to the production of hoof defects. Wet, unhygienic conditions and poor bedding also contribute to what is often a herd problem. Bacteria such as *F.necrophorum, A.pyogenes* and spirochaetes may infect the lesions.

Clinical signs

Lameness depends on the number of feet involved. Affected animals tend to walk on tip-toe, with "paddling" or "goose-stepping" gait, and are reluctant to rise and move and may sit on their haunches. Lateral claws, especially of hind feet, are most commonly affected. The affected claw is warm, painful and the primary lesion is usually apparent. Severe pain occurs when abscesses develop at the coronary band and the leg is often held off the ground. Cellulitis may occur in the limb and reach the carpus or the hock. The heel and coronary band become swollen and blue-black in colour, with multiple sinus formation. Septicaemia and bacteraemia can occur and secondary abscesses may occur elsewhere, e.g. in brain, spine and liver. Bone and joint involvement may be seen. Rarefaction of the third pharangeal bone may occur. Alteration in joint spaces and new bone formation may also be noted.

Affected sows should be assessed for humane slaughter. Those too lame to transport, unable to bear weight on the limb or recumbent, should be humanely destroyed on the spot.

Treatment

Improve hygiene and management. In particular, ensure that slats have pencil edges and are at least 100 mm wide. Pigs should be run through foot baths containing 5-10% formalin (2-3 times a week. Paring septic hoof lesions, poulticing, and bandaging help, but are rarely economic. Amputation of the affected claw may be carried out. Inject with antibiotic such as tetracycline, ampicllin and use of a spray, e.g. tetracycline on local lesion. Ensure that biotin level of ration is adequate.

2.   Laminitis.

Occurs mainly in boars and heavily pregnant or recently farrowed sows. Sometimes associated with post-parturient fever, the signs of which can mask the laminitis.

Clinical signs

Stiffness, reluctance to move, affected animals walk on the front of carpi, and are recumbent for long periods. Claws are warm and tender. Pulsation of digital arteries is prominent.

Treatment

Corticosteroids, anti-histamines. Reduce feed and, if fever, give a broad-spectrum antibiotic parenterally.

3. Overgrowth and deformity of claws

Claws are not identical in size or shape. The lateral claws are slightly larger and broader. This is especially evident in the hind feet of pigs over 6 months of age. The toe is curved in the lateral, and pointed in the medial claw. Overgrowth is mainly seen in pigs over 1 year. The commonest causes are keeping pigs on muddy ground or on very deep litter with insufficient exercise. Boars, especially those kept in small pens, are often affected. Generally it only affects the main claws, but sometimes the accessory claws may also be affected. When a single claw is overgrown, it often results from a change in weight bearing secondary to some painful lesion. Gross deformity is less common and is usually congenital and may occur in one or a number of claws in the same pigs.

Reference

Kornegay, E.T., Bryant, K.L., Notter, D.R. (1990). Applied Agri.Res. 5, 327-32???.
Toe lesion development in gilts and sows housed in confinement as influenced by two size and location
Wells, G.A.H. (1984). In Practice 6, 43-53. Locomotor disorders of the pig.

Adventitious Bursitis

Bursitis is common on the hocks of pigs which have been reared on hard floors from birth. Bursae which are soft and fluctuating may give rise to pain and lameness. They occur most frequently in white pigs and are associated with lesions of the claws. There is no association with infection. Trimming may be required at slaughter.
The condition can be prevented by housing on deep bedding, either straw or sawdust.

Reference

Smith, W.J., Smith, M. (1990). Proc. IPVS. 11, 300. Adventitious bursitis of the hock, results of a study examining the epidemiology and development.

Proliferative osteitis

Proliferative osteitis of the femoral greater trochanter and the humeral medial condyle may cause lameness in sows. Sows with greater trochanter osteitis are usually first parity gilts after weaning, and found in the dog-sitting position and only rise with pain and discomfort Those with humeral medial epicondylar lesions are often recumbent and when made to rise do so with reluctance and have a marked forelimb lameness. There is a hard enlargement medial and proximal to the distal humerus.
Lesions of the greater trochanter appear as a haemorrhagic mass in the surrounding muscle 1-3 cm laterally and caudally from the trochanter which is

346

covered with osteophytes and may be relatively radiolucent. The proximal end of the humerus has similar roughening of the medial condyle and in late cases extensive enlargement and damage to the elbow joint may occur, and fractures may develop.

Affected animals should be assessed as to their ability to be transported for slaughter and slaughtered humanely on site if unable to rise or to put weight on all four feet.

The condition may be reduced in its severity by care with the management of recently-weaned gilts which should not be penned on slippery floors with older animals or in large groups. Calcium and phosphorus intake during lactation should be maintained.

Reference

Blowey, R.W. (1992). Vet.Rec. 312-315. Proliferative osteitis of the femoral greater trochanter and humeral medial epicondyle as a cause of lameness in sows.

Teat necrosis

Teat necrosis may occur in neonatal pigs, appears as a black scab on each necrotic teat and affected piglets may reach 20% in some affected herds. It results from floor abrasion and is greatest on heated concrete floors with no bedding. A genetic predisposition has been identified. Teats which were necrotic in neonates may not develop in pubertal and farrowing gilts. Prevention involves using rubber matting or bedding in farrowing pens or placing bandage or plastic skin on the undersides of neonatal gilts.

Teat damage

May result from piglet biting, and if so, piglet's teeth may be clipped. Ends of teats may be cut off by sharp expanded metal floors.

Vulval damage

Vulvas may be damaged in neonates by being cut off in perforated floors and in sows during farrowing through normal tears or by damage against farrowing crate bars. Recently damage by rats which bite the vulvas of tethered sows has been seen. Animals are found with eroded vulvas and pools of blood. Vulva biting in sows has become a problem where loose housing is practised. It occurs when there is queueing for food or when heavily-pregnant sows on restricted rations are mixed in large groups. Increases in the number of times such sows are fed daily, reduction of group size to 10 and stabilisation of groups may reduce it.

Other injuries

Fighting may lead to severe scratching and cuts, sharp fittings may also lead to cuts and kennelled sows may push through narrow doors and damage their shoulders. Pressure sores may develop when thin sows are penned on concrete and localised abscesses may occur on the skin particularly at injection sites and over the tail head and shoulder. Lesions in the backs of sows housed outdoors may be caused by crows or magpies which peck them.

Ear, Flank, Tail Biting and Penis Sucking

These vices all occur as a result of poor husbandry conditions and can be prevented by improving ventilation, reducing humidity, reducing group size and the size variation within a group and by providing straw bedding, play chains, increased trough or feeder space or using single space feeders.

Once these vices have begun, affected pigs may have to be removed from a group or, conversely, the animal carrying out the damage may have to be removed. These conditions may occur even under apparently ideal conditions of husbandry.

Ear biting can lead to the loss of the whole ear or to necrotic crumbling lesions, particularly on the lower part of the pinna. They should be distinguished from the necrosis found in salmonellosis and other septicaemic diseases. Cervical lymph node enlargement may occur.

Flank biting must be distinguished from lesions of pig pox, trauma from rough pen fittings, and exudative epidermitis.

Tail biting is the most common and potentially the most serious of the vices. The tail may be chewed to the root and pigs may excavate a cavity in the perineum. Death frequently follows. Less severe damage frequently leads to local infection and to pyaemia with abscess formation, endocarditis and paralysis from spinal abscesses. *A.pyogenes* is the organism most frequently incriminated.

Affected pigs should be assessed, penned separately if injuries are not severe, and sent for slaughter as soon as possible. Others should be killed humanely.

Penis sucking. Least serious vice, results in a pendulous prepuce and may result from premature weaning or failure to adapt to drinkers.

Guide to the Differential Diagnosis of Pig Diseases

This section is intended as a guide to the notes on individual conditions. It is in the form of a list of the more common conditions seen in particular age groups of pig and takes no account of the conditions most likely to occur in individual husbandry systems. Conditions which are common will be marked thus*.

Disease of young piglets (Neonatal Morbidity and mortality) 0-7 days

Unless 24 hour weaning is practised, the piglet is nearly always on the sow at this point in its life.

1. Dead at birth "born dead"

Page

a) Aborted. (Born before term)

Fever in sows caused by infectious disease*	
Enterovirus*	22
Aujeszky's Disease	64
Parvovirus	18
Fusarium	228
Erysipelas	202
Leptospirosis	98
Carbon monoxide	336
Brucellosis	105
Toxoplasmosis	253
PRRS*	58

b) Born at term

Mummified piglets	
SMEDI	25
Parvovirus*	18
Aujeszky's	64
PRRS*	58
Freshly dead	
Delays in parturition* (in membranes with non-expanded lungs)	
Congenital abnormality*	293
Fever in the Sow*	
Fusarium poisoning	228
Carbon monoxide poisoning	336
Vitamin A deficiency	279
Toxoplasmosis	253
Leptospirosis	98
Aujeszky's Disease	64
Inclusion body rhinitis	53
Parvovirus*	18
Chlamydia	222
PRRS*	58

2. Dead after cleaning membranes

Hypoglycaemia*	267
Crushing by sow *usually secondary)	

Disease of piglets 7 days - weaning

The age of weaning varies, but is commonly 21 days or more. Some of the conditions which appear in this age group may also occur in weaned pigs, especially thos weaned at less than 21 days of age.

Diseases of Weaned Pigs

A number of conditions occur most frequently after weaning or are seen in their most characteristic form in the recently-weaned pig up to slaughter weight.

(g)   Skin lesions

Diseases of Adult Animals

These will depend very much on the husbandry conditions and type of enterprise. An adult animal is considered as one which is retained for breeding or has been bred before.

(a)   Nervous signs

357

(h)   Reproductive conditions

INDEX

Page

Cryptosporidium 251
Cyanocobalamine B12 290
Cystic Kidneys 294
Cystic Lymph Nodes 295
Cysticercus cellulosae 244
Cystitis and pyelonephritis in sows 217
Other cystitis 216
Cytomegalovirus (IBR) 53
Demodectic Mange 260
Deoxynivalenol (vomitoxin) 230
Dermatophilus sp. 224
Dermatosis vegetans 298

DIFFERENTIAL DIAGNOSIS 348
Dwarfism 296
Dysentery 140
Ear Biting 347
ECTOPARASITES 256
Eimeria spp 248
Electrocution 335
Encephalomyocarditis 26
Endometritis 324

ENDOPARASITES 236
Enterococcus *(Streptococcus durans)* 213
Enterovirus infections 22
Enzootic pneumonia 160
Eperythrozoonosis 107
Epidemic Diarrhoea 36
Epiphyseolysis 341
Epitheliogenesis imperfecta 300
Ergot poisoning 232
Erysipelas 202
Escherichia coli - General 116
　　　Mastitis 315
　　　Xyaria 219
　　　Neonatal diarrhoea 123
　　　Oedema Disease 131
　　　Post-weaning diarrhoea 127
　　　Septicaemia 122
Eubacterium suis (see *Actinomyces suis*) 217
Euthanasia 11
Exudative epidermitis (Greasy Pig Disease) 199
Fasciola hepatica 244
Fat deficiency 279
Flank biting 347
Flies 260
Foot and Mouth disease 89
Foot lesions in baby pigs 343
Foot lesions in older pigs 343
Foot rot 343
Frost bite 335
Fumonisin toxicity 234

FUNGAL DISEASES 226
Furazolidone poisoning 340
Fusarium poisoning 228,230
Gastric Torsion in sows 329
Gastric Ulceration 325
Gastritis 328
Getah virus 95

NOTES

NOTES

NOTES

NOTES